The Nutrition Debate:

SORTING OUT SOME ANSWERS

the Nutrition Debate:

SORTING OUT SOME ANSWERS

Joan Dye Gussow, Ed.D. and Paul R. Thomas, M.S., R.D.

Bull Publishing Company
Palo Alto, California

Copyright 1986
Bull Publishing Co.
P.O. Box 208
Palo Alto, CA 94302

ISBN 0 – 915950 – 66 – 9

Interior and Cover Design: Michelle Taverniti

Distributed in the United States by:
Kampmann & Company, Inc.
9 East 40th Street
New York, NY 10016

Library of Congress Cataloging in Publication Data

The Nutrition debate.

Consists, primarily, of articles reprinted from various sources, but
includes some previously unpublished materials.
1. Nutrition. 2. Diet. 3. Food. I. Gussow, Joan Dye. II. Thomas,
Paul R., 1953 –   . [DNLM:
1. Nutrition — collected works. QU 145 N9734]
TX355.5.N86 1986   613.2   86 – 21616
ISBN 0 – 915950 – 66 – 9 (pbk.)

To Joan's husband and Paul's parents:
With thanks from each of us for the
first three decades.

Table of Contents

Prologue: Is This Book for You? — Words to Decide By *viii*

Introduction: In Which We Expand on Our Assumptions *2*

1. The Recommended Dietary Allowances: Eating by the Numbers? *18*

What is the Future of the Recommended Dietary Allowances? *by Bette Caan and Sheldon Margen* • Recommended Dietary Allowances — Definition and Applications *by the Committee on Dietary Allowances* • Recommended Dietary Allowances: Are They What We Think They Are? *by Alfred E. Harper* • Trends in Dietary Standards and Their Impact on Public Health Programs *by D. Mark Hegsted* • The RDAs Are Not For Amateurs *by Ruth M. Leverton* • Some Problems with Nutritional Analysis Software *by Anne Rogan and Stella Yu* • The RDA's and Public Policy *by Ross Hume Hall* • The RDAs and the Food Industry: Some Interpretations and Recommendations *by Myron Brin* • Recommended Dietary Allowances and Third World Populations *by A.R.P. Walker and B.F. Walker* • Hearings on the Adequacy and Usefulness of the Recommended Dietary Allowance Standards *by William T. Thompson* • The Relationship Between Nutrients and Cancer *by the Committee on Diet, Nutrition, and Cancer* • Recommended Dietary Allowances: Scientific Issues and Process for the Future *by the Food and Nutrition Board* • Afterword *by Joan Gussow and Paul Thomas*

2. Food Guides: Simplifying the Numbers *62*

The Four Basic Food Groups cartoon *by Lynda J. Barry* • A Program for America . . . , *General Mills advertisement* • Suggested Revisions of the Basic 7 *by Olive Hayes, Martha F. Trulson and Fredrick J. Stare* • Food and Health *by Jean Mayer* • Editorial: Teaching Tools *by Helen D. Ullrich* • Teaching Tools *by Ruth M. Leverton* • Spontaneous Classification of Foods by Elementary School-Aged Children *by John L. Michela and Isobel R. Contento* • Evaluation and Modification of the Basic Four Food Guide *by Janet C. King, Sally H. Cohenour, Carol G. Corruccini and Paul Schneeman* • Updating the Basic Four *by Patricia Hausman* • Chuck the Basic Four? *by Stephen Clapp* • Why

iv

We Need Nutrition Guidelines *by Joan Dye Gussow* • The Hassle-Free Guide to a Better Diet *by the U.S. Department of Agriculture* • The Handy Five Food Guide *by Janice M. Dodds* • Considerations for a New Food Guide *by Jean A.T. Pennington* • What Kind of Food? *by Colin Tudge* • Afterword *by Joan Gussow and Paul Thomas*

3. Dietary Goals and Guidelines: A Progressive Jump or Jumping the Gun? *110*

What Foods Should Americans Eat? Better Information Needed on Nutritional Quality of Foods *by the General Accounting Office* • Summary of Dietary Recommendations Made for Healthy Americans by 10 Federal, Professional, and Health Organizations *by Patricia M. Behlen and Frances J. Cronin* • Dietary Goals — A Progressive View *by D.M. Hegsted* • Finding a Common Language to Educate and Plan *by D.M. Hegsted* • Food and Nutrition Policy: Probability and Practicality *by D. Mark Hegsted* • Do We Know Enough to Eat? *by Joan Gussow* • Are Professionals Jumping the Gun in the Fight Against Chronic Diseases? *by Robert E. Olson* • Dietary Goals — A Skeptical View *by A.E. Harper* • Establishing and Implementing Dietary Goals *by Gilbert A. Leveille* • Statement of the American Medical Association • Toward Healthful Diets *by the Food and Nutrition Board* • Nutrition Dilemmas — What's the Truth? *by Katherine Clancy* • How the 'Experimental Imperative' Subverts a 'Public Health Perspective' *by Michael Jacobson* • Diet Related to Killer Diseases Dialogue *between Jerome L. Knittle and Hubert H. Humphrey* • Afterword *by Joan Gussow and Paul Thomas*

4. Animals and/or Vegetables: Asking the Right Questions about Meat *156*

Man's Benefactor *by Harlow J. Hodgson* • Like Driving a Cadillac *by Frances Moore Lappé* • Rainforests and the Hamburger Society *by James Nations and Daniel I. Komer* • Meat and Poultry Inspection: The Scientific Basis of the Nation's Program *by the Committee on the Scientific Basis of the Nation's Meat and Poultry Inspection Program* • Antibiotics in our Food Supply *by Environmental Nutrition Newsletter* • Modern Meat *by Orville Schell* • Meat Hunger *by Marvin Harris* • The Red Meat In Our Diet — Good or Bad? *by Delia A. Hammock* • Meat and Nutrition *by the American Meat Institute* • The Far Side cartoon *by Gary Larson* • Are Vegetarians Healthier Than the Rest of Us? *by Bonnie Liebman* • Are You a Semi-Vegetarian? *by Joel Gurin* • Afterword *by Joan Gussow and Paul Thomas*

5. Health, Natural and Organic: Foods or Frauds? *208*

The Far Side cartoon *by Gary Larson* • Can Crunchy Granola Bring New Meaning to City Life? *by Julie Baumbold* • Testimony Before the Federal Trade Commission *by Max Huberman* • Statement before the Federal Trade Commission *by Annette Dickinson* • Natural and Organic Food Claims and Health and Related Claims *by the Federal Trade Commission Staff* • The Top 25 'Superfoods' *by Denise Foley* • Natural? Organic? What Do They Really Mean? *by Vernal S. Packard, Jr.* • Silent Fall • Scientific Agriculture at the Crossroads *by Thomas H. Jukes* • A Rose (Natural) is a Rose (Organic) is a Rose? *by Barry Commoner* • The Organic Alternative *by Joan Dye Gussow* • Eating 'Natural' Gains Popularity *by Charlene C. Price* • Health Food Stores Investigation *by Simon P. Gourdine, Warren W. Traiger, and David S. Cohen* • Why Health Foods Cost So Much *by Paul Obis* • Afterword *by Joan Gussow and Paul Thomas*

6. Nutritional Supplements: To Pill or Not to Pill, Is That the Question? *268*

Vitamin Usage: Rampant or Reasonable? *by John L. Stanton* • Supplementation Patterns of Washington State Dietitians *by Bonnie Worthington-Roberts and Maryann Breskin* • Promises Everywhere *by Victor Herbert and Stephen Barrett* • 'I've Been Taking Vitamins For Years . . . ', *Hoffmann-La Roche, Inc. advertisement* • Sure a Well-Balanced Diet is a Key to Good Health . . . , *Lederle Laboratories advertisement* • Truth in Advertising: Does It Apply to Vitamin Supplements? *by Denise Hatfield* • Fishing for Health *by Bonnie Liebman* • More Physicians Are Recommending Diets that Contain Fish . . . , *R.P. Scherer Corporation advertisement* • Cabbage, Brussels Sprouts, Carrots, Cauliflower, Spinach and Broccoli vs. Cancer, *PharmTech Research, Inc. advertisement* • Letter to the Federal Trade Commission About the Daily Greens Supplement *by Michael F. Jacobson and Bonnie F. Liebman* • Vitamin Supplementation—A Practical View *by Willard A. Krehl* • Vitamins and Supplements: Are They Really Needed? *by Paavo Airola* • Who May Benefit From Supplementation? *by the Council for Responsible Nutrition* • Quantitative Evaluation of Vitamin Safety *by John N. Hathcock* • Vitamin Supplementation—A Skeptical View *by Alfred E. Harper* • The Task of Nutritional Science *by Arthur J. Vander* • Vitamins: Is the Public Swallowing a Necessary Pill? *with David B. Roll* • A New Approach to Vitamin Supplementation *by Susan Male Smith* • Are All Vitamin/Mineral Supplements the Same? • The Pill Perplex *by Jim Schreiber* • Vitamin E: Natural? Mixed? Synthetic? *by Paul Huff* • Foods and Nutrients *by Walter Mertz* • Afterword *by Joan Gussow and Paul Thomas*

7. Food Safety: Is it Really Safe at the Plate? *342*

Cartoon *by Jim Tomasewski* • The Role of Nonnutritive Dietary
Constituents *by the Committee on Diet, Nutrition, and Cancer* •
How Are Food Additives Tested? *by Michael F. Jacobson* • Is There a
Food Safety Crisis? *by Edwin M. Foster* • Diet and Cancer — Round 2
by Janet Hopson and Joel Gurin • Ability to Conduct Health-Hazard
Assessment of Substances in Seven Categories of Select Universe *by
the Steering Committee on Identification of Toxic and Potentially
Toxic Chemicals . . .* • Food Security in the United States: A
Nutritionist's Viewpoint *by Joan Dye Gussow* • Risk and Reason *by
Cathy Becker Popescu* • Living With High-Risk Systems *by Charles
Perrow* • Staying Alive in the 20th Century *by William F.
Allman* • Pesticides and Food: Public Worry No. 1 *by Chris
Lecos* • Prevention in America: The Experts Rate 65 Steps to Better
Health, *a survey by Louis Harris and Associates* • Dealing With the
Hazards In Your Life *by Michael Jacobson* • Overview: Pollution and
the Food Chain *by Joan Dye Gussow* • Afterword *by Joan Gussow
and Paul Thomas*

Epilogue *406*

Prologue:
Is this Book for You?
—Words to Decide By

I t is probably always advisable to begin a book by putting into print at least some of the authors' underlying assumptions. "Where are these people coming from?" you have a right to ask. "Where do they think they are going?" We will try to answer these questions very briefly in this Prologue. In the next section (the Introduction) we will explain them in more detail. Although some authors might worry that giving the plot away ahead of time would discourage potential readers, we like to think that when you know what we have in mind, you won't be able to resist reading on.

Four beliefs underlie this book. First, most people don't really know what to worry about in the field of nutrition — even if they have read a great deal on the subject. Therefore, they don't know what questions to ask or what sorts of answers they hope to receive.

Our second assumption is that it requires more than the results from scientific research to answer most of the eating questions people need — or at least want — to have answered. Most practical nutrition questions are policy questions, e.g., What should I eat? Scientific data, however conclusive, must be interpreted to be useful. And most interpreters need practice in helping the public make practical use of the known facts.

Third, information needed to make use of those "known facts" is often hard to find and even harder to pull together — and is not all found in the standard nutrition literature. Sometimes first-rate discussions of the real issues in nutrition turn up in books and articles written by people from other fields, who bring fresh viewpoints to food-related issues.

Finally, we would argue that while nutrition is good to pay attention to, there are other things that are also important to our health — peace of mind being one of them. The exaggerated importance given to dietary specifics by those of us with a vested interest in the field risks making people frantic without helping them, since much of what is happening to our food supply seems both uninterpretable and outside our control.

Those are our assumptions. In a moment we will begin to expand on them. Before we do, however, we will take a paragraph or two to tell you what sort of book they have led us to produce. This is a book in which people with very different points of view on what we see as some of the real issues in nutrition are allowed to lay out their most convincing arguments. Because, as we said earlier, information on all sides of many important issues is not readily available in the standard nutrition literature, the book includes both old and new materials taken from a variety of sources — testimony, letters, unpublished speeches, little read newsletters, and books from other fields — in addition to professional journals.

In laying out these controversial issues, we have come to our own conclusions about which positions are most valid — taking into account all of the relevant facts. However, other than providing a little road map at the beginning of each chapter, we have tried to stay out of the controversies ourselves. Where we could not, we have included among the arguments for your consideration a piece by one of us.

At the end of each chapter, we try to highlight what we believe are some of the most important things for you to take note of. Again, however, remember that we are trying to stimulate thought. Our best hopes for this book will have been fulfilled if you do not agree with our conclusions — or even with our questions — and decide to investigate further.

Introduction —
In Which We Expand
on Our Assumptions

Now that you've decided to go on reading, we want to put some detail into the assumptions we have just laid out.

Assumption I: Most People Don't Know Which Nutrition Issues to Worry About

In his introduction to a recent book entitled *The Medical Wars*, writer Stephen Barrett says that the issues raised by the book's author are on the minds of "most thinking persons who are concerned about their health." Judging from the table of contents, the issues he believes occupy health-minded people include Love Canal, Masters and Johnson's sex therapy, the effectiveness of orthomolecular medicine, prefrontal lobotomies and electroshock therapy, and some other more mundane issues such as the effects of sugar, fats, cholesterol, fiber, food additives, etc., on health.

The notion that such issues weigh on the minds of most health-minded thinking people must be put up against the consistent finding of public opinion polls that at any given moment most Americans have a hard time remembering exactly what they ought to be worrying about. To pick a poll at random, a report published in *Public Opinion* during the 1984 election campaign found that a larger proportion of the people sampled knew that Walter Mondale had used the phrase "where's the beef?" (to criticize Gary Hart) than knew whether inflation had gone up or down in President Reagan's first term.

The amount of attention given by the public to these unequally important issues is, to some extent, a reflection of the relative attention given to them by the media. A wise man once commented that trying to find out what is going on by reading the papers is like trying to find out what time it is by watching the second hand of a clock. Television is even less informative. After all, starvation in Ethiopia was widely reported in the newspapers for at least a year before that one evening when 30 seconds of TV footage on wasted children suddenly generated an outpouring of American concern.

The elusiveness of the public's attention is necessarily sobering to people like us, who are attempting to write a book they hope even laypeople might be interested in. Even more sobering to any writer may be the finding that only 15% of the population in 1980 *ever read for pleasure*. (It is comforting to us to know that some people will be assigned to read this book for class; we are even optimistic enough to hope they will find some pleasure in the reading.) It would be an intimidating challenge to identify those issues that are of burning interest to all thinking people concerned about nutrition.

3

However, we think we *have* identified some of the real issues that must be confronted in deciding what to eat. Typically, these are not the issues discussed in nutrition department seminars. Knowing how zinc is absorbed from the small intestine is unquestionably important for the nutrition professional, but it doesn't really help the ordinary eater decide what to eat.

The questions plaguing the average eater are very different: Is it worth paying extra for bread free of preservatives? Do I need to take a vitamin supplement? Why do people give up meat and should I? These kinds of questions — the sorts of questions to which there are no *right* answers — are not really "scientific" questions, and hence are not often dignified by scientific debate. Yet without an honest debate about such questions by those who produce the data on which such answers must be based, there is little hope that ordinary people can make really wise food choices out there in the marketplace jungle. One cannot pick intelligently through the 12 – 15,000 items in the supermarket without a plan. Answering such questions requires understanding a series of policy issues that underlie them — the real issues in nutrition. It is these "policy" issues, and the questions they raise, that are the subject of this book.

To begin to explain more what we mean by a policy issue as opposed to a scientific question, we will go on to Assumption #2.

Assumption #2: Scientific Research Alone Cannot Provide Answers to Many of the Questions Eaters Want Answered

One often comes across statements made by scientists deploring the public's ignorance of the scientific method. Consider the following statement by the President of the Institute of Food Technologists (1985 – 86): "As the food supply has become ever more nutritious, safe and convenient it has also become more complex. This has made it ever more incomprehensible to those who lack the background and training to understand how and why the changes that are being made really are improvements." (Food Technology, July 1984, page 10)

What is worth noting about such a statement is that it has two parts. One part says that there is too little public understanding of modern science and technology; the other part says that if the public did understand science, it would think the way the speaker does. This argument assumes that because ordinary people misunderstand (or know nothing about) the methods of science, they are easily led into error by those (usually non-scientists) who choose to give them false or half-true information. The motives of such people are very often presumed to be greed or political power — or both.

It is true that most people do not really understand the methods of science. It is equally true, however, that a good deal of the "truth" we need in order to decide, for example, whether what has happened to the food supply is really an improvement, is not part of the output of what most people think of as science. Let us give you an example.

Several years ago, one of us became interested in the question of whether food advertising on television misled children. To address this question, an ad was invented for a hypothetical product, a "pink substance consisting of 50% sugar and 50% cereal grains, welded together into a flake by destructive high heat processing and suffused with artificial color and flavor, anti-oxidants, and a few added vitamins and minerals." The question was: Would an ad for such a product be misleading if children who saw it were convinced by the ad that the product in question was a breakfast cereal?

In testimony before a federal judge one of us (J. G.) pointed out that she did not believe such a product was a breakfast cereal, but thought it very likely that those who manufactured and advertised such a product believed that it was. Such a disagreement, she wrote later, is not resolvable through what is typically thought of as scientific research; data derived from controlled scientific experiments cannot help us decide whether something that is half sugar can be called a cereal:

"Such interpretational problems can only be resolved by attempting to reach some sort of understanding of where products like pink corn flakes — and ads for such products — fit into the whole system whereby children and their parents acquire and consume food and thereby attain or lose health. It is only thus that one can come to understand whether such products are part of the solution or part of the problem; and only when we have made that decision can we decide whether or not we wish (ultimately arbitrarily) to define pink corn flakes as 'cereals,' as 'nutritious,' and as 'part of a good breakfast'."

In short, most arguments both inside and outside of the profession are less about data, than about what data mean and what we ought to do about them. The thought may be troubling to some, but this book is dedicated at least partially to the proposition that for many issues of importance to the ordinary eater, what is conventionally called scientific research can answer many fewer of our everyday questions than we have come to expect. (You who are students may have intuitively realized this when you mastered some details about the body's use of vitamin D, for example, only to realize that your new knowledge didn't help you decide whether it seemed a good idea to fortify children's cereals with vitamin D.)

5

This does not mean that science cannot produce useful data, only that the data must be fitted into larger world views before they are meaningful. Science does not usually even *intend* to help us assess the everyday relevance of all the bits of information it turns up; we are unfair to scientists when we ask them to give us meanings as well as facts.

Let us consider, because it is an issue that comes up in the first chapter of this book, the establishment of a Recommended Dietary Allowance for a nutrient — vitamin A for example. One major question of interest to scientists is — has been for years — just how can we exactly determine the 'requirement' for vitamin A? What is the minimum amount required to prevent the otherwise healthy human from developing any known deficiency symptoms? And, since all individuals will not need exactly the same quantity, what is the actual range of differences between individuals?

Now it turns out that even under experimental conditions involving volunteer subjects willing to participate in often tedious experiments for a long period of time, it is much harder than one might imagine to figure out just how much vitamin A is needed to prevent deficiency in the individuals being tested (who do not, of course, include examples of the entire range of sexes, ages and sizes that humans come in). Yet, even if you assume that this amount could be determined with great exactness, even if you assume that the experimenters could come up with a number representing the quantity of vitamin A the average person needs in order to avoid deficiency symptoms, you still haven't really answered the question of how much vitamin A ordinary people ought to be advised to *consume*.

The problem is not simply how to calculate from the experimental figure the amounts appropriate to all those other ages and sizes not included in the experiment (although that *is* a problem). The ultimate problem comes in deciding what the nutritional *goal* is, and that turns out to be a policy (or philosophical) problem rather than a scientific one. Should the amount recommended be just enough to prevent deficiency symptoms? Or should it contain a small additional safety factor on the assumption that we want to provide some sort of "guarantee" of adequacy? Or, in light of new data showing a lower risk of some types of cancer among people who eat large amounts of foods containing vitamin A and carotenes, should we set the allowance even higher?

The answers to these questions take one well beyond the basic scientific data; those data remain the same no matter how disparate the answers they give rise to. This is because the answers have everything to do with the philosophy of the scientist making the recommendation. Consequently, these sorts of philosophically-based judgment calls arise in relation to all sorts of scientific issues.

Just how confusing such problems can become for the eating public is perfectly illustrated in an exchange that took place at a Senate hearing on food safety. Two well known scientists, Dr. William Lijinsky of Oak Ridge National Laboratory and Dr. John Weisburger of the American Health Foundation were testifying in regard to the safety of added nitrites in the food supply. Here, verbatim, is their exchange with Senator Patrick Leahy of Vermont.

Senator Leahy: Do we run a greater risk from the addition of nitrites to food than from what occurs naturally, generally in the United States, in vegetables and other substances?

Dr. Lijinsky: Yes.

Dr. Weisburger: There I would say categorically 'no'.

Senator Leahy: OK. I understand the answer. I am no better off than before I asked the question, but I understand the answer."

Both these scientists were working from a common data base — they knew the relevant experiments, but they obviously operated from different beliefs about which data were relevant. Their opposing conclusions are what help keep science honest but they leave the average person no better off than Senator Leahy was as a result of that exchange.

Yet the average person must decide every day which of the available edible substances he or she will incorporate into his or her own flesh. This means that nutrition professionals in contact with the eating public, need to understand how to think about these issues and how to translate into rational dietary advice the scattered bits of data nutrition science provides. Most sciences, it should be recognized, are not subjected to an equivalent public clamor for practical answers.

Now let's take a minute to examine the word *policy* which we have used a number of times. It is a very vague word that most often comes up when the government does (or does not do) something it feels the need to explain. "That's part of our policy toward (insert name of country)."

Our favorite clarification of the word comes from a book called *Evolutionary Economics* by Kenneth Boulding. A policy, Boulding explains, is a guideline — a decision that helps determine future decisions. "I decided to shave this morning," he writes, "though this is not very much of a decision, because I have a policy of being clean shaven, and my beard grows fast enough so that in order to sustain this policy I have to shave every morning. If I had a policy of growing a beard I would not shave in the morning." (Kenneth E. Boulding. *Evolutionary Economics.* (1981). Beverly Hills, CA: Sage Publications, Inc. Page 170.)

The purpose of policies, including ones much larger than whether or not to be clean shaven, is to "economize the decision-making process." If your policy is not to eat breakfast, you do not have to decide every single morning when you roll sleepily out of bed whether you ought to eat. A policy saves time and energy.

However, Boulding points out, policies should not be rigid. You may decide one lovely summer morning that you will eat breakfast, even if it is your policy not to do so. It may be your policy to have breakfasts on weekends — but one Saturday morning you may decide to go out and play tennis instead, in which case you may skip breakfast and eat brunch after the match. You can disregard your own policy, but having one helps you and others to predict what you are going to do in a given situation.

Now to return to the example we used earlier, a decision about *how* high to set the RDA for vitamin A becomes a policy decision, rather than a scientific one, the minute the decision makers have to decide which goals other than avoidance of deficiency symptoms must be taken into account in setting an allowance.

Over time, the RDAs — as the only specific nutritional standards we have — have been incorporated into all kinds of government programs. They are goals for the school breakfast and lunch programs. They are used for meal planning in hospitals and other institutions as well as in the military. They are used as a basis for nutritional labelling, for evaluating food surveys and so on.

If an RDA committee decides that the quantity they will settle on as the RDA for vitamin A is *just* enough to prevent deficiency symptoms, as opposed, for example, to a perhaps more generous allowance useful in planning food supplies for groups of people (the original purpose of the RDAs), that will be a policy decision, not a scientific one. And it will therefore be a decision that will affect all the numbers the committee comes up with for the other nutrients. You can see, then, how important it is to distinguish between policy decisions and scientific ones.

Sometimes professionals fail to acknowledge how much policy has to be made where scientific matters are concerned. They would like to believe that all the questions that arise when we must make decisions can ultimately be settled with scientific certainty. This is why great difficulties for the educator always arise at the interface between science and policy, where those who must give answers to the public are confronted with indignant scientists who say "We still don't know enough. We can't yet answer that."

Two good examples of this sort of dilemma turn up in our chapters on the Goals and Guidelines and on Nutritional Supplements. Much of the controversy over Dietary Guidelines is really over *how* certain the science relating specific dietary components to specific diseases must be before public-health related policy decisions can be made. The supplementation argument is a different one. Although the practice of regularly taking supplementary nutrients — vitamin and mineral pills — has become increasingly widespread in this country, even among highly educated people, many nutrition professionals have tended to treat this practice (at least officially) as if it were entirely irrational. So the public — which is looking for serious advice — gets ridiculed or denounced and turns for advice to untrained people who are happy to profit by recommending supplements for all the ills afflicting the human race.

Unfortunately, there is very little science to turn to to resolve this problem. This is because the question of what are *optimal* levels of nutrients is hard to research and has not been part of the official research agenda. Indeed, there is scarcely science enough at the moment to support the RDAs. Moreover, the crass commercialism, fraud and deception in the supplement field has understandably deterred many scientists from looking seriously at the issue of supplementation.

Despite the lack of solid knowledge about levels of nutrients optimal for health, there are ways of thinking about this issue that will enable eaters to make rational decisions and help nutrition practitioners be useful to them. However, as you read through the selections in Chapter 6, you will find that our sources are varied and often unconventional — which brings us to Assumption number 3.

Assumption #3: The Professional Publications Nutritionists Normally Read Don't Cover All Sides of Many Controversial Food Issues

If you would like to test for yourself the truth of this assertion, you might skim the major nutritional journals for the last five years and see what they have to say about the issues we are discussing in this book. (If you don't know which journals they are, ask a nutritionist or dietitian.) We think you will find very little to help you decide whether to take supplements, whether the food supply is safe (and what *safe* means) or why people concerned about their health and the health of the planet might want to be vegetarians.

There are several reasons for this situation. At least two of them are relatively simple. First, the purpose of many journals is to help scientists communicate with each other about their work. Therefore, most of what they publish are research papers in which an investigator has developed a hypothesis, set up an experiment, and then collected and analyzed those data to decide whether

9

they support or disprove the hypothesis. Since science proceeds in very small steps, the articles published often represent the growing tip of a small area of research — whose implications only those people knowledgeable in that particular area will fully understand.

If a journal does carry "arguments" over conclusions, they will usually appear in widely separated issues — since the publication delay for most journals is very long. And this is the second reason why the content of most journals has so little to do with current public controversies. Journals are not really current in the way the press tries to be.

Submitted research papers are peer reviewed, which means that they are sent out to other scientists who comment on whether the paper is worth publishing, and if so, whether changes ought to be made. If changes are required, the paper is returned to the original author(s) for modification, after which the paper is resubmitted and eventually published. Obviously an issue that is "hot news" to the public — the 1984 alarm over the contamination of grain products with EDB, for example — comes and goes too fast to be dealt with in the pages of a journal, even if the editors thought it was appropriate.

Usually, however, they would not think it appropriate — which brings us to some of the more complicated reasons why journals so frequently don't publish articles helpful to eaters (or even eating instructors). The issues where a substance like EDB is concerned often have to do with how persistent it is, how it gets into the produce, at what level it is found in processed flours if grain is treated with it, and so on. These are not nutrition science questions. Therefore, even if studies dealing with such issues were done, they would be considered more suitable for journals covering topics like toxicology, cereal science, or environmental pollution than for nutrition journals. This is a reflection of the fact that nutrition at the level of the eater touches on so many scientific disciplines.

Therefore, when a public scare like the EDB contamination comes up, nutrition professionals are usually no more equipped *by their professional reading* to deal with the public's questions than are ordinary newspaper readers (even though they have had more practice judging scientific evidence). Our chapter on Food Safety is intended to give you a framework for thinking rationally about these poison-of-the-week kinds of problems when you cannot — as most people cannot — get hold of all the relevant scientific data.

Another and even more serious reason why many important and controversial questions are never dealt with in professional literature is because all professions tend to arrive at a set of shared convictions that only certain topics are worth serious examination.

10

Where topics do not "fit," busy professionals sometimes settle for "conventional wisdoms," since we feel we don't have time to check out everything for ourselves.

One of our favorite observers, Phillip Slater, has written a whole book about science's tendency to limit the things it will attend to at any given time. The alternative to ignoring things, as he points out, is "unbearably worse — a million psychotic piebald beggars scrambling over each other to get in the gate and be heard." Science has something like the equal time problem on television. "Like the networks, science can only afford to give a hearing to its own establishment and the loyal opposition." And while it is commonly assumed, he goes on to say," . . . that scientists have a single standard of evidence that they apply uniformly to all events that come to their attention, this is pure fantasy. . . . Some events get in the door on their own say so. Others arouse a storm of objections and get dragged off to the laboratory to be given the third degree." (Philip Slater. *The Wayward Gate.* (1977). Boston: Beacon Press. Pages 45, 51)

Because popular nutrition seems to be afflicted with more than its share of "psychotic piebald beggars," "unconventional" topics in nutrition often tend to be dismissed *without* serious questioning; standard points of view about such topics are often repeated without any careful examination. An interesting way of demonstrating this to yourself is to take a statement about some unconventional topic that appears in the professional literature as accepted "truth" and try to locate sources for the reported facts.

Many of the easiest to trace examples of such agreed-upon certainty are related to subjects on the "faddist" fringe. Organic agriculture is one of these. When we first came into the field of nutrition, anyone who asked a sympathetic question about organic agriculture or organic foods was likely either to be labeled a faddist, or judged a sentimental fool blind to the wonders of modern agriculture.

We once came across the statement in a lead article of a major journal to the effect that organic foods were more likely than other foods to be contaminated with salmonella, since organic farmers used manures for fertilizer. We were skeptical of the salmonella claim, since we understood that the manure used in organic farming was usually handled so as to destroy dangerous microorganisms. Since the author of the article was not an expert on organic agriculture, we looked to see where her information had come from. She had cited an article by another author who was also not an expert on organic agriculture. So we looked to see what *that* author's source was; it was an anonymous pamphlet from the Food and Drug Administration.

We finally tracked down the original source; it was a Dutch study in which raw sewage was sprayed on cropland to test how

11

long it would take the soil micro-organisms to destroy the salmonella in the sewage. Clearly such an article could provide no information at all about whether organic produce was or was not wholesome; indeed since raw sewage is universally considered dangerous for food crops, the research was designed specifically to examine circumstances under which its hazardousness might be reduced.

Even though the cited article did not support the claim that salmonella is likely to occur on organic produce, please observe that we are not denying the possibility that salmonella *might* occur there; the point is that no evidence has been provided one way or the other. (There *is* published evidence that salmonella frequently contaminates conventional meat and poultry products—but it is not cited to warn against their consumption.) The point is that when topics are out of favor, even experts may get careless about making sure they have data to support their statements.

Let us give you a specific recent example. In an article from the April 1983 issue of the *Journal of the American Dietetic Association* entitled "Nutrient and food supplement practices of lacto-ovo vegetarians," authors Marsha Read and Diane Thomas wrote the following: "Research indicates that particular subgroups of the population are more vulnerable to the aforementioned sales pitches [for food supplements] than others. These include the elderly, pregnant women, the sick, the poor, and athletes (7)."

Now for a reason we will mention shortly, we were somewhat skeptical of this statement so we looked up citation 7. It was "Herbert, V.: The health hustlers, In Barrett, S., and Knight, G., eds: The Health Robbers. Philadelphia: George F. Stickley, Co., 1976." So we went to Herbert's chapter to see what evidence he had that the elderly, pregnant women, the sick, the poor and athletes are more vulnerable to supplement sales pitches. On page 100 of *The Health Robbers* we read, " 'Health food' rackets cost Americans over a billion dollars a year. The main victims of this waste are the elderly, the pregnant, the sick and the poor." But there were no citations.

This is not a criticism of Read and Thomas — they correctly quoted the author they correctly cited. Many people are not so careful. A recent article in the prestigious *British Medical Journal* reporting on a survey of medical citations, showed that errors of citation in different journals ranged from 8% to 46%, and in the *British Medical Journal* itself "seriously misleading" misquotations ran to 10%. So you should always check citations you have reason to doubt. (You ought to check out *our* citations too, as they occur in the introductions and afterwords to each chapter. We've removed the citations from the readings themselves because we have cut so extensively. But since we have provided full references to all the articles, we urge you to go back and look at the complete originals — with their footnotes — whenever your doubts or your curiosity leads you to do so.)

But what this exercise mainly shows is that when you read only the standard nutrition literature you are likely to find yourself increasingly embedded in a set of shared assumptions about what constitutes a legitimate nutrition problem, and about which nutrition "facts" don't need careful examination. Therefore, in order to decide if the assumptions are correct or whether the "facts" are really facts, it is important that you remain skeptical, read widely, read outside your own area of immediate concern, and follow your nose when a question arises. Always ask "how do they know that?"

Since so much of what you read will be many steps removed from the basic data, you should, whenever you can, go back and look at the basic data. However, sometimes — as was the case with a student of ours who went to check out the assertion that the elderly bought health foods — you will find that there haven't been any studies, only assertions. And sometimes — as happened when a colleague of ours tried to check up on the toxicity of Vitamin A — you will find that there are 20,000 citations, and you won't have time to check up on even one tenth of them to see which ones provide useful information. Then you will either have to do a study yourself (as our student did) or you will, more often, have to decide whom to believe.

How will you make that decision? We are often told that we should judge the credibility of an author by whether she or he has a degree in nutrition or an allied field, and whether he or she is attached to a prestigious educational or scientific institution. This presents an immediate difficulty since many of the most prominent people in this field have M.D. degrees, which M.D.'s agree do not *guarantee* competence in nutrition. Many other experts in the field of nutrition have PhD's in nutrition science, reflecting the fact that they are well trained in biochemistry and metabolism and skilled in carrying out basic research in the field. But they themselves would not necessarily claim to have enough knowledge of food or of human eating behavior to allow them to put the data they generate into a perspective useful to eaters.

However, the most daunting problem in reaching a decision about whom to believe is that most of the big fights in nutrition — like the one over the postponement of the 10th edition of the RDA's — find equally credentialled people on both sides of the dispute. This is why we believe it to be one of this book's virtues that it presents many voices.

The idea of writing a book made up of many voices — not a book of readings, precisely, but a book that uses readings to conduct arguments — was emotionally appealing to both of us. The

13

reason for this emotional appeal was unclear, however, until someone reminded us that this is how real life presents itself.

All of us experience the world not as one authoritative voice, giving us one view of reality, but as a din of opposing voices each giving us a little (or perhaps none) of the truth. Our task is to sort these voices out. As educators we consider it our role to help people sort out truth from half and quarter truth, to put together satisfying and intellectually honest pictures of what the facts are and what the facts demand of us.

It is satisfying neither to professionals nor to the general public to act as if controversies do not exist. To pretend consensus often requires that you shut out much of what the world is telling you. Our chapter on Nutritional Supplements, for example, shows that there is a real conflict between the facts that: 1) nutritionists tend as a group to tell people to get their nutrients from foods; and 2) nutritionists often take supplements themselves. Anyone who denounces supplement taking as a consequence of "ignorance and misinformation" is shutting his eyes to the fact that many nutritionists (who are presumably *not* ignorant about nutrition) take supplements.

Therefore you must learn to think for yourself. Be skeptical of everything you read, test it against sources you have good reason to trust, and, if you intend to *use* information — to teach or make eating choices on the basis of it — ask yourself how it fits into the framework of human eaters over time and around the world. One develops wisdom by being open and receptive to the great truths, which often come when one is thinking about seemingly unimportant or unrelated things.

This argues for being well rounded and for attempting, at all times, to recheck our biases. All of us have such biases. What is essential is that once in a while we ask ourselves, "What if I'm wrong?" and require of ourselves that we prove all over again why we believe as we do about certain issues.

Therefore, we don't worry that we're exposing you to the reality that important nutritionists disagree about important things. We're concerned only that we may not have been fair, may not have exposed you to the best statement of each position or may have left out altogether one or another telling argument. Therefore, we ask you to send us, for our second edition, articles or ideas you think we ought to have included in this one.

Our belief that an inflated sense of the importance of one or another position has helped contribute to the contentiousness of the field leads us to our fourth and last assumption.

Assumption #4: The Details of Nutrition Science are Probably Less Relevant to Health Than You Believe They Are

Those of us who sometimes in the past have felt nutrition didn't get the respect it deserved, always found comfort in repeating that old saw "you are what you eat." However, in the face of what appears to be a public stampede in the direction of "proper" food and "adequate" exercise, we would urge all our readers — those learning to teach others about nutrition and those who simply wish to think clearly for themselves about the relevant issues — to keep a sense of perspective about the importance of food to health. You are not *only* what you eat!

Consider Figure 1, a chart showing the relative importance 103 experts in public health assigned to various personal activities and exposures in terms of their effects on health. As you can see, the first nutrition behavior, "Not eat(ing) too much fat," ranks 20th in the opinion of the experts and gets an overall importance score of 7.82 on a scale of 1 – 10. In other words, these experts believe what you eat is important, but that it is less important to your health than whether or not you avoid getting involved with drugs or tobacco products, which rank second and first respectively on this list, with importance scores well over 9.

We are surely not prepared to tell you, as you embark on a book about nutrition, that nutrition is *not* important to your health. It surely is (as is reflected in the fact that 9 of all 39 items are nutritional ones). But the experts agree that it may be more important to *worry* less (7th) than to *eat* less (21st). "Feeling happy with life" turns out to be more important than lowering sodium or sugar intake — probably even more important than eating your vegetables like your mother told you.

We believe that one secret to feeling happy with life is feeling competent to make informed choices about everyday activities — to feel that you are not being fooled. Therefore we would like to think that by helping you make your way through the minefields of food-related misinformation out there, we may be contributing not only to your knowledge of nutrition issues, but to your feelings of competence and well being.

Figure 1. Experts' Weighing of Thirty-nine Health and Safety Factors for Adults

Thinking about the overall health of the general population, how important is it for adults to . . .

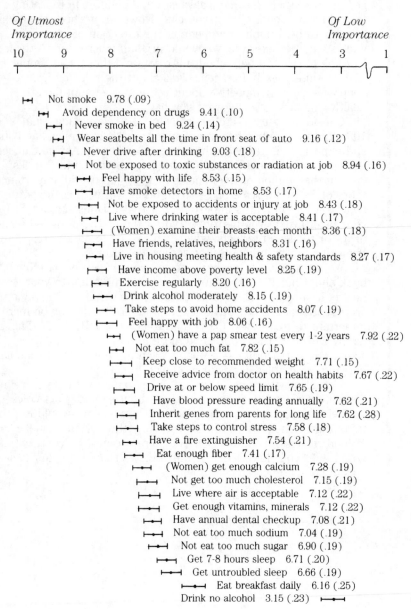

Of Utmost Importance ... *Of Low Importance*

| 10 | 9 | 8 | 7 | 6 | 5 | 4 | 3 | 1 |

Not smoke 9.78 (.09)
Avoid dependency on drugs 9.41 (.10)
Never smoke in bed 9.24 (.14)
Wear seatbelts all the time in front seat of auto 9.16 (.12)
Never drive after drinking 9.03 (.18)
Not be exposed to toxic substances or radiation at job 8.94 (.16)
Feel happy with life 8.53 (.15)
Have smoke detectors in home 8.53 (.17)
Not be exposed to accidents or injury at job 8.43 (.18)
Live where drinking water is acceptable 8.41 (.17)
(Women) examine their breasts each month 8.36 (.18)
Have friends, relatives, neighbors 8.31 (.16)
Live in housing meeting health & safety standards 8.27 (.17)
Have income above poverty level 8.25 (.19)
Exercise regularly 8.20 (.16)
Drink alcohol moderately 8.15 (.19)
Take steps to avoid home accidents 8.07 (.19)
Feel happy with job 8.06 (.16)
(Women) have a pap smear test every 1-2 years 7.92 (.22)
Not eat too much fat 7.82 (.15)
Keep close to recommended weight 7.71 (.15)
Receive advice from doctor on health habits 7.67 (.22)
Drive at or below speed limit 7.65 (.19)
Have blood pressure reading annually 7.62 (.21)
Inherit genes from parents for long life 7.62 (.28)
Take steps to control stress 7.58 (.18)
Have a fire extinguisher 7.54 (.21)
Eat enough fiber 7.41 (.17)
(Women) get enough calcium 7.28 (.19)
Not get too much cholesterol 7.15 (.19)
Live where air is acceptable 7.12 (.22)
Get enough vitamins, minerals 7.12 (.22)
Have annual dental checkup 7.08 (.21)
Not eat too much sodium 7.04 (.19)
Not eat too much sugar 6.90 (.19)
Get 7-8 hours sleep 6.71 (.20)
Get untroubled sleep 6.66 (.19)
Eat breakfast daily 6.16 (.25)
Drink no alcohol 3.15 (.23)

16

The weight for each factor is the mean importance rating given by 103 experts using a 1-to-10 scale. Given in parentheses is the standard error of the mean. An indicator of the variability of individual ratings around each mean is graphically displayed as a band or range consisting of ± two standard error values.

1

The Recommended Dietary Allowances: Eating by the Numbers?

W ell before nutrition became a science, millennia before the nutrients were isolated from foods, people told each other what to eat, and some of the advice was pretty good. After all, if traditional diets hadn't been nutritionally complete, no one would have lived long enough to make them traditional. It was only yesterday in planetary time, little over half a century ago, that scientists decided they knew enough about the food substances responsible for keeping people alive and healthy to set out a series of nutritional goals based on numbers. In our country these were called the Recommended Dietary Allowances (RDAs).

When the two of us learned about the Recommended Dietary Allowances in school, we learned which amounts of which vitamins and minerals, and how much protein, a "reference" man or woman was supposed to get each day (students today learn different numbers than we learned because the RDAs have been revised since we went to school). And when we had learned these numbers, we kept a 7-day record of our own diets, looked up the nutrients in a food composition table, and checked to see whether we had "met" the RDAs. That was wrong!

That's not what the RDAs are supposed to be used for, as the selections that follow make clear. Just what the RDAs are and are not good for, whether they are too high because we are such a rich country, or, as some people argue, too low because we are overcautious, or whether they are simply the best that can be done in an imperfect world is what the selections that follow are all about.

Early in the chapter we have included excerpts from the official booklet on the 1980 RDAs, explaining what the committee that set these Recommended Dietary Allowances thinks they are for. We have done this to let you see that some of the public confusion over the RDAs comes about because even the scientists do not agree on just what they are intended to be.

In 1980, the RDAs were intended to meet the needs of almost all healthy people. In 1985, an RDA committee proposed a change in definition to "adequate to prevent deficiency." The furor that resulted from that and other proposed changes caused the National Academy of Sciences to postpone the 1985 RDAs. So keep in mind as you read that these are not "scientific" definitions, but simply opinions of different groups of scientists about what dietary standards ought to be.

Whatever definition is used, the actual RDAs are presented as numbers in a table, and as anyone who has ever done research knows, numbers are slippery. When the sloppy reality of biological research gets translated into exact numbers, the numbers begin to take on a life of their own — they tend to acquire a certainty and precision they were never intended to have.

This false sense of certainty is increased in the case of the RDAs by the fact that these precise looking numbers are laid out in the RDA booklet itself for specific age and sex groups, thus seeming to indicate that they are designed to serve the needs of particular members of the population, even though the committee itself says they are not. (No wonder then that our teachers ignored all those warnings about the RDAs being for groups, and had us check out our diets against the RDAs, no wonder that we ignore the warnings and have our own students check out their diets, much less painfully, on the computer.)

The remoteness of these numbers from reality is increased even further when they are translated into the USRDAs — a sort of simplified, amplified version of the RDAs designed for use on food labels.

The quantitative aspect of the RDAs has made them an obvious target for computerization (computers *love* numbers). Now we can calculate food composition almost effortlessly and let the computer tell us what percentage of the RDA (or the USRDA) our diets or our sample menus provide. Is this a boon or a bane to nutrition education? If the RDAs are not for amateurs, as one of our selections argues, are they for the average computer user? Tempting as it is to make little puns about bites and bytes, can a computer, turning out numbers faster than we could, tell us what we need to know about dietary adequacy?

Other issues will also be raised by the selections in this chapter. Perhaps the most surprising suggestion you will read is that the very existence of the RDAs has helped to degrade the American diet. Many will not find the argument convincing; we hope you will at least find it a thought-provoking reminder that most of us do not, day by day, eat by the numbers. We eat foods. The best the numbers can do is help us avoid, or perhaps correct, serious errors in food choices.

The very first (1941) version of the Recommended Dietary Allowances consisted of 3 sheets of almost letter-sized paper stapled between gray paper covers, the front one of which was decorated with a bright yellow yardstick. The contents included not only recommended intake levels for 8 nutrients plus calories, but a day's menu that met the nutrient recommendations at a cost (in Chicago prices) of 32¢ a person. In the brief excerpt that follows, Berkeley's Professor Sheldon Margen and nutritionist Caan explain the origins of this first set of recommendations.

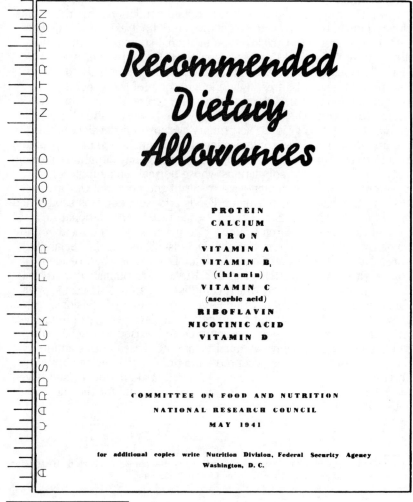

From *Recommended Dietary Allowances, May 1941,* National Research Council. National Academy Press, Washington DC. Used with permission.

WHAT IS THE FUTURE OF THE RECOMMENDED DIETARY ALLOWANCES?*

Bette Caan and Sheldon Margen, M.D.

Historically, for religious, cultural or health purposes, various dietary laws have existed. The main intent of these laws was to prohibit use of adulterated and spoiled foods or to maintain designated cultural standards. More formal recommendations of dietary intake, particularly of specific nutrients, had to await the development of so-called "scientific nutrition."

A primary precondition of these recommendations was the estimation of human nutrient requirements which did not exist until the early 1920's. The first effort to develop nutritional standards was made in 1935 by the Technical Committee on Nutrition of the League of Nations. This agency limited its recommendations essentially to energy and protein needs. Interestingly enough, some of the general principles in use today, particularly the use of a reference individual, and some of our concepts regarding energy needs were quite clearly enunciated by this group. The primary purpose for developing these dietary allowances was to determine the amount of food that people required, so that it could be supplied in emergency situations, particularly warfare, and for populations whose normal food supplies had been cut off. In 1941, mainly as a result of the potential U.S. involvement in the war, a Committee on Foods and Nutrition was established within the Division of Biology and Agriculture in the National Academy of Sciences Research Council. The primary demand for this group came from the Council on National Defense. The "official" beginning was a National Nutrition Conference for Defense led by President Roosevelt on May 26, 1941. The first RDA's were published by the Food and Nutrition Board which came into existence this same year. Subsequently the RDA's have undergone a number of revisions, with a new edition coming out approximately every five years, . . . In one way or another they have been and continue to be used as the official guidelines for practically "all nutritional enterprises in this country. They have served as the accepted yardstick for feeding the armed forces; they have unified concepts of nutritional allowances and have stimulated research to determine the requirements for the various nutrients." . . .

What is the Future of the Recommended Dietary Allowances? Speech by Bette Caan and Sheldon Margen. Edited portions used with permission.

And here, speaking for itself, is the Committee on Dietary Allowances for the 1980 RDA's. This excerpt from the 1980 edition points out the intended function of the allowances, some of the difficulties that arise in estimating them, and some of the ways the committee believed these numbers ought and ought not to be utilized.

RECOMMENDED DIETARY ALLOWANCES — DEFINITION AND APPLICATIONS*

Committee on Dietary Allowances, Food and Nutrition Board.

Recommended Dietary Allowances (RDA) are the levels of intake of essential nutrients considered, in the judgment of the Committee on Dietary Allowances of the Food and Nutrition Board on the basis of available scientific knowledge, to be adequate to meet the known nutritional needs of practically all healthy persons.

RDA are recommendations for the average daily amounts of nutrients that *population groups* should consume over a period of time. RDA should not be confused with requirements for a specific individual. Differences in the nutrient requirements of individuals are ordinarily unknown. Therefore, RDA (except for energy) are estimated to exceed the requirements of most individuals and thereby to ensure that the needs of nearly all in the population are met. Intakes below the recommended allowance for a nutrient are not necessarily inadequate, but the risk of having an inadequate intake increases to the extent that intake is less than the level recommended as safe.

RDA are recommendations established for *healthy* populations. Special needs for nutrients arising from such problems as premature birth, inherited metabolic disorders, infections, chronic diseases, and the use of medications require special dietary and therapeutic measures. These conditions are not covered by the RDA.

RDA are intended to be met by a diet of a wide variety of foods rather than by supplementation or by extensive fortification of single foods. RDA have not been set for all recognized nutrients. (Estimated

---

*Recommended Dietary Allowances, 9th Edition. National Academy Press, Washington, DC, 1980. Used with permission.

safe and adequate intakes have been set for some nutrients in this edition). Therefore diets should be composed of a *variety* of foods that are acceptable, palatable, and economically attainable by the consumer using the RDA as a guide to assessment of their nutritional adequacy.

Estimation of Recommended Dietary Allowances

The *ideal* method in developing an allowance would be to determine the average requirement of a healthy and representative segment of each age group for the nutrient under consideration, then to assess statistically the variability among the individuals within the group, and finally to calculate the amount by which the average requirement must be increased to meet the needs of nearly all healthy individuals. Unfortunately, experiments on man are costly, they must often be of long duration, certain types of experiments are not possible for ethical reasons, and, even under the best conditions, only a small number of subjects can be studied in a single experiment. Thus requirement estimates often must be derived from limited information. . . .

With limited information about requirements, about the variability of requirements, and about factors that influence the utilization of ingested nutrients, allowances for many nutrients cannot be estimated directly from the available scientific knowledge; judgment must be invoked in interpreting and extrapolating from the available information.

It is necessary to recognize these problems in order to understand why recommendations for nutrient allowances may differ from country to country and why the allowances for some nutrients exceed the presumed requirement by a much greater proportion than those for others. On the whole, those who accept responsibility for estimating allowances tend to select the higher of alternate levels when there is little evidence that small surpluses of nutrients are detrimental; on the other hand, consistent uncompensated deficits, even small ones, will lead to deficiencies over a long period of time. . . .

Application of Recommended Dietary Allowances

In considering the use of the RDA for a variety of purposes, certain limitations must be kept clearly in mind:

RDA should be applied to population groups rather than to individuals. RDA were devised as standards or guides to serve as a goal for good nutrition on the basis that, in population groups consuming a varied diet providing the RDA for all nutrients, there would be few individuals suffering from nutritional inadequacy. RDA are estimates of acceptable daily nutrient intakes in the sense that the needs of most healthy individuals will be no greater than the RDA. The basis for estimation of RDA is such that, even if a specific individual habitually consumes less than the recommended amounts of some nutrients, his diet is not necessarily inadequate for those nutrients. However, since the requirements of each individual are not known, it is clear that the more habitual intake falls below the RDA and the longer the low intake continues, the greater is the risk of deficiency.

RDA should not be used as justifications for reducing habitual intakes of nutrients. In developing RDA, no effort was made to relate them to what, for reasons other than strictly nutritional ones, may be considered desirable intakes. For example, a diet that provided merely the recommended dietary allowance for protein would be unacceptable to most people in countries where animal products are an important part of the diet.

In planning diets, it is usually not possible to supply all the recommended nutrients at exactly the allowance levels. Intakes of some nutrients will exceed the RDA standard when the diet provides just the recommended quantities of others that are in low concentration in the food supply. For example, animal products that are naturally high in protein are important sources of several trace nutrients; to meet the allowances for some of the trace nutrients it may be necessary to exceed the allowances for protein and other nutrients. . . .

In addition to the limitations discussed above, the following points should be recognized: (1) RDA have not been established for all the essential nutrients, (2) many foods have not been analyzed for all these nutrients, and (3) interactions of various types between nutrients and other food constituents may affect the bioavailability of some nutrients and hence the usefulness of some information about food composition. . . .

When the RDA are used as the basis for estimating food requirements and meal patterns for [feeding programs,] . . . the RDA should be met with a wide variety of foods. Nutritional deficiencies are encountered primarily in populations that select from a limited variety of foods. It has not been possible to set RDA for all the known nutrients. RDA serve, rather, as a guide such that a varied diet meeting RDA will probably be adequate in all other nutrients. Therefore, it is important to plan a diet to meet the RDA with a wide variety of foods rather than to depend heavily on a more limited selection fortified only in nutrients for which an allowance has been set (cereals, juice substitutes, etc.).

The foods selected must be palatable and acceptable so they will be consumed over long periods of time in the required quantities. . . .

It is well established that individual foods are not nutritionally complete. A basic principle of nutrition education is that foods can be grouped according to patterns of nutrient distribution. Nutritional adequacy is best assured through the use of a wide variety of foods con-

25

taining complementary patterns of nutrients. It is neither necessary nor advantageous to make any food nutritionally balanced, except for meal replacements or for therapeutic purposes.

In setting standards for new products that may displace the traditional products, it is more appropriate to use the nutrient composition of the food displaced as a guide for fortification than to use a standard derived from the RDA. . . .

Typically the Journal of the American Dietetic Association *publishes articles analyzing and discussing each new edition of the RDAs. This article by the Chairman of the 1974 RDA Committee, Dr. Alfred Harper, lays out the justification for setting up numerical dietary standards to serve a variety of purposes. Be particularly attentive while reading this piece to Dr. Harper's sections on "Differences of Opinion" and "Limitations of Allowances." The first explains why "judgment" is always involved in making recommendations — even after all the scientific data are in hand. The second makes it clear how difficult it may be to interpret nutrient intake data, however carefully they may be collected.*

RECOMMENDED DIETARY ALLOWANCES: ARE THEY WHAT WE THINK THEY ARE?*

Alfred E. Harper, Ph.D.

Historic Background: Definition of Allowances

. . . Lydia J. Roberts, who chaired the first Committee . . . stated that . . . the Recommended Dietary Allowances . . . were meant to be "goals at which to aim in providing for the nutritional needs of groups of people."

From the beginning, the Recommended Dietary Allowances, except that for energy, have been recommendations for levels of intake of nutrients sufficiently in excess of average nutritional requirements to meet the needs of nearly all of the population — a public health or statistical concept. They are intakes that, on the basis of the available

*Alfred E. Harper: "Recommended Dietary Allowances: Are they what we think they are?" Copyright The American Dietetic Association. Reprinted by permission from *Journal of the American Dietetic Association*, Vol. 64: 151, 1974.

scientific evidence and in the judgment of the Committee developing them, are compatible with maintenance of the health of most people. As Dr. Roberts emphasized, they are not amounts required by all individuals; they are not absolute nutritional standards; they are not recommendations for an ideal diet, as many assume. They are "goals at which to aim in providing for the nutritional needs of groups of people." Yet, the term "Recommended Dietary Allowances" connotes to many people recommendations for the ideal, best possible, diet. Such terms as "acceptable nutrient intake" or "acceptable levels of nutrient intake" are probably more descriptive of the original concept and less open to misinterpretation.

This brings us to the phrase "goals at which to aim," a second source of misunderstanding and a phrase that should be examined critically. . . . The Recommended Dietary Allowances were not intended to be goals for the amounts of nutrients that should be present in some vaguely defined ideal diet. They were to be goals in the sense that they were estimates of amounts of nutrients great enough to meet *the physiologic needs of most people,* quite independently of the amounts that could be provided readily from the available food. This is clear from reading about the objectives of the original Committee. . . .

Value Judgments

The logical starting point for estimating allowances for nutrients other than those that are consumed solely for their energy content is to assemble information about estimated requirements. However, requirements differ with age and body size; among individuals of the same size owing to differences in genetic make-up; with the physiologic state of the individual — growth rate, pregnancy, lactation; and with sex. They may also be influenced by a person's activity and by environmental conditions. . . .

. . . The initial problem in estimating an allowance is to establish values for average requirements. If sufficient data are available from human experiments, an average requirement can be calculated. If not, information . . . about minimum nutrient intakes of individuals in good health may have to be used.

Even when knowledge of human requirements is available, agreement about the criterion for judging when the requirement has been met may still be a problem. The requirement for a nutrient is the minimum intake that will maintain normal function and health. For infants and children, the requirement may be equated with the amount that will maintain a satisfactory rate of growth; for an adult, with the amount that will maintain body weight and prevent depletion of the nutrient from the body as judged by balance studies or the maintenance of acceptable blood and tissue concentrations. For some nut-

27

rients, the requirement may be assessed as the amount that will just prevent the development of specific deficiency signs, an amount that may differ by several fold from that required to maintain maximum body stores. A substantial element of judgment is involved in deciding where, between these extremes, the requirement has been met. . . .

From Requirement to Allowance

To derive an allowance from a requirement, variability among the requirements of individuals must be considered. The ideal way to do this is to determine the variability of the individual values used in estimating the average requirement. Assuming that individual requirements fit a statistically normal distribution pattern, 95 per cent of the population should have requirements that fall within plus or minus twice the standard deviation of the average requirement. . . . Thus, if an allowance is set at two standard deviations above the average, that amount should be sufficient to meet the needs of 97.5 per cent of the individuals in a population. For many biologic measurements, this is from 30 per cent to 40 per cent above the average.

The probability that human requirements are skewed, as some would have us believe, to cover a range tenfold or more above the average seems highly unlikely. Were this common in biologic systems, biologic measurements would not show the consistency they do. . . .

Differences of Opinion

With such problems, it is perhaps not surprising that there are differences of opinion about the validity of values for requirements and allowances. It is not overly difficult to obtain agreement on the selection of the scientific literature pertinent to requirements and, where there are enough values for individual requirements, an estimate of variability can be made mathematically. However, because of the paucity of information about requirements for some nutrients and because of differences of opinion concerning the criteria of nutritional adequacy for others, "in the judgment of the Committee" is the key to understanding why there may be differences of opinion on a value for the requirement and in extrapolating from the requirement to an allowance.

Few would fault the procedure of review by a committee, with further review of committee recommendations by consultants, before reaching conclusions. However, a psychologic element enters here. The evidence must be culled (I prefer this word to the modern one, "collated"—a vague term used so widely by administrators and committees); some of the information must be discarded out of hand because of its inadequacy; some must be given greater weight, some less; this requires judgment. And collective judgment—be it committee

28

judgment, corporation judgment, or public judgment — can result in an action that would not be taken by any individual alone. A committee with a majority of optimists may be confident that a low allowance is fully adequate while one with a majority of pessimists will feel that a high allowance is inadequate. A single dominant consultant or member of the organization charged with making the decision may influence the judgment of a majority of others. Committee judgments are far from infallible; differences among the United Kingdom, Canadian, FAO/ WHO, and U.S. recommendations testify to this. It is well to keep in mind that the best efforts of a conscientious committee — which I assure you this one was — do not create data to fill the many existing voids and do not eliminate human fallibility.

Despite obstacles, Committees on Dietary Allowances derive values that are useful guides for practical nutrition. But what do they mean and what are their limitations?

Limitations of Allowances

If all members of the population group have intakes equal to or in excess of the allowances, the likelihood of any individual having an inadequate intake is small. Even if an individual has a low intake on one day, this is not of particular concern if it is compensated by a high intake on another. The Committee concluded that if intakes fluctuated, but average intakes over five to eight days met the allowances, there was little cause for concern.

However, if the average intake of a population exceeds the average allowance, it is not valid to assume that all members of the population have adequate intakes. Intakes, like requirements, vary among individuals and, for various reasons, some persons may have low intakes even when the food supply is more than adequate. . . .

On the other hand, if intakes of some nutrients are habitually less than the allowances, it does not necessarily mean that an individual consuming such amounts has an inadequate diet. The Recommended Dietary Allowances, except that for energy, are estimated to exceed the requirements of most individuals in a population. Nevertheless, with no way of predicting whose needs are high and whose are low, it does mean that the farther habitual intake falls below the allowance, and the longer the period of low intake, the greater is the risk of deficiency.

Criticisms Refuted

Two opposing criticisms of the Recommended Dietary Allowances, both of which I find disturbing, are voiced frequently. The first relates to statements that the allowances are not meaningful because they are   29 excessive. I would re-emphasize that many such statements result from a misunderstanding of the objectives of the allowances. They are not requirements; *they are recommendations directed toward insuring the nutritional health of groups.* They must, therefore, be high enough to meet the needs of those with the highest requirements and, hence, must exceed the needs of most people.

On the other hand, some allowances may be higher than they need to be. Committees given the responsibility for developing the Recommended Dietary Allowances, when in doubt, tend to select the higher of alternative values because there is no evidence that small surpluses of nutrients are harmful, whereas small deficits, over time, lead eventually to depletion and deficiency. If allowances are unrealistically high, observations that many diets fail to meet the high allowances raise unnecessary concern about the adequacy of the food supply. Some eminent nutritionists have concluded that if there is no evidence that the health of the population is at risk when the allowance for a nutrient is not met, one should probably examine critically the allowance rather than the diet. This is a sound reason for regular revision of the Recommended Dietary Allowances.

The other criticism that disturbs me even more represents the other side of the coin; it is the assumption that the Recommended Dietary Allowances are inadequate and do not represent the amounts of nutrients that should be provided by an ideal diet. We do not know the ideal nutrient intakes for longevity, resistance to chronic diseases, and maximum physical and mental performance in old age. While it may be true that requirements for these differ from those for a satisfactory rate of growth and for prevention of depletion of a nutrient from the body, there is no evidence to support such views. For energy, there is evidence that more is not better — and there is reason to question whether this does not hold also for protein for older age groups. Vitamins A and D in excess are toxic.

Proposing unrealistically high intakes of nutrients, on the assumption that if meeting needs is good, exceeding them is better, is like doing a cost-benefit analysis without being able to quantify the benefit — it is a meaningless exercise. Decisions concerning nutritional recommendations based on opinion rather than on scientific evidence and judgment are grist for the food faddists' mill. We should be aware that, although we do not have methods for proving absolutely what is true, we are able to detect what is false — and the more we discard what is false, the greater is the probability that what remains approaches truth. This has been the objective of successive Committees on Dietary Allowances.

Another, not uncommon, assumption that disturbs me is that bulletins in which the Recommended Dietary Allowances are presented are sociopolitical documents. As I have emphasized, they are scientific documents, developed to the best of the ability of those concerned with their preparation; nevertheless they are also documents that have social and political uses. This makes it critical that they be as scientifically sound as possible. If allowances were to be adjusted or modified for social or political reasons, the recommendations would soon lose their value — both as guides for dealing with nutritional problems and as a source of information for those dealing with social and political problems. With the current danger of the food supply becoming limited, and with the likelihood of even greater limitations in the future, it is especially important that allowances be based on realistic estimates of physiologic needs and that we do not allow ourselves the luxury of proposing high allowances just because the amounts of nutrients currently available in the food supply are in excess of nutritional needs. . . .

Dr. Mark Hegsted, a long-time student and critic of the RDAs here expands on some of the difficulties pointed out by Dr. Harper, difficulties that arise when the RDAs are used for interpretation of survey data. The problems are severe enough, he argues, to warrant discarding the RDAs altogether, and coming up with something new.

TRENDS IN DIETARY STANDARDS AND THEIR IMPACT ON PUBLIC HEALTH PROGRAMS*

D. Mark Hegsted, Ph.D.

I've been concerned about dietary standards for a long time. My thesis . . . is . . . that, although the RDAs have had an eminent history, they've run out of usefulness. It's time to discard the RDAs and develop a whole new system.

First, they've become so complicated. The first recommendations were based on ten nutrients. Now the list is up to thirty and these are set for 17 age/sex groups, and that works out to 500 age/sex/nutrient specific recommendations. . . . We simply don't have adequate information to do that. So 80 – 90 percent of the recommendations are really guesstimates. The RDAs don't even consider items such as fat, cholesterol, sugar, and dietary fiber. Further, we may have to consider factors in foods that are anticarcinogenic — they may be more practical than some of the essential nutrients. So if we continue with this format of adding new materials that are either nutrients or important

*"Trends in Dietary Standards and their Impact on Public Health Programs," by D. Mark Hegsted, Ph.D. *Currents: The Journal of Food, Nutrition & Health,* 1:2 – 4, Spring 1985.

in nutrition, it's perfectly clear that the RDAs will get even more complicated.

If the RDAs were really to be taken literally, it would mean that each member of the family would have to eat a different diet. There really isn't any evidence that such measures are necessary, and even if they were, it isn't practical or sensible. For example, try to imagine a restaurant that would provide a different menu for 17 different age/sex groups.

Next, we have learned, I think, that some nutrients can't really be considered in isolation. The best example is iron. We know that iron requirements depend on the form of iron in the diet, i.e., whether there's meat in the diet, how much vitamin C there is in the diet, and how much inhibition of iron absorption. As we learn more about other nutrients, these kinds of interactions are going to become more important, and dealing with each nutrient in isolation is not really a very sound practice. The current RDA system has difficulty dealing with this level of complexity.

Another criticism of the RDAs is that the bulletin says these are to be met by food. Yet several of the RDAs are so high that we all recognize that that's not possible. There is either something wrong with the philosophy or with the levels.

One of the ideas that fosters this kind of complexity is the attitude among many investigators that we needed all these standards in order to evaluate dietary survey data, e.g., the nutritional requirements of children are different from adults and so on.

With regard to that, I can only say that I think it's becoming clear at present that none of us really knows how to evaluate dietary data. This is partly because the data are so poor. There is considerable evidence that the dietary surveys seriously underestimate food intake. I think that the national dietary surveys may have yielded more misinformation over the past 20 or 25 years than they have real useful information.

There are other things that we have to recognize: one, nutrient deficiencies in this country are not a major public health problem. That's not to say that everybody is adequately fed in terms of essential nutrients, but the number of serious problems that we can identify, related to classical nutritional deficiencies, are minimal. That has to mean that the average diet Americans are eating provides a reasonably decent supply of essential nutrients, otherwise there would be deficiencies. This is true even though the national surveys indicate very large proportions of the populations consume much less than the RDA.

. . . All the survey data we have indicate that all age and sex groups after infancy eat about the same mix of foods. That is to say, the "nutrient density" of their diet is about the same regardless of the group you look at. That's obviously what one expects. You put some food on the table, the children, you and your grandmother and everybody selects what they want, with the amount depending on their energy needs. On the average, this means the same proportions. Though nutritional requirements of children, adolescents, teenagers, and men and women are different, if they eat a nutritious diet, the difference in total food intake covers the difference in absolute nutrient needs. I think what we need are some guidelines that tell us how to feed a family or a population or a group of people.

In contrast to the apparent adequacy (I'm not saying it's optimum), but the *apparent* adequacy of our average diet with regard to essential nutrients, it's perfectly clear that the average American diet does not protect against the chronic diseases such as heart disease, cancer, stroke, diabetes, and hypertension. These are the public health problems — these are the problems that nutritionists ought to be more concerned about. Our primary concerns should be with fat (the amount and type), cholesterol, sugar, salt, dietary fiber, and perhaps some of the vitamins which may protect against cancer, for example.

As for the chronic diseases, they are, in fact, just that. They have a long generation time, and it's perfectly clear that good nutrition, say for children, must protect their health and guard them against what's coming down the line in twenty or thirty years. Dealing with each age/sex group as an independent problem really doesn't make any sense when we deal with the chronic diseases.

Finally, I think we have to recognize that we've always had two different types of food standards. One is like the RDA in which we have attempted to specify absolute intakes for different individuals. The other type defines acceptable concentrations in the diet. I think we would all agree that children probably can tolerate less toxic material than adults, but we don't specify absolute amounts for different age and sex groups. Rather, we specify concentrations in the diet; but, because children eat less than adults, they consume smaller amounts of toxic material. When we establish nutritional standards for animals, we don't specify a different level for a one hundred pound pig and another for a two hundred pound pig. They may all be in the same pen, and all, more or less like the family, eat out of the same trough. It obviously makes more sense to define nutritious diets for pigs than it does to specify intakes for each pig.

We all recognize that large infants that grow rapidly eat a lot more food than little infants that don't grow rapidly; but we don't try to develop a different formula for each type of infant. Rather, we develop a diet, a formula that's nutritious, now based more or less on the composition of breast milk . . . .

So I think we need a better set of standards — standards that define a nutritious diet for Americans. I think we all agree that we need to teach people how to eat, beginning in childhood, but that we can't expect children to eat much different from their families. All our experience tells us if we want to modify diets, we have to deal with the family and, if possible, with the community. I will argue that the dietary standards have to be feasible and reasonable and acceptable.

33

Such is not the case with the RDA.

Now, one of the problems with the standards set by the RDA is that they essentially attempt to define zero risk. A human that eats 18 milligrams of iron is an exception. And, at least with our current diets, it's not reasonable to expect all women to eat as much as 18 milligrams of iron simply because there are some few who need that amount. Similarly, while it is true that people with cholesterol levels of 300 to 350 may well be at risk, we know we can't get every American to eat the kind of diet that would be protective for those people at very severe risk. . . .

The first principle in establishing dietary standards should be, "If it ain't broke, don't fix it." That is, the evidence should be substantial before we recommend major changes in the American diet. Second, the recommendations should consider food supplies and current dietary habits. Recommendations which few people will accept have little use. And third, our major concern should be the dietary practices which are relevant to the chronic diseases — not changes in intake of essential nutrients. I do not insist that every age/sex group should eat exactly the same diet if sufficient evidence indicates otherwise; but the standards should be consistent with the fact that effective nutrition programs deal with the family and the community, not the individual.

Dr. Ruth Leverton tried for many years to apply the RDAs in government programs. We have included here one of her comments on the difficulty of doing so — especially in a way that would satisfy the committees that developed the allowances.

THE RDAs ARE NOT FOR AMATEURS*

Ruth M. Leverton, Ph.D., R.D.

. . . My discussion here will focus primarily on the more obvious pitfalls encountered when the Recommended Dietary Allowances are translated into food guides or other patterns for desirable eating, used to evaluate food consumption data, and employed to develop food plans and menus at different cost levels.

The Recommended Dietary Allowances form a valuable tool for interpreting food consumption data and planning diets in terms of

*Ruth M. Leverton, Ph.D., R.D.: "The RDA's are not for amateurs." Copyright The American Dietetic Association. Reprinted with permission from *Journal of the American Dietetic Association*, Vol. 66:9, 1975.

selected nutrients. But, like any tool, they have areas of greatest use-*ful*ness, of partial or peripheral usefulness, and of use*less*ness. They can be misused and often, like survey data or computer programs, they are expected to provide more or different information than they were ever designed to give.

The Recommended Dietary Allowances, as a tool, can be used too specifically or too broadly. For instance, undue significance may be placed on small differences between an intake of a nutrient and the allowances for that nutrient. At the other extreme, comparison of the nutritive value of food intakes with the Recommended Dietary Allowances is often erroneously extrapolated into a judgment of the nutritional status of the subjects.

One of the greatest challenges in applying the allowances is to find a way to report the results that is acceptable to the scientists who developed them. A major hurdle has been the dichotomy represented by the Food and Nutrition Board's insistence that they were intended for use only when dealing with *groups* of people, but at the same time, the Board's willingness to give . . . *individual* figures for twenty-four age-sex groups plus those for pregnancy and lactation. Such specificity implies research data that do not exist. . . .

It is well known that the Recommended Dietary Allowances are set high enough "to maintain good nutrition in practically all healthy people in the United States" and "are designed to afford a margin sufficiently above average physiological requirements to cover variations among practically all individuals in the general population." It follows, of course, that malnutrition cannot be assumed to occur "whenever the recommendations are not completely met."

If this last statement is observed, then one pitfall lies in trying to make a value judgment as to what would be an intake level, lower than the Recommended Dietary Allowances, at which a person could be considered at risk or that malnutrition was imminent. In the Department of Agriculture's nationwide food consumption surveys, we labeled as "poor," a diet that supplied less than two-thirds of the allowances for one or more nutrients. It seemed probable that such a level could be nutritionally inadequate over an extended period. This overall criterion is open to criticism because the margin of safety that was included in the Recommended Dietary Allowances differed for different nutrients. However, the margins of safety for the various nutrients have never been stated in quantitative terms — nor has a figure been given for the basic requirement to which a margin of safety was added. There are times when a general, descriptive term of overall diet quality, such as "good," "fair," or "poor," is useful. However, in developing or using one, we must be aware that we are going counter to the way the Food and Nutrition Board thinks the Allowances should be used. . . .

. . . Allowances for calories are relatively rigid because, of course, they include no margin of safety. They have been reduced significantly in successive editions of the Recommended Dietary Allowances. In contrast, the allowances for the nutrients are generous and include margins of safety to allow for individual differences. Use of allowances that overstate the need for nutrients, when planning and evaluating diets, may result in unnecessary modification of diets and food expenditures, as well as unwarranted concern about "shortages" of nutrients. The shortages will be exaggerated even more by the use of the U.S. RDAs of the Food and Drug Administration.

The energy-nutrient dilemma is illustrated by the 1968 allowances for four age groups of men, and for women from eighteen to seventy-five-plus years. Men in the eighteen-to-twenty-two-year-old group have a caloric quota of 2,800; for women in the same age group, the quota is 2,000. However, allowances for vitamin A activity, folacin, vitamins B_6 and B_{12}, calcium, and phosphorus are the same for both sexes. Even when the caloric quota for older women drops to 1,750, the allowances for five of these six nutrients remain the same as for the men with a 2,800-kcal quota. The allowance for vitamin B_{12} is increased for the oldest age groups at the same time the caloric allowance is reduced.

Thus women must eat foods of much higher nutrient density (the ratio of nutrient content to caloric value) than the men. We have been accustomed to saying that when a homemaker prepares nutritious meals (meeting the allowances) for her husband and children, she, too, will have an adequate diet, but she must eat smaller servings so as not to exceed her caloric allowance. Smaller servings, however, will not provide for the higher nutrient density she needs. . . .

Then there is the pitfall of failing to read the text that accompanies the table of Recommended Dietary Allowances. The allowances are set forth as "levels of intake." This means the allowances are meant to be ingested. Yet, it is not uncommon to find overall food supplies or market orders evaluated in terms of the Recommended Dietary Allowances with no margin for losses in processing, storing, and preparation.

A common fallacy is to assume that if a diet provides the recommended allowances, the needs for all nutrients have been met. Reading the fine print in the table, we find the statement: "The recommended allowances can be attained with a variety of common foods providing other nutrients for which human requirements have been less well defined." Of great concern in this regard is the use of the Recommended Dietary Allowances as the basis for fabricated, contrived, or synthetic foods. Such products may not be reliable replacements for traditional foods if only the nutrients for which there are allowances have been added.

An entire paper could be written on the pitfalls of placing unwarranted weight and faith in figures that are only averages. Failure to recognize and respect the limitations of an "average" figure is a fault common to many professional workers in many fields. "Average" is the easiest statistic to develop and probably the most misused. It is a great simplifier, but the oversimplification it breeds is misleading and often a disservice to its users. Averages have their uses, but we must be sure we know their limitations.

. . . I believe it all adds up to the fact that effective application of the Recommended Dietary Allowances requires understanding, skill, restraint, and even tolerance. I feel their existence, controversial as they are, has been a potent factor in coordinating and directing dietary planning and nutritional teaching. Food and nutrient needs and how to supply them are not a simple science. We have been pressured to make our subject simple so that everyone can be a specialist. The science of food and nutrition cannot be taught in ten easy lessons. It is a horrendous pitfall to think that caring enough, trying hard enough, having enough innovative approaches, and giving the facts enough "charisma" will result in everyone wanting to and being able to become a specialist, an authority in the science of food and nutrition.

On the other hand, wise food selection and the nutritional reasons why, as one component of the science of food and nutrition, do lend themselves to popular teaching on a nationwide scale. Food selection can be taught in broad terms for those who want simplicity or in specific terms for those who want details.

The RDA's are not for amateurs!

> *Whatever the pitfalls inherent in using the RDAs, those nutrition professionals who had to use them to assess or plan diets quickly recognized the computer as an ally. It could do better and more quickly what they had been used to doing painstakingly by hand. In the article excerpted here, from a special issue of the* Journal of Nutrition Education *devoted to computers in nutrition, Rogan and Yu offer a few warnings about the increased opportunities for misues that the computer's quickness permits.*

SOME PROBLEMS WITH NUTRITIONAL ANALYSIS SOFTWARE*

Anne Rogan and Stella Yu

Use of nutrient data can be complex and problematic. Indeed, articles and advertisements related to nutrient analysis software programs in popular computer journals may evoke the image of a number-eating dragon. This dragon feeds on information regarding an individual's size, shape, age, and exercise and eating habits; consumes these data in a split second; and expels hundreds of personalized tidbits of information related in some way to the dietary and exercise practices of the individual. With such technological power comes the potential for serious problems, including misuse of information by pseudo-nutritionists, inappropriate use of information by legitimate professionals, and misinterpretation of information by lay audiences. As nutrition educators, we must train ourselves and other health-related professionals to recognize these problems and to prevent them.

Potential Misuse by Pseudo-nutritionists

The nutrition software dragon provides any owner of a computer with a tool that can generate nutrition information in a variety of forms. Our fear is that we are entering a stage of "nutrition quackery" in which some irresponsible entrepreneurs will exploit the public through the use of computers. It is conceivable that health food stores, health spas and clubs, and nontraditionally educated "nutrition consultants" could use these programs as a way of documenting the need for their services and nutrition products. . . .

---

*"Some Problems with Nutritional Analysis Software", by Anne Rogan and Stella Yu. *Journal of Nutrition Education;* 16:65–66, June 1984. Used with permission.

Output Interpretations

Printouts of the nutritional analyses are indeed impressive in appearance. Many nutrient analysis software programs list the protein, carbohydrate, fat, vitamin and mineral content — as reported by USDA publications, depending upon the data base — for individual foods consumed during a day; most programs also provide nutrient totals for the entire intake. Printouts often provide the Recommended Dietary Allowances (RDA) based on the individual's sex and age, and usually compare the estimated nutrient intakes with the RDA.

In most of the programs, these results appear without any interpretation. Interpretation of results becomes the burden of the software package users, who may or may not be informed about appropriate use of the RDA. Users may interpret an attainment of 80 – 100% of the RDA for all nutrients as satisfactory or, what is more likely, they may view any intake less than 100% as an indication of the need for various and sundry protein, vitamin and/or mineral supplements. We would not expect most consumers to know that the RDA were not established to provide nutrient requirements for a specific individual, or that for most nutrients, the RDA may exceed an individual's actual nutrient requirement. Indeed, it is extremely difficult, even for the professional, to make definitive statements regarding the nutritional adequacy of any individual's diet based on a nutrient analysis of any meal or set of meals. . . .

Nutrition educators have an important task ahead: controlling the dragon. We must increase our knowledge of nutrient data and our understanding of the problems which accompany the educational use of information generated by nutrient analysis software. We must also educate ourselves as well as other health-related professionals to the potential benefits and pitfalls of nutrient analysis software. However, our ultimate goal should be to foster changes in the development of nutrient analysis software so that these programs function as useful tools with sound educational purposes rather than as unruly beasts.

> *Ross Hall is a biochemist and author of a 1974 book,* Food for Nought, *critical of what he considered the unexamined effects on our food of the forward march of technology. Here he questions the unintended effects of reducing nutrition to numbers on the quality of our food supply.*

THE RDA's AND PUBLIC POLICY*

Ross Hume Hall, Ph.D.

Central Planning vs Personal Initiative

"The recommended intakes are intended for the use of planners" so begins the Handbook on Human Nutritional Requirements published by the Food and Agricultural Organization (FAO) of the United Nations . . . We might ask, planning for whom? And, who is doing the planning and for what purposes?

James D. Grant, Deputy Commissioner, Food and Drug Administration (FDA), Washington, provides a partial answer: ". . . manufacturers in the food industry have introduced an amazing array of new foods or different forms of traditional foods. In this way, an alert and inventive industry is responding to consumer demands by the application of a creative and a well-developed sense of what appeals to consumers. In this role, industry has a distinct responsibility to make products that are not only pure and safe, but also nutritionally wholesome from the standpoint of public health." . . .

Lord Kelvin, the eminent nineteenth century British physicist once remarked that it wasn't science unless it could be measured. His comment tended to dismiss a large part of biological science as non-science, a slight that biologists have been trying to rectify ever since by putting their sciences on a mathematical basis. But, when dealing with biological phenomena numbers can be quite insidious, and like the siren's song that lured Ulysses to the rocks, they can trap and destroy the unwary. The main problem with numbers is that, although they can be paraded through computers with mathematical precision, they really have no meaning if they are not based on biological reality. . . .

Consider a room full of people engaged in multiple conversation. How would you reduce the complex sociological interaction, all the subtleties to mathematical formulae? About the best you could do

*"The RDA's and Public Policy," by Ross Hume Hall, Ph.D. *The Ecologist and Entropy,* Volume 1, November-December 1977. Used with permission.

would be to count the numbers of people, note their sex, age and a few other countable parameters — none of which would record the social complexities inherent in the situation. In short, *when a complex biological phenomenon is reduced to numbers much is lost, so much so that the numbers may have little significance.*

Nourishment is a very complex biological phenomenon in which one life form gives up its life and is converted into another life form. People eat food that at one time was either a living plant or animal and all its biological complexities resident in that living (ex) flesh are transformed into the unique complexities of the human consumer. Science has not had much success in defining precisely the nature of this phenomenon and except for an understanding of the principles, the details remain hazy. How then can we go about assigning numbers to something as nebulous as nourishment and should we even try? Might as well try to measure precisely the dimensions of a cumulus cloud. . . .

Reduction of nourishment to numbers actually has had a long history. In 1813 Sir Humphrey Davy, the famous British chemist, observed: "If the organs of plants be submitted to chemical analysis, it is found that their most infinitive diversity of form depends upon different arrangements and combinations of a very few of the elements." Sir Humphrey was greatly impressed by the power of the then new techniques of analytical chemistry to reveal the innermost secrets of living matter. Life science subsequently developed in the nineteenth century using analytical chemistry as its basic tool and by the middle of the century chemical analysis had shown that all living organisms consisted of fat, carbohydrates and protein. It seemed a reasonable conclusion to believe that nourishment represented a conversion of these basic substances of the eaten into the eater. Biochemical studies of this century have clearly shown the mechanism of how it happens, but, still this body of facts provides only a partial understanding of the phenomenon of nourishment . . . the more advanced studies now being carried out on body metabolism are revealing incredibly complex relationships between nutrients and cell viability. . . .

A Mature Nutrition Idea

The 1940s represented a coming of age of public acceptance of nutrition scientists. . . .

It was during the war (1940) that the Food and Nutrition Board within the National Academy of Sciences — National Research Council, Washington, was established. One of its first concerns was to define, in accordance with the latest information, the recommended dietary allowances (RDA) for some of the known dietary essentials of people of different ages. . . .

41

The Coming of the RDAs

The new government nutritional policy worked out beautifully for food manufacturers because it fitted into their already established technology of food fabrication. They began to list the analytical values of selected nutrients on their labels, impressively calculated in percentage RDAs. Government law required only declaration of a short list of nine nutrients. If the product was intrinsically short of one item on the list, it was easy to fortify with the absent member. Products such as Hostess Cup Cakes were now advertised for children as snack cakes with body-building vitamins and iron. The body-building vitamins consist of three of the B vitamins, all technically easy to add. . . .

There Is No Scientific Basis for Setting Exact RDAs

The scientific basis for setting the RDAs for humans is not exact and is open to political and economic persuasion. If this kind of subjective decision-making were confined to a laboratory exercise it would have no major impact, but it is not. It is decision-making that strikes at the heart of the quality of nutrition for an entire nation. Let us not make the mistake, however, of believing that if the RDAs could be set precisely that all would be well with American nutrition *because the whole premise of the RDAs shatters when it runs into human biology.*

Human biology is an integrative process, everything happening at once, each process in perfect relation with all others. And, human nourishment is nature's way of tying human biology directly into the fundamental relationships of life. The adding machine premise of the RDAs is incapable of giving any hint of those relationships. . . .

The overall policy of the food industry is now becoming clear — it is the institutionalization of the feeding of a whole nation. The technology for doing this has been available for some time but in order to make the policy palatable, the public and its political leaders have to be persuaded that the food it receives is nutritious. *The RDA concept provides that rationale.*

> *Testimony now from what might be thought of as an interested observer. Dr. Myron Brin is a nutrition scientist who works for a manufacturer of vitamins used in supplements and food fortification. Isn't it possible, he asks, that the RDAs are lower than they ought to be for optimum health?*

THE RDAs AND THE FOOD INDUSTRY: SOME INTERPRETATIONS AND RECOMMENDATIONS*

Myron Brin, Ph.D.

... It is often not fully appreciated that the studies upon which certain RDAs are based were carried out in a laboratory setting with pure nutrients rather than food. This also results in inherent errors, because pure nutrients are more fully absorbed by human subjects, while the vitamins which occur in food are usually bound, and, therefore, may not be completely or equally available to all people, and from all food products. Therefore, corrections should be made upward for absorption. Another item is that the RDAs are developed from the nutrient intake level necessary to prevent acute deficiency signs. It would be more constructive it seems to us, to establish RDA levels from a premise of maintaining optimum health, including functional and behavioral health, rather than prevention of acute disease... I make these statements because the science of nutrition has developed a large body of information in the last 25 years demonstrating that serious biochemical and metabolic changes occur in man during the process of nutrient depletion and long before overt clinical signs appear.

The RDA bulletin states that they are set at levels of the average need to prevent deficiency signs plus two standard deviations, in order to cover 97.5% of the population which is presumed healthy. Yet for a large number of the vitamins or minerals there is no data base or other way to calculate the average allowance, not to speak of calculating a standard deviation. The data are just not available. Thus, the RDAs in those cases are only estimates of need and in fact may be gross underestimates. To extrapolate these data from one sex to another or to different age groups, therefore evolves into a matter of educated guesses on the part of the professionals undertaking this task.

---

*"The RDAs and the Food Industry: Some Interpretations and Recommendations," by Myron Brin. Testimony before the U.S. House of Representatives Committee on Science and Technology, July 13, 1978. *The Scientific Adequacy and Usefulness of the Recommended Dietary Allowance (RDA) Standards*, pages 396–407.

43

. . . It is perfectly reasonable that the RDAs do not reflect optimum intake to maintain optimum health, since they may be too far toward the conservative end of the intake level. . . .

Some Practical Applications of the RDA

To assume that people in the United States are now getting full RDAs of their nutrient needs by proper self-selection of mixed diets is unfounded as exemplified by findings of the major nutritional surveys. These surveys have been carried out by experts in the U.S. Departments of Agriculture (USDA) and the Department of Health, Education and Welfare (HEW), as well as innumerable surveys done in local communities by various investigators at universities and medical schools. Also, to assume that education alone will cause people to change their dietary habits rapidly in order to consume their full need of all nutrients is really moot, since it must be put into a practical time frame. We feel that it is becoming more and more unlikely because of the marked increase in the cost of food relative to income — the protective foods are more expensive than ever — the costs of meat, fish and vegetables are out of sight. Less expensive food can be made more nutritious by proper enrichment, however. . . .

Chemical Diets Versus Food

Man can survive, grow and develop on purely chemical diets as shown in studies of total parenteral nutrition in premature and other children during their growing years. In adults and the elderly, body weight can be controlled by what is put in the vein to maintain a state of health, by all diagnostic criteria. The same is accomplished by oral feeding of chemically elemental diets. However, this mode of nutritional maintenance is not acceptable for people generally, because people eat food and not chemicals, and that is the way it should be. It would be foolhardy, though, to overlook the fact that upon eating, the body digests the food into its chemical components, which only then are reconverted to energy or tissue. We must, therefore, be sure that our food choices contain these chemical components. However, to say that the addition of synthetic nutrients to foods reduces their value and is to man's detriment is wrong, because in fact there is worldwide experience to demonstrate that these nutrients are not only equivalent to those found in nature in foods, but often are more readily biologically available than the nutrients which occur naturally. . . .

Summary

We believe in the scientific concept of the RDAs and we recognize the public service dedication of the members of the Food and Nutrition Board Subcommittee on RDA. However, we feel that in some cases the RDAs are on the conservative side and need liberalization for the benefit of the public health. At this point in time there are the resources in the United States to provide all of the micronutrients to all people at very low cost.

Are the RDA's too low? Quite the contrary say two British nutritionists who have worked extensively in poor countries. Isn't it possible, they ask, that the RDAs are much higher than they need to be simply because we are so rich?

RECOMMENDED DIETARY ALLOWANCES AND THIRD WORLD POPULATIONS*

A. R. P. Walker, D.Sc. and B. F. Walker

The recent publication in the United States of amended Recommended Dietary Allowances (RDA), and in the United Kingdom of corresponding data, makes absorbing reading to those of us living in juxtaposition with different ethnic groups accustomed to very contrasting intakes of nutrients. It is appreciated that these allowances relate primarily to populations in Western contexts, and are designed to meet the needs of virtually all healthy persons. Understandably, allowances are far higher, perhaps double, compared with physiological needs. However, the fact is that large segments of all less privileged populations — the huge bulk of the world's inhabitants — unquestionably have low intakes, often far lower than the RDA of many important nutrients. To workers engaged in research among such populations, questions repeatedly obtrude, such as "Do these low intakes really matter? At what low levels of intakes are malnutritional stigmata evoked which are accompanied by higher than average morbidities and mortalities? To what extent do habitually low intakes

*"Recommended Dietary Allowances and Third World Populations," by A. R. P. Walker, D.Sc., and B. F. Walker. Copyright *The American Journal of Clinical Nutrition*, 34:2319–2321, October, 1981. American Society for Clinical Nutrition. Used with permission.

prejudice physiological processes such as pregnancy and lactation?"
Apart from situations where exceptionally low intakes prevail, the relevant knowledge available is nowhere near adequate.

School pupils consuming Third World diets (usually containing allowances far lower than RDA) grow slower than pupils on Western diets. Does such behavior, ipso facto, denote the presence of inferior health? Although the risks of low weight-for-age postulated remain to be established, many workers believe that growing children should be fed to reach their maximum growth potential. Yet, studies are lacking which define the disadvantages or advantages, past, present, or future, which are linked with the slower or the faster growth of pupils. There appears to be no knowledge of the *current* state of health of the children who were used 35 years or so ago in the establishment of the Boston and Iowa reference standards. Which particular percentile of weight-for-age of the pupils used have had the best track records, in the course of the years, regarding occurrences of obesity, hypertension, diabetes, coronary heart disease, etc., — the 10th, 30th, 50th, or 70th percentile, or which? Conceivably, slower than average growth could be beneficial. Because of shortage of basic knowledge many doubt that for good health all children everywhere should conform to American norms.

RDA for pregnancy and lactation, respectively, include daily intakes of 96 and 86 g of protein, and 1200 mg of calcium. The supplying of additional allowances for these processes is plausible. Yet even among Western populations no critical studies appear to have affirmed that prowess in lactation is regulated by levels of intakes of nutrients. Among developing populations, it is virtually out of the question for the RDA for pregnancy and lactation mentioned to be attained. Notwithstanding, approaching 100% of Third World mothers lactate successfully, usually for prolonged periods, and seemingly without obvious prejudice to themselves. Among some groups of poor rural Asian mothers the average period is 20 months. That Asian and African mothers are able to perform this, albeit yielding a somewhat reduced volume of milk (750 to 800 ml), is truly remarkable. There is so much in this field that requires clarification.

As to calcium intake — black mothers in South Africa, although accustomed to a quarter or so of RDA for pregnancy and lactation, have been found to display satisfactory calcium homeostasis (cortical dimensions of metacarpal and humerus). This was found to be obtained even when pregnancies were very numerous and lactations long. In later life, the Gilbertian situation is such that black mothers have less severe osteoporosis than far better circumstanced white mothers who have had few children and barely significant lactational experience. Black mothers, moreover, have one-tenth of the frequency of hip fractures found in white mothers. It is ironic that white women, to reduce or offset bone resorption at late middle-age are being en-

46

joined to ingest an extra 800 mg calcium daily, despite their already habitually high intakes of the element.

In general discussions on these and related topics, the commendable experiences of less privileged populations are either ignored or given scant consideration. Do physiological requirements differ according to whether a population is primitively living or developing, or whether it is developed? In the United States, there are significant proportions of populations, young and old, who have calcium intakes of the same order as those of the South African blacks mentioned. Of the segments of Americans who are accustomed to large shortfalls from RDA, do they or do they not manifest unequivocal deficiency stigmata of clinical significance?

From our vantage point, we would advocate a measure of reorientation of nutritional research endeavor. It is not so much that we have misgivings over the relevance of RDA to Third World populations, but rather that we are concerned over the lack of knowledge concerning the effects of the nutritional situations which will inevitably prevail in the not so distant future. Because of increases in population, and because obviously there are limits to increases in food production, the huge bulk of the world's inhabitants will ultimately be *compelled* to consume a largely vegetarian diet. Surely, rather than aiming to produce faster growing or taller children, or of seeking to learn of what *more* can be added, with advantage, to the already luxus diets of most Western populations, we should be concentrating on studying the converse. Namely, knowledge must be acquired of the relatively low levels of nutrient intakes, for young and old, which are compatible with good health and well-being, and which are consistent with satisfactory accomplishments of physiological processes and of performances of everyday tasks of life. . . .

Now another piece of testimony. This time it comes from a food supplement manufacturer, William T. Thompson. Under the circumstances he might be expected to agree with Dr. Brin that RDAs are set too low. What he has to say may therefore surprise you.

HEARINGS ON THE ADEQUACY AND USEFULNESS OF THE RECOMMENDED DIETARY ALLOWANCE STANDARDS*

William T. Thompson

. . . Since I am not a nutritionist or biochemist, I will not presume to comment on the merits of the RDA as tools for the use of scientists. I will instead address a trend that has become increasingly pronounced during the sixteen years that I have directed my family's company, sixteen years during which I have witnessed the mounting public interest in and awareness of nutrition. During that period the RDA have been translated into U.S. RDA's and have consequently been transformed from a relatively arcane and little known scientific device to a widely debated and highly visible labeling tool for use by the general public in assessing the nutritional desirability of a large number of foods. In the process, the RDA have been altered from an academic analysis of data to an official pronouncement of the U.S. Government. They have ceased to be perceived as DIETARY allowances to be achieved by the averaging of the variability in several days' or weeks' consumption of whole foods, and have come to be perceived as necessary DAILY intakes, capable of identification and compression into one ounce of cereal or one tablet of a supplement or one spoonful of orange powder dissolved in water. Most striking, they have shifted from RDA viewed as a statistical concept for judging the adequacy of diets of large groups of people to a specific recipe for individual foods and food replacements. We have begun to engineer food analogs to the specifications of the RDA, and we then use the RDA as a measure to determine whether the resulting foods are "nutritious", thereby creating a closed loop which ignores the incredible complexity and richness of real foods and permits constructed analogs of food to appear to serve the full purpose of traditional nourishment. These new functions

*"Hearings on the Adequacy and Usefulness of the Recommended Dietary Allowance Standards," by William T. Thompson. Testimony before the U.S. House of Representatives Committee on Science and Technology, July 13, 1978. *The Scientific Adequacy and Usefulness of the Recommended Dietary Allowance (RDA) Standards*, Pages 450–467.

of the RDA, as a basis for the U.S. RDA, have, I believe, many unfortunate, undesirable and unintended side effects, the most important and most damaging of which is the misuse and manipulation of the U.S. RDA's by the American processed food industry to present engineered food analogs as being nutritionally equivalent to, or even superior to, the basic and traditional foods that are being replaced.

Debates about food have always sparked controversy, in part because food is such a personal topic, but at least until recently, we as a society shared a common understanding about what food *was*. Our concept of food was largely limited to that huge variety of commodities — meats, fruits, grains, vegetables, seeds, nuts, dairy products, etc — which over the millenia man has depended upon for nourishment and to which his physiology has been adapted. When the first RDA committee met in 1941 it began with the fundamental assumption that, given a food supply made up of such "ordinary foods", it would be possible to use the admittedly scanty available scientific information on human nutritional requirements to establish guidelines for other nutrition professionals to use in evaluating the multitudinous diets based on those foods. It was taken for granted that a diet made up of "natural foods" would supply a myriad of nutrients, both known and unknown, in addition to the few vitamins and minerals for which standards had been set. The standard allowances were never viewed as more than indicators of the total nutritional quality of the food used.

Since the time the first RDA committee met, however, we have experienced a revolution in the growing, processing, and distribution of food; and in consequence, American eating habits have changed almost beyond the recognition of our grandparents. The "ordinary food" of 1941 is not the "ordinary food" of 1978. Had the members of the original RDA committee entered a time capsule in 1941 and re-emerged today, most of the products on an average supermarket shelf would be unfamiliar to them, since many of today's "ordinary foods" have been literally created from scratch in the past three decades. Eating patterns have shifted sharply from diets composed of basic, raw, whole foods prepared at home to diets composed of processed, fabricated, constructed foods prepared away from home. We have, as a society, too willingly embraced "new and untested eating patterns", and these patterns have penetrated not only throughout our urban areas but equally into the rural communities and the smallest independent towns in the country. This fact was brought home to me recently when I visited the farm my family owns and has operated for over 30 years in the middle of Missouri.

The farm lies on the Gasconade River, about ten miles from the little town of Vienna, Missouri, population 505, in Maries County in the foothills of the Ozarks, near Jefferson City. You'd be hard pressed to find a place more middle of the Midwest, in all ways, than Vienna, Missouri. There are only two markets in Vienna: the Cash Market and Dave's.

49

Less than 20 years ago, relatively little of Vienna's food passed through either market. People grew their own vegetables, raised their own cows and chickens, slaughtered their own pork, gathered berries, nuts, mushrooms and wild spring greens. Today, like the rest of America, they harvest their corn from produce shelves and pluck their chickens from refrigerated bins. The chickens for sale at Dave's market are not even locally grown, but are purchased from out of state and available fresh only on Wednesday. The cereal shelves at Dave's look like the cereal shelves in Marina del Rey, with the staple cereals of yesteryear relegated to a small section, dwarfed by 58 frontings of Fruit Loops, Honey Comb, Total, Sugar Corn Pops, Cookie-Crisp, Capt'n Crunch, Cracklin' Bran, Product 19, Cocoa Puffs and Fruit Brute. Juices which used to be home-squeezed are now bought in bottles or frozen concentrates or replaced entirely by fabricated analogues such as Tang.

More and more foods in our markets are being replaced, in other words, by what my wife calls "food-like products" — branded, fabricated, fortified, television advertised creations of man's ingenuity. Such products were admittedly filtering into our food supply long before nutrition labeling came on the scene, but their most explosive growth has occurred since nutrition labeling made it possible for them to be portrayed as the nutritional equivalents — or even the nutritional superiors — of real food. . . .

. . . Products are being portrayed as superior foods when in fact they are merely inferior vitamin/mineral supplements. As food analogs, these fabricated products have the drawback of providing only a limited number of nutrients, contained in a base of highly refined carbohydrates, with the abundance of accessory nutrients and other compounds present in real foods totally absent. As nutrient supplements, these products masquerading as "conventional foods" have the same drawback of providing only a limited number of nutrients, at a cost of almost twice as much as equivalent nutrient supplements in traditional forms. . . .

It was . . . hoped, at one time, that nutrition labeling would spur an unprecedented burst of research into the actual nutritional values of common foods, and into the natural variability of nutrient content under many conditions of cultivation and processing. Instead, the US RDA has been used predominantly as the measure of nutrients *added* to foods. Its potential as a spur to food composition research has not been realized. It is critical that food composition research be given a high priority, for it is only through understanding the marvelous complexity of real foods that we can fully appreciate the potential impoverishment of our food supply as fabricated products continue to proliferate. The rationality of utilizing a selected number of nutrients as indicators of total nutritional value depends importantly and fundamentally on the assumption that the foods measured will also contain myriads of nutrients other than the standards. By focussing on a limited number of nutrients, and by relying on fabricated foods as a source of these nutrients, we are decreasing the natural diversity of our diets. The 58 cereals available in Dave's Market are not really 58 different cereals. They are 58 different *products* constructed from a handful of refined grains and sugars, plus added vitamins, minerals, flavorings, and colors, differentiated by a plethora of names and colorful packages and "free" premiums. This apparent diversity *of products* masks a galloping homogenization and standardization of our food supply. The decrease in real diversity of the foods we eat causes a decrease in the degree of insurance that can be provided by eating a "wide variety of commonly available foods."

Clearly this is not what the [National] Academy of Sciences and the RDA committees had in mind when the standards were formed, nor is it what the FDA had in mind when it condensed the N.A.S. RDA into the U.S. RDA. . . .

The next excerpt is from the National Academy of Sciences' massive 1983 volume entitled Diet, Nutrition, and Cancer. *It illustrates vividly what can happen when the nutritional quality of the food supply is judged solely on the measured nutrients it contains.*

THE RELATIONSHIP BETWEEN NUTRIENTS AND CANCER*

Committee on Diet, Nutrition, and Cancer

Changes in the Food Supply

. . . The daily per capita intake of nutrients during certain years between 1909 and 1976 . . . based on food disappearance data reported by Page and Friend (1978), show that if nutrients alone are measured, the food supply appears to have undergone little overall change during this period. There has been a slight decline in total calories available for consumption, essentially no change in total protein, and a moderate increase in total fat, balancing a similar decline in total carbohydrate. The available supply of most of the vitamins and minerals mea-

---

*"Section A: The Relationship Between Nutrients and Cancer. *Diet, Nutrition and Cancer*, 1983, pp. A1 – A15. National Academy Press, Washington, DC. Used with permission.

sured has remained essentially unchanged. The exceptions are iron and vitamins B_1, B_2, and niacin, which have increased, and magnesium, which has decreased. The increases probably reflect the enrichment of a variety of flour-based products. Since magnesium is lost during the refining of flour, as are a number of trace minerals, the decline in magnesium intake might reflect a general decline in trace minerals, especially those derived from whole grains.

However, these figures on the availability of a limited group of nutrients tend to obscure the extensive changes that have taken place in the food supply during the past 50 years. Some of these can be seen by examining the changes that have occurred in the contribution of various food groups to total calories. For example, the percentage of calories derived from grain products has been halved. . . . Most of this change can be attributed to a decline in per capita intake of flour: from approximately 131 kg per capita in 1909 to 63 kg in 1976. The intake of fat has also changed. . . . Although total per capita fat intake increased only 27% during this period, fat as a percentage of calories increased by 35%. There was also a 56% increase in the intake of separated fats, most of them from vegetable sources. In other words, as attention shifts from nutrients to food groups and from there to specific food substances, it becomes increasingly evident that there have been extensive changes in the composition of what is actually available to eat. . . .

. . . There have been continual shifts in the numbers, types, and varieties of available foodstuffs. Even when the kinds and amounts of foods consumed in the past can be accurately determined, their chemical composition remains unknown and may have changed significantly over the decades. For example, a frozen pizza made with imitation cheese, tomato extender, and soy-protein "pepperoni" is composed of a very different collection of chemicals than the apparently similar product made 10 years earlier with mozzarella cheese, tomato paste, and meat sausage.

The proportion of manufactured products in the average diet has been increasing, especially in developed countries, but the detailed composition of many of these products is not known. Manufacturers often consider it proprietary information. . . .

52

In late 1985 the Food and Nutrition Board held a workshop to discuss, in light of future RDAs, many of the same problems we have highlighted in this chapter. Issues that emerged from that workshop, and from the controversy over the delay in the 1985 RDAs, were summarized by the Board in the article from which these brief excerpts were taken.

RECOMMENDED DIETARY ALLOWANCES: SCIENTIFIC ISSUES AND PROCESS FOR THE FUTURE*

Food and Nutrition Board

. . . Some Scientific Considerations in the Preparation of RDAs

Fundamental Scientific Considerations
Some of the fundamental scientific issues requiring resolution are summarized below.

Definition. Does the definition of the RDAs apply only to the prevention of deficiency diseases or generally to promotion of growth, maintenance of good health, and the reduction of risk of other diseases? What are the physiological indicators of *good* health? Can *optimal* health be defined?

Purpose. What is the purpose of the RDAs? Given their multiple uses, is it feasible to use the same allowances for different purposes (e.g., for food and nutrient labelling as well as for interpreting food consumption survey data to predict nutritional risk), or should different nutrient recommendations be developed for different applications?

Criteria. In light of recent advances in nutrition, what criteria are appropriate for establishing RDAs? For example, are measures of functional capacity and evidence that certain dietary factors may lower the risk of chronic diseases appropriate for inclusion among the criteria? What type, consistency, and strength of evidence are required for establishing RDAs, for modifying current RDAs, and for determining

---

*"Recommended Dietary Allowances: Scientific Issues and Process for the Future." Food and Nutrition Board statement, National Research Council — National Academy of Sciences, 2101 Constitution Ave., N.W., Washington, DC 20418, January 1986. National Academy Press, Washington, DC. Used with permission.

whether to develop an RDA for a nutrient or whether a provisional recommendation or a safe and adequate range would be more appropriate? In the absence of evidence indicating a deficiency or other adverse effect in the population, how much weight should be given to the average dietary intake of a nutrient as a criterion for determining nutrient allowances?

Data Base. Which data base would be most appropriate, considering the purpose and definition of the RDAs? For example, what is the relevance of data from controlled clinical trials or epidemiological data linking food consumption to such variables as birth weight or morbidity? What types of data serve as the basis for nutrient allowances developed by other national and international organizations? . . .

Population Subgroups. Are the current age and sex groupings for the RDAs scientifically the most valid and logical? For example, since the majority of data on human nutrient requirements are derived from experiments in young adults, can they be extrapolated with confidence to estimate the nutrient needs of infants and the elderly? Should the age and sex groupings for the RDAs be reexamined in light of knowledge about physiological breakpoints that are characterized by significant changes in growth rates, e.g., during infancy? What are the implications of current concepts about physical activity levels and patterns of weight gain during pregnancy for nutrient and energy needs? What is the effect of supplementation on pregnancy outcome and consequently on nutrient needs?

Application. Can the data on which the RDAs are based be used to determine nutrient allowances for individuals, or only for groups? Should meeting the RDAs through the usual diet be a major criterion for establishing an RDA? Can the RDAs serve as a foundation for diets that are feasible and within reach of the general population? If not, what guidance can be given about food fortification or nutrient supplementation, and what are the health implications of nutrient intakes that are consistently above or below the RDAs?

Specific Nutrients
Many scientific issues pertain to specific macro- and micro-nutrients. [One] that require[s] particular attention [is] outlined below. . . .

- *Vitamin C:* What physiological parameters should be considered in establishing the RDA? Absence of clinical signs of scurvy? Maintenance of a certain size body pool? Avoidance of behavioral abnormalities or psychological manifestations associated with vitamin C deficiency? Other considerations? What is the effect of maintaining different sizes of vitamin C body pools (e.g., 1,500 mg, 900 mg, or 600 mg) on specific health indices of vitamin C nutriture? What is the

54

significance of observations that vitamin C enhances iron absorption, and what weight should be given to data suggesting enhanced iron absorption but not necessarily enhanced iron storage in omnivores? Are vitamin C requirements of smokers higher than those of non-smokers? Can the antioxidant and antinitrosating potentials of vitamin C be quantified, and are they relevant to establishing an RDA? Is there documented evidence of benefit or risk associated with the current average vitamin C intake (i.e., approximately 80 to 100 mg/day), which is higher than the current RDA? Is epidemiological evidence linking vitamin C-containing fruits and vegetables to lower cancer risk sufficiently definitive and relevant for consideration in establishing an RDA? . . .

General Considerations for the Future
A number of procedural considerations were identified. [One of] the most important [was] the following: . . .

- The process for developing the RDAs should be open for discussion among scientists, health practitioners, and other users. Throughout the study, periodic attempts should be made to obtain input from additional scientific experts outside the committee and from other users of the RDAs. . . .

Purposes and Uses
. . . The RDAs . . . might be designed with at least the following purposes and uses in mind.

Safety and Quality Assurance. The allowances might be designed to protect the public from excessive as well as deficient nutrient intake, and the RDA report might include information about the strengths and limitations of the data on which the RDAs are based.

Dietary Assessment. The steps leading to the establishment of the RDAs (e.g., estimating the average requirements and their variances) might be explained in a manner that enables nutritionists to make reliable estimates of the percentage of the populatio at risk for deficiency and toxicity. . . .

Public Education. The report might contain guidance on the use of the RDAs for making food choices to prevent deficiency, protect against toxicity, and reduce the risk of diet-related chronic diseases.

Nutrition Research. In the process of developing the RDAs, attempts might be made to identify specific needs for research to improve the scientific basis for establishing RDAs. . . .

Scope of Work and Expected Outcome

The following are some important considerations pertaining to the nature and scope of work for developing the RDAs:. . .

- Consideration might be given to the feasibility of developing RDAs for food factors other than essential nutrients (e.g., carotenoids, dietary fiber, cholesterol, and different components of fat) or for essential biological constituents (e.g., omega-3 fatty acids, which are essential to the brain) that are available only through the diet.
- Biological and common environmental and social factors that contribute significantly to the variability of dietary requirements in the general population might be identified. These factors include, but are not limited to, age, sex, reproductive status, genetic background, bio-availability of nutrients in specific foods and in different types of diets, drug-nutrient interactions, use of nutrient supplements, occupation, activity, stress, and physical disabilities.
- Where data permit, an *average physiological requirement* and an estimate of its variance, as well as an average *upper safe level* according to each category of criteria, might be established. Thus, attention might be given to determining if it is appropriate to establish a single RDA or a series of allowances for each nutrient, depending on the intended use. . . .

Afterword

There you have them—some of the real issues where the RDAs are concerned. When we went to school little appeared in our books suggesting that those official-looking numbers we had to memorize were associated with any controversy. Yet obviously they are. What you conclude from all this is up to you. But there are certain points we'd like to emphasize.

Notice, to begin with, that these impressive numbers are usually based on a small amount of data, drawn often from a single age group and extrapolated to the entire population made up of people of all ages, sexes and conditions. Yet, as Leverton observes, the figures are presented in terms of particular age-sex groups, a specificity that "implies research data that do not exist." (You may recall our discussion in the Introduction about the difficulty of doing such research.) This leaves lots of room for interpretation—and disagreement.

Committees that establish RDAs must first make judgments about the adequacy of scientific data, and then about the meaning of those data. If the population shows no obvious signs of deficiency with regard to a certain nutrient, can the average intake of that population be used to estimate the recommended allowance?

Is "no obvious signs of deficiency" the desired end point? Or are we looking for something more?

As we discussed in the Introduction, it is not merely that "we do not know the ideal nutrient intakes for longevity, resistance to chronic diseases, and maximum physical and mental performance in old age." We don't even agree about what we mean by "adequate" intake. Is adequate vitamin C nutrition the amount that will produce tissue saturation or simply the amount necessary to prevent scurvy in experimental settings?

Notice the interesting question the Walkers ask. Is rapid growth of children to their full genetic potential a good idea? Does it lead to long and healthy lives? If it does not, then what measures other than growth do we use to measure the nutritional well-being of children? In animals it has long been known that high quality diets fed in amounts smaller than the animals might spontaneously eat can lead to longer lives and less degenerative disease. Should we act on that observation with respect to humans? *Could* we? Or should the RDAs take into account new data suggesting that higher levels of some nutrients may help prevent degenerative disease?

The noted biologist René Dubos once wrote that although the RDAs were derived from studies made on normal people, "It is now realized . . . that there are enormous individual differences, some caused by genetic constitution, and others caused by the past history of the particular person, as well as by the occupation and ways of life of that person." What is "adequate" for all these people? "Nutritional science would greatly benefit," Dubos continues, "from the development of functional tests designed to measure the ability of the organism to develop scar tissue, and produce antibodies, to generate phagocytic cells, to correct tissue damage, to modify behavior, in brief to make adequate biological and psychological response, to various life situations." (René Dubos. "The Intellectual Basis of Nutrition Science." *Nutrition Today.* 14:31–34, July/August 1979)

We noted in the introduction to this chapter that *any* definition of the RDA is arbitrary, based on the opinions of the committee members about what a "recommended allowance" ought to be. What we now see is that any definition of adequacy that promises merely to prevent known deficiency disease, is accepting a criterion with which many people would disagree. It is something like the difference between defining health on the one hand as the avoidance of disease, and on the other — as the World Health Organization has proposed — as "a state of physical, mental and social well-being and not merely the absence of illness or infirmity."

So we need to keep reminding ourselves that even though these numbers are *based* on scientific observation and experimentation (albeit limited), they are the product of a process that

57

is not scientific but judgmental.

All of the authors in this chapter who address this topic acknowledge that. Actually, it's self-evident. If no judgment were involved, all recommended allowances — at least for those of us in rich countries — would be exactly alike, and those for the U.S. population would not differ from one edition to the next unless new studies had markedly changed the data base. In fact, our allowances differ in many respects from those of even our closest neighbor, Canada, and they have changed from edition to edition in the U.S. even when there were few or no new experimental data.

Different committees, in short, consider the available data and come to different conclusions. What accounts for these differences? Are they the result of industry pressures, or "politics" as some people charge? Is our calcium requirement so high because we have a powerful dairy industry? Do we resist urging a lower intake of animal protein, despite the fact that our present intake far exceeds the RDA, because powerful meat interests have put pressure on the committee? Are the RDAs for certain nutrients higher than they need to be, and too high for many people to get on an ordinary diet, because of the influence of those who make — or use — fortification nutrients? Or do we maintain higher than necessary recommendations because of pressure from advocacy groups who fear cuts in government programs if nutrient allowances are lowered?

The answer to all those questions is probably "no." But those questions cannot really be answered. To conclude that there is industry or consumer bias in a committee's decisions would require that we make another set of judgments — based on even less objective evidence than there is to support the RDAs themselves — on the motives of the committee. As Dr. Hegsted once noted, neither the public nor the nutrition community as a whole really knows how committee judgments have been made.

One need not question the integrity of the decision makers, however, to insist that these numbers are not "objectively" arrived at, if by the term *objective* we mean that no considerations except data-based ones have been taken into account. While Dr. Harper insists that the Recommended Dietary Allowance bulletins should not be viewed as socio-political documents, he himself notes that the "optimism" or "pessimism" of a committee may affect its judgment. Since it is not clear what an RDA committee might be optimistic or pessimistic *about*, we must interpret him to mean simply that every scientist comes to such a task with his/her own world view, that will affect, as we said in the Introduction, his or her reading of the available (and surprisingly scanty) data. That the committee rather than a single individual makes the judgment at least helps to keep the numbers from representing merely one individual's particular interpretation.

There is at least one "world view" that can be assumed to affect most scientists serving on committees that set RDAs for the U.S., namely the abundance of the U.S. food supply. As the Walkers suggest, the very fact that high levels of most nutrients are so readily available to most people in the U.S. has probably tended in the past to produce a mental predisposition toward setting levels much more than minimally adequate. To check this out you might want to compare the U.S. allowances with each other over time, or compare them with the Food and Agriculture Organization (FAO) allowances for countries with a less abundant food supply.

Another bias that is probably inevitable for the scientists who set the RDAs is a growing isolation from the practical aspects of their recommendations — from the fact that these recommendations are often being used to answer the question, "What should we *eat*?" You may remember our telling you earlier that the very first RDAs included a day's menu which met the nutrient recommendations. Over time, this food emphasis has been increasingly lost, so that many people who are trying to use the RDAs in the everyday world find it difficult to construct diets that meet recommended levels of all the different nutrients.

As Hegsted notes, "If the RDAs were really to be taken literally, it would mean that each member of the family would have to eat a different diet." Not only is such an outcome unlikely, it is difficult to imagine how humans could have gotten themselves into a situation where ordinary food shared from the family pot would not adequately nourish the family — especially in a country which is relatively rich in both food and the resources to acquire it.

In the beginning, RDAs applied to only a small group of indicator nutrients — "indicator" meaning that if your diet contained those nutrients in the amounts specified, you could assume that your other nutritional needs were met. Today there are RDAs for a long list of nutrients, and the notion has arisen that the goal is to somehow construct a diet containing appropriate quantities of each of them. It is therefore interesting that the participants in the workshop planning the next edition of the RDAs urged the committee, before issuing the new allowances, to see whether the proposed allowances could be met by ordinary foods.

Although we did not intend to include it when we began this book, the article by the Food and Nutrition Board addressing some of the broader issues that must be considered in designing new RDAs shows that many of the problems identified in this chapter will be dealt with in future editions. Among the most difficult questions are those of how the RDAs should be used by government agencies who have historically made use of them as standards for food programs and indicators of nutritional status in surveys. What percent of the RDA must be met by what percentage of the individuals in a survey before one can assume that most people are adequately nourished? When any given individual calculates his or her dietary intake, what percentage of how many nutrients can fall below the RDA without suggesting that that individual is at risk?

These are, of course, precisely the problems that trained nutritionists will need to resolve — with, it is to be hoped, the help of the new RDA committee. But the need to *interpret* not only in setting, but in *using* the RDAs, is precisely why Rogan and Yu express concern about the widespread use of computer analyses by those not trained to understand what those print-outs mean!

Once we move beyond specific numbers, consideration of the RDAs reveals fundamental differences in points of view. Contrast Brin's view of nutrition — the delivery of certain chemicals to the body — with Ross Hall's view of nourishment as "a complex biological phenomenon in which one life form gives up its life and is converted into another life form." People who hold such differing views of the process (neither of which can be proved "true") would find it hard to talk together about dietary requirements.

Taken together with Harper's statement that we don't know what an optimal diet consists of, these very different interpretations illustrate once again that reactions to the RDAs reflect philosophies of science as well as of life. Harper believes we are able to detect what is false, even though "we do not have methods for proving absolutely what is true." He is reminding us here of the scientific method which — contrary to popular understanding — is based on hypothesizing explanations for phenomena and then setting up experiments to *dis*-prove them.

Anyone with a taste for burrowing in the literature can discover for themselves, however, that many testable hypotheses regarding optimal levels of nutrients have seldom if ever been tested, once again partly because we have not been able to agree upon the end points we are testing for. Even more daunting is the fact that some of the agreed-upon end points, extending life span for example, are essentially untestable in humans (see Chapter 6).

Can we use the RDAs? They are the only standard we have for planning meals for institutions, for assessing nutritional status in dietary surveys, even for deciding whether our individual diets may be lacking something essential.

Can we use the USRDAs to choose nutritious foods from the grocery shelves? If you believe Brin, you can. If you believe Hall and Thompson, you can't. Leverton and Hegsted too worry about the effect of extensive fabrication and fortification on the perception of nutritiousness, and about the tendency of the RDAs, as they come to include more nutrients, to lead us to forget other components of food possibly relevant to health, for which there are no RDAs.

Before we all became conscious of the desirability of avoiding excess sodium, we might have told you to take the RDAs with a grain of salt. Now we'll simply warn you not to let the attractive certainty of the numbers substitute for clear and careful thought.

2 Food Guides: Simplifying the Numbers

As Leverton explained in the previous chapter, the RDAs are not for amateurs — or for the housewife planning family meals. This means that professional nutritionists need some device that can translate nutrient needs into foods for those who are not professionals. It seems simple enough at first to group foods according to the nutrients they contain, but the selections you are about to read will show you that arguments over the RDAs are no more heated than arguments over the best way to translate all those numbers into food groups.

After all, the RDAs may be judgment calls, but the fact that they are numbers makes them seem pretty objective, and awfully definite. Different countries may come up with somewhat different numbers, but there is no real debate about which nutrients are essential.

There are, however, disagreements about which foods are essential. And when the micrograms and milligrams get translated into foods, livelihoods and lifestyles are suddenly threatened. How foods get grouped (and they can be grouped in a surprising variety of ways as you will see) affects how many servings of what kinds of foods nutritionists will recommend, and those recommendations will affect the jobs of people who produce and sell certain kinds of foods. Food groups are definitely not neutral!

The food grouping system that is probably most familiar to most of us is called the Basic Four. It may seem to you — as it did to us when we first had to learn the Four Food Group system in school — that this particular arrangement (meat, milk, fruits/vegetables, grain products) was handed down from on high, like Moses' tablets. To enlighten you, we are including in this section a bit of history of why and how we came to move from seven to four food groups. Were the reasons for the change educational? Was a four-food-group system easier to teach than a seven-group system? Was the reason for the change political? Did meat producers provoke the change in order to promote meat consumption? You will have to decide for yourselves.

The most important argument, perhaps, is the one that centers about the nutritional usefulness of the system. Does the Basic Four work? Does it really help people select an adequate diet? Some nutritionists think that with a few modernizations the guide is just fine, educationally and nutritionally. Others think it is fatally flawed. The first group has tried to fix up the Basic Four by making changes; the second group has tried to think about altogether new classifications that would be nutritionally and educationally sound, and useful, for the last decades of the 20th century and beyond. We hope you enjoy the debate.

NUTRITION EDUCATION*

Food and Nutrition Board, National Academy of Sciences

For nutrition education programs, it is customary to group foods according to the nutrients for which the foods are major sources. Guidelines are usually provided to illustrate how nutrient needs can be met by selecting from among a relatively few groups of foods. Such food groupings and food guides are useful for illustrating the essential elements of a basic diet, but it is important that such guides be adapted and modified imaginatively to meet the needs of individuals and families with different levels of income, cultural patterns, and lifestyles. The RDA for nutrients can be obtained from a wide variety of food combinations and dietary patterns — any of which can be adequate, provided that care is exercised in food selection.

*"Nutrition Education," *Recommended Dietary Allowances*, 9th Edition, 1980, page 14. Food and Nutrition Board. National Academy Press, Washington, DC. Used with permission.

ERNIE POOK'S COMEEK*

Lynda J. Barry

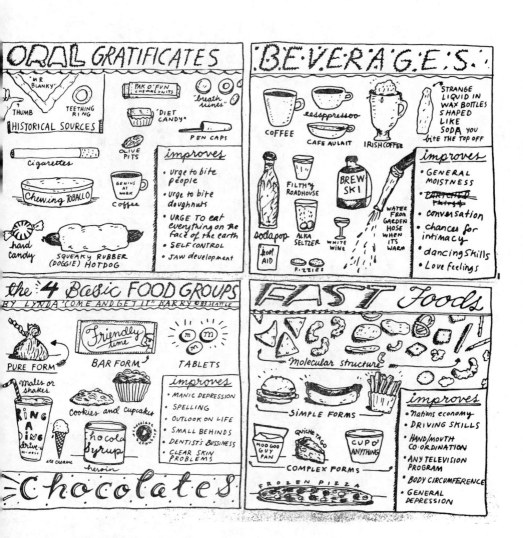

Here—from a Wheaties advertisement in the Philadelphia Inquirer *for July 4, 1943 — is the food guide Americans used during World War II. As you can see it has seven groups, three for different kinds of fruits and vegetables, one each for cereal products, meats and milk, and an extra one for fats.*

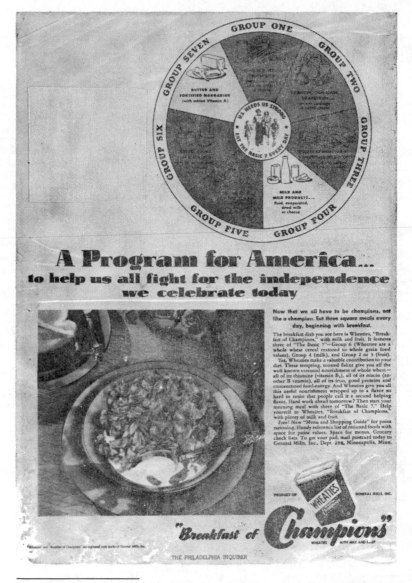

From "A Program for America . . . to help us all fight for the independence we celebrate today." The Philadelphia Inquirer, *July 4, 1943. Used with permission.*

> *In this landmark article, the first published proposal for a four-food-group system for the U.S., faculty from the Department of Nutrition at the Harvard School of Public Health laid out the arguments in favor of having fewer than seven food groups.*

SUGGESTED REVISIONS OF THE BASIC 7* AS FEW AS TWO *FOOD GROUPS CAN BE USED AS A NUTRITION GUIDE*

Olive Hayes, Martha F. Trulson, D.Sc., and Fredrick J. Stare, M.D., Ph.D.

Food charts and posters are familiar tools in nutrition education. The desirable goal of such tools is to achieve maximum simplicity consistent with scientific facts, available foods, and acceptable food patterns in the country in which they are to be used.

It is questionable whether the Basic 7, the most widely used nutrition education tool of this kind in the United States, achieves this goal of maximum simplicity. Although it has undoubtedly been useful in nutrition education, it is complicated and its effectiveness is probably curtailed accordingly.

The Basic 7, as we know it today, was announced in 1943 as part of the National Wartime Nutrition Program of the Agricultural Research Administration of the United States Department of Agriculture. . . . It consists of a collection of foods which are apportioned to seven groups on the basis of their major contribution to the nutrient value of the diet and their function in the American dietary. Its aim is to promote variety in food consumption and to provide a plan whereby even the individual who knows nothing of the science of nutrition can select a diet adequate in protective foods. . . .

Criteria for Judging Effectiveness of Teaching Aids

Two criteria by which one may judge the effectiveness of a teaching aid are validity and simplicity. It is impossible to teach effectively from a tool that is inaccurate; it is difficult to teach from one that is complicated or cumbersome. Questions can be raised regarding both these

Received for publication May 26, 1955. Presented at the 35th annual meeting of the American Dietetic Association in St. Louis, on October 19, 1955.

aspects when we examine the Basic 7 chart. One could argue that a person might habitually select green and yellow vegetables of such low vitamin A content that the total daily intake of this vitamin would fall below desirable intakes. Or one might pose the questions, "What is meant by a serving? How large or how small should these servings be?" Also, it should be recognized that even exact compliance with the food guide may not produce an adequate diet as regards calories. Therefore, it must be emphasized that the seven groups are suggested as "cornerstones" for building an optimal diet, and it is expected that the individual will use additional foods, if necessary, to adjust his caloric intake to his caloric need. Failure to do so might well result in an inadequate diet, since adequate calories are necessary for growth and maintenance.

Unfortunately, such defects are inherent in any simple teaching device. To attempt to remove them might destroy the effectiveness of the tool by destroying its simplicity. Although the Basic 7 plan cannot be made more valid without losing its simplicity, cannot a plan be made more simple without losing its validity? One might well ask why seven groups are necessary; why not two, three, four, or five?

Figure 1. Scales of a Balanced Diet — Suggested Two-Group Plan for Revision of Basic 7

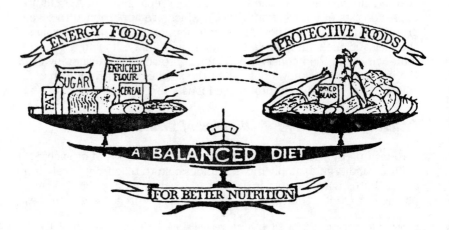

Food Guides of Other Countries

Several other countries have adopted guides of good nutrition. It is interesting to note that none of these countries have found it necessary to use seven groups. Yet they all follow the Basic 7 method of classifying foods into groups on the basis of their major contribution to the nutritive value of the diet. . . .

In some of these countries the need for nutrition education is greater than in others, and personnel and facilities for nutrition education are variable. Possibly their greater needs and fewer educational resources in comparison to those in this country, have led them to adopt simpler food plans.

Scales of a Balanced Diet

The American diet is an abundant one and to develop a guide to good nutrition from such an array of foods is not an easy task. It might be argued that this complexity of diet is the reason for a complex food guide. Yet there is no great virtue in having seven groups if a lesser number would serve the purpose as well.

As few as two food groups can be used to construct a nutrition guide. These groups might consist of merely the energy foods and the protective foods. They might be portrayed on balance pans of a set of scales, rather than on a wheel or circle (*Fig.* 1). In one pan are placed the energy foods (cereals, grains, potatoes, sugars, and fats); the other pan would contain protective foods (meat, fish, poultry, eggs, legumes, milk and its products, fruits including citrus, and vegetables including green leafy and yellow). Since all of the energy foods listed, except sugar and fat, may also serve as protective foods if used in sufficient quantities, these foods are shaded and an arrow is shown leading to the pan of protective foods. Similarly, since some of the protective foods can also serve as energy foods, this is also indicated. Thus an attempt is made to portray the concept that a balancing of energy foods with protective foods is necessary in a balanced diet, but that a balanced diet is possible by having some of the low-cost energy foods serve as protective foods and vice versa.

One advantage of such a two-group plan is that the hands may be utilized in teaching; each hand might represent a food group and any sub-groups of five or less could readily be counted off on the fingers of each hand.

This two-group plan might be a useful one, particularly if nutrition education has been limited. In such circumstances, the individual is not quite sure of the degree to which food affects his health and many times the words "protein" and "vitamins" mean little or nothing to him. He is ready to learn the most elementary facts about nutrition,

69

such as: (a) food affects his health to a large extent; (b) his diet should be balanced; (c) such balancing is achieved by using both energy and protective foods; and (d) some energy foods may function as protective foods and vice versa.

Proposed Protective Shield

A second educational food plan is suggested in which the emphasis is on protective foods. This may be more applicable to a country with an abundant and varied food supply such as the United States, where the primary problem of nutrition education is to guide people to greater knowledge and increased use of the protective foods. For this purpose a chart of four groups is proposed. It might be set up as a shield bearing the caption "Protect Your Health with Protective Foods" (*Fig.* 2). The four groups are: (a) enriched or whole grain bread, flour, cereals, and potato; (b) meat, poultry, fish, eggs, and legumes; (c) fruits, including citrus, and vegetables, including green leafy and yellow; and (d) milk, cheese, and ice cream. The chart is essentially a regrouping of the foods in the Basic 7, rather than an omission of foods.

Figure 2. Shield for Health — Suggested Four-Group Plan for Revision of Basic 7

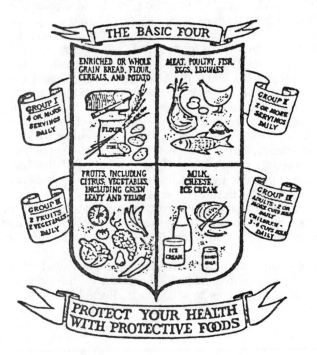

Group 1: Enriched or Whole Grain Bread, Flour, Cereals, and Potato

This group should be accompanied by the notation "four or more servings daily." These foods serve as important sources of energy and because of the quantity in which they are frequently eaten, they also provide protein, iron, and B-complex vitamins. . . .

Group 2: Meat, Poultry, Fish, Eggs, and Legumes

This group should be accompanied by the notation, "two or more servings daily." It is the major contributor to the protein, vitamin, and mineral content of most American diets. Animal protein foods are readily available in this country and their use should be encouraged. However, the importance of cereal protein in low-cost diets should not be underestimated, and when consumed with milk or the protein of leafy vegetables and fruits provides good nutrition. . . .

Group 3: Fruits, Including Citrus, and Vegetables, Including Green Leafy and Yellow

This group should be accompanied by the notation, "select two fruits and two vegetables daily," thereby suggesting an adequate intake of vitamin A and ascorbic acid and an increased intake of iron. No less than three food groups are used to accomplish this purpose in the Basic 7. Potatoes, the main item in Group 3 of the Basic 7, are grouped with bread, flour, and cereals in this proposed four-group plan. . . .

Group 4: Milk, Cheese, and Ice Cream

This is the same as Group 4 of the Basic 7. The major contributions of this group are protein, riboflavin, and calcium. It may be argued that this group could be combined with other protein foods, on the basis of their major nutritive content. But milk has a slightly different function in the American diet than do the other protein foods; one is not apt to regard milk and meat as substitutes for one another in the same way that one regards meat and eggs or potato and bread. Also if one accepts the Recommended Dietary Allowances of the Food and Nutrition Board, milk must be given separate emphasis. This is particularly necessary with regard to calcium and riboflavin. . . .

Therefore, it is felt that keeping milk and its products in a separate category is wise, especially if the teaching program is oriented toward children. Also, the food groups should be in accordance with the available food supplies and dietary customs of the country for which a guide is planned. Since this country has large supplies of dairy products the population can obtain these foods regularly.

It might be suggested that butter and fortified margarine should be included in the Basic 4 because of their contribution to the diet other than calories, particularly vitamin A and possibly essential fatty acids. This may have been the basis for their inclusion in the Basic 7. 71

Yet butter and margarine . . . are an integral part of the American diet, and there is no nutritional reason to urge an increased intake. Indeed, as regards fats in general, there is evidence suggesting that less calories from fat might be a desirable change for the American dietary to make.

It is felt that the four-group food plan may be the most effective teaching aid for use in the United States. By use of this plan an individual may be guided to a selection of foods which is balanced in respect to all nutrients except calories, and as stated previously, the average consumer in this country does not appear to need encouragement in selecting high energy foods in order to insure an adequate caloric intake. . . . Thus it may be stated that the proposed four-group plan appears to be as valid as the current seven-group plan and is clearly a much simpler chart. A school child can and will remember four groups more easily than seven.

A unique way of teaching nutrition to school children might be to serve their lunch on plates or trays partitioned into four segments, each segment bearing a picture of a basic food group. Such a procedure would represent a daily learning experience without expenditure of classroom time and would be an especially effective measure in schools where the children are allowed free selection of foods. Many other methods of incorporating a food guide into nutrition education can be utilized. The diversity of such methods depends on the initiative and skill of the worker as the very simplicity of the four-group plan would be an assurance of success in most situations. . . .

> *Although his Harvard colleagues proposed a four-food-group
> system in 1955, Professor Jean Mayer, then a Harvard faculty
> member too, was still objecting to it as a teaching tool 20 years
> later. He believed that the Basic Seven gave "a much more sat-
> isfactory grouping of foods that contain similar nutrients."*

FOOD AND HEALTH*

Jean Mayer, Ph.D.

Source of Nutrients

The key to good nutrition is a varied diet containing as high a proportion as possible of fresh, unprocessed, or minimally processed (canned
and frozen) foods; the greater the diversity of such foods, the fewer
the chances that any nutrients will be missing. To facilitate thinking
about the different types of foods and their contributions to good
nutrition, foods have often been grouped into certain categories. The
"basic seven" classification was popularized during World War II. More
recently a "basic four" classification has been introduced: the milk
group, the meat group, the bread-cereal group, and the vegetable-fruit
group. The basic four system is not satisfactory. There is no reason,
for example, to classify potatoes and spinach together. It would make
more sense to group together the main sources of animal protein and
good quality vegetable proteins (milk, meat, fish, eggs, peas, and
beans), and separate starchy fruits (bananas) and roots (potatoes)
from green, leafy vegetables and other fruits. . . . The "basic seven"
classification . . . gives a much more satisfactory grouping of foods that
contain similar nutrients. It must be noted, however, that even the
"basic seven" do not cover "fabricated foods" like cocktail cheese
puffs, imitation cream, vegetable-protein "bacon" chips, or the complex
convenience foods like TV dinners and frozen or canned, completely
prepared main dishes, such as stews, lasagna, or pizza, which have become so popular in the past decade. The only way in which these can
be described adequately is through comprehensive nutritional labeling. . . .

The seven food groups are: (1) leafy, green, and yellow vegetables;
(2) citrus fruits, tomatoes, raw cabbage, and salad greens; (3) potatoes
and other vegetables and fruits; (4) milk and milk products; (5) meat,

---

*"Food and Health," by Jean Mayer. *Health,* © 1974, p. 135. Van Nostrand Reinhold Co.,
Inc. Used with permission.

poultry, fish, eggs, dried beans and peas, and nuts; (6) bread, flour, and cereals; and (7) butter and fortified margarine.

Nutritionists generally recommend that a person eat one serving of food from each of the basic seven groups every day. Other foods may be added to the seven as desired, depending on eating habits and activity. . . .

In a world of increasingly processed foods, are food guides still useful at all? Mayer suggests that some sort of system based on nutrients will be required to deal with these new products. In this editorial from the Journal of Nutrition Education, *Editor Ullrich seems to agree. But Leverton suggests that for the public, generalities may make better teaching tools than specifics.*

EDITORIAL: TEACHING TOOLS*

Helen D. Ullrich, M.A., R.D.

How would your diet rank if you checked yesterday's intake against the daily food guide of four groups of foods? Where would you put the pizza or the tacos? One, two, or all groups?

If you are putting your nutrition know-how into practice, you probably ate the foods that supplied all the nutrients you needed but didn't necessarily choose the recommended number of servings from each of the food groupings. If we teach with a tool we can't even apply consistently to ourselves, maybe it is time to figure out a new tool.

When food groupings were first used in the 1920s to guide people in their choice of food . . . very little was known about nutrition. The word protein was only used by scientists. Minerals were substances in the earth, and vitamins were a mystery. As nutrition knowledge progressed, it was still felt that people ate food, not nutrients, so the choice of food rather than nutrients was taught.

In the 1970s the scene has changed. Protein is a household word. Food is advertised not by the food group it falls into, but because it contains protein, energy, minerals, or vitamins. While some nutrition educators hate to admit it, the vitamin jar appears on many dining

*"Editorial: Teaching Tools," by Helen Ullrich. *Journal of Nutrition Education*, 2:80, Winter 1971. Used with permission.

tables. Maybe it is time we started stressing the nutrients the body needs and where they can be found. A grouping of foods by nutrient content seems to make more sense in today's world.

To develop a teaching tool or guide which is generally useful is not an easy task. All levels of knowledge need to be considered. Perhaps there should be a regrouping of foods which can be expanded as knowledge increases. As Hill and Cleveland point out, it took four years to develop the four food groupings, and it has been revised twice since.

There are many people in all parts of the world who spent a great deal of time and effort trying to devise a simple teaching tool. In some countries, a grouping of three kinds of food is used. These groups are named protective, body building, and energy foods.

We would like to make this journal an open forum for ideas as a new teaching tool. No idea is too far out. Accounts of historic decisions are also requested. Please be brief so we can include lots of ideas. Perhaps from the suggestions, a new valuable tool can be devised.

TEACHING TOOLS*

Ruth M. Leverton, Ph.D., R.D.

I am accepting the invitation offered in your editorial in the Winter, 1971, issue to comment on teaching tools and food guides.

You suggest that it is time to find a new tool when we as nutritionists "teach with a tool we can't even apply consistently to ourselves." Could it be that we as nutritionists have so much detailed information that we cannot tolerate generalities? Food guides are developed for the general public, not for the professional nutritionist.

You also suggest that, "A grouping of foods by nutrient content seems to make more sense in today's world." This has always been the basis for USDA, as well as many other, guides. Allocation of mixed dishes such as pizza or casserole dishes to one or more food groups in a guide will depend on their basic ingredients. Serving size needs to be considered too.

Before we "throw the baby out with the bath water," I suggest that we consider the meaning and purpose of a *guide* as contrasted with a *guarantee* of nutritional adequacy. Rigid rules of "eat this and that" would be needed in order to guarantee an adequate intake. . . .

---

*Letter: "Teaching Tools," by Ruth M. Leverton. *Journal of Nutrition Education*, 3:51, Fall 1971. Used with permission.

. . . The minimum servings listed form the *foundation* for a good diet. They provide a substantial share of the RDAs. . . . Minimum servings (based on average choices from nationwide food consumption studies) need to be supplemented by nutrients from additional servings of the same types of foods as well as foods not listed in the four groups.

I am looking forward to the open forum you invite on the subject of food guides. It will be most profitable, however, if our objective is clearly stated. Is it to guide or to guarantee? If it is to guarantee, will we need to regiment people's food "choices"?

If nutritionists can't or don't use the Basic Four, can children? Is the four-food-group system something children can readily understand? Here two educators examine this question by asking children how they spontaneously classify foods.

SPONTANEOUS CLASSIFICATION OF FOODS BY ELEMENTARY SCHOOL-AGED CHILDREN*

John L. Michela, Ph.D. and Isobel R. Contento, Ph.D.

. . . . Nutrition educators commonly have held that nutrition education should be conducted in a manner to be understood and effectively acted upon to bring about desirable eating practices. Accordingly, nutritionists through the decades have designed for public education various food guides which "convert the professional's scientific knowledge of food composition and nutrient requirements for health into a practical plane for selection by those without training in nutrition." The Basic Four or the Four Food Groups, which is the guide currently used with all age groups, is especially popular for use with children inasmuch as it provides relatively specific instructions assumed to be understandable to children. . . .

. . . There is some evidence that suggests that children may have difficulty understanding a classification system that places foods into groups largely on the basis of their nutrient composition as is the case with the Basic Four system. . . .

---

*"Spontaneous Classification of Foods by Elementary School-aged Children," by John L. Michela, Ph.D. and Isobel R. Contento, Ph.D. *Health Education Quarterly*, 11:57–76, Spring 1984. Reprinted by permission of John Wiley & Sons, Inc.

One likely reason for children's difficulties in understanding nutrient-based classification of food is insufficient cognitive development. The act of classifying is a mental operation carried out on cognitive representations of objects and depends on the abstraction and retention of clear criteria. Children at lower levels of cognitive development are unable to make consistent use of criteria as abstract as nutrient composition. . . .

Our review and analysis suggest the need for research on the bases for classification of foods that children actually use and on the changes in food classification with increasing cognitive development. Professional, logical, and common-sense analyses of the entire domain of food suggest a multitude of possible bases for classification of foods other than nutrient composition, including various effects of foods upon sense organs (flavor, odor, appearance, texture); food preference; biological origins of foods; health effects; and social and cultural conventions. . . .

In sum, no prior research tells how elementary school-aged *children* classify foods *spontaneously* when an *encompassing* set of food stimuli is presented.

Method

Sample

Participants were children from two urban and three suburban public schools in two metropolitan centers in the American northeast. There were 115 participants in all — 59 female and 56 male; 16 blacks, 20 Hispanics, and 79 white. They appeared to be mostly middle class with a few from lower socioeconomic classes. They ranged in age from 5 to 11½ years. . . .

Interviews

The interviews on children's food classification systems were conducted individually, usually in some unused room in the cooperating school. The child was presented with pictures of 71 foods, 11 of which were mixed foods such as sandwiches or spaghetti and meat sauce, and the remainder were single food items, e.g., milk. The child was then instructed to classify the foods into groups containing foods that were alike in some way or should be in the same group for any reason. We emphasized that "we are interested in which foods you think should be put in the same groups and why. . . ."

Results

The main categories formed by the children as labeled and reported to the interviewer are shown in Table 1. It can be seen that all the children formed a sweets group; 50% a fruits group; 50% a vegetable group (only 25% formed a combined fruit and vegetable group while the remainder classified both fruits and vegetables with meals); 48% a drinks group; 24% a dairy group; and 20% a breads and grains group. While there is obviously some correspondence here with nutritionists' classification of foods, major departures from the Basic Four scheme include the presence of groups of sweets and of drinks, and the low frequency of classifying fruits and vegetables or breads and grains together in the same group.

Table 1. Major Food Categories Formed by Children

Groups Formed	*Percent of Children Forming Each Group*
Sweets	100
All sweet items = 1 group	70
Two groups: desserts, candy	30
Meat and Fish	70
Meats and fish alone	34
Meats and fish with stews, sandwiches	36
Fruits	51
Vegetables	50
(Fruits and vegetables together)	25
Drinks	48
(Milk in drinks group)	36
Dairy	48
Milk, cheese, yoghurt	24
Cheeses only (milk, yoghurt in other groups)	24
Breads	32
Grains	
Breakfast cereals only (no other grains or bread)	19
Starches (rice and noodles)	30
Starches and breakfast cereals	6
Breads and grains	20
Meals	
Breakfast	41
Lunches	24
Dinners	30
Snacks	25

Note. Percentages are calculated over the total sample of 115 children.

Next, a classification scheme was developed for the criteria that the children reported they had used in forming food groups. This scheme is shown in Table 2. . . .

Table 2. Criteria Used by Children to Classify Foods

Classes Formed	Members	Frequency
1. Traditional semantic categories	e.g., fruits, meats, vegetables, breads, candy, desserts, and others	100
2. Functional categories		140
	breakfast items	47
	lunch items	28
	dinner foods	35
	snacks	29
	main course foods	1
3. Nutritional quality		49
	"junk" foods	26
	"nutritious" foods	11
	good/bad	9
	healthy foods	2
	cavity foods	1
4. Taste/texture		38
	sweet or sugary foods	29
	crunchy/crisp	3
	hard/soft	3
	slimy	1
	fatty/greasy	1
	cold/hot/wet	1
5. Food unknown or never tasted		18
	pinto beans	8
	beets	5
	bagels	5
6. Preference	like/dislike	1
7. Miscellaneous		7
	foods made with milk	1
	party foods	1
	things that will melt	1
	baked things	1
	foods that go in the refrigerator	1
	foods to eat when it is cold outside	1
	salty things	1

Note. The maximum frequency in each class is 115, and frequencies add up to more than 115 because children each used more than one criterion for classifying foods.

Most of the children (100 of them) used traditional semantic categories as criteria for placing foods into groups (e.g., fruits, breads, vegetables, etc.). Many (28–47 also used functional criteria (i.e., meals versus snacks) to place foods into groups (e.g., dinner foods, snacks). Criteria denoting evaluations of the nutritional or healthful quality of the food items were also used by a sizable number. Sweetness as a criterion was tabulated in the next category only if the child actually used the word "sweet" to describe the group (as opposed to using words such as dessert or junk foods to describe them). It was striking that the criterion of food likes or dislikes was used by only one child, and that none of the children used nutrient terminology in describing the basis for classifying foods (e.g., "high protein foods"). The numbers in Table 2 add up to more than 115 because some children used more than one criterion for classifying foods. . . .

Discussion

The present research cannot rule out the possibility that children at any of the cognitive developmental levels have the *capacity* to learn abstractly about nutrients and existing food grouping systems. Nevertheless, we know that usually they did not use the Basic Four system in our grouping task. For example, further analysis of our data tells that the specific food "milk" was classified with the appropriate Basic Four group, "dairy products," by only 30% of the children, while 42% classified milk with "drinks" as a food group and another 18% classified' milk with "foods served with meals." Further, children never placed beans in the meat group, nor potato chips in the vegetable group but always with pretzels and/or crackers. We will suggest that it may be much more practical to use naturally occurring conceptualizations as the basis for instruction about foods and nutrients, even when the goal is to foster more sophisticated understanding.

> *If one faithfully uses the Basic Four, does one end up with a diet that meets nutrient needs? Finding that the answer was "no," Janet King and her colleagues set out to revise and update the standard.*

EVALUATION AND MODIFICATION OF THE BASIC FOUR FOOD GUIDE*

Janet C. King, Ph.D., Sally H. Cohenour, Carol G. Corruccini and Paul Schneeman

Evaluation of Guide and Menus

Food guides have been used by nutritionists since the 1920s as a device for teaching how to plan adequate diets and to make wise food selections. The guide currently in use is the Basic Four Food Guide which was published by the United States Department of Agriculture (USDA) in 1956 and was based on the 1953 Recommended Dietary Allowances (RDAs). . . . We questioned, therefore, whether the Basic Four remains a useful guide for selecting a well-balanced diet . . . . Our objectives were two-fold: first, to compare the nutrient content of published menus based on the Basic Four guidelines with the current RDAs; and second, to modify the food guide if any of the nutrients provided by just the foods in the Basic Four guide fell below two-thirds of the allowance.

Twenty different full-day menus for adults published as examples of well-balanced diets based on the Basic Four were selected for analysis. Only those menus providing all four food groups in the amounts specified by the Basic Four were used. The nutrient content of each menu was calculated. . . .

The foods in each menu were divided into two groups: the Basic Four foods and the supplemental foods. The Basic Four foods included the minimal number of daily servings recommended by USDA: two 2–3 oz servings of meat or meat alternates, two servings of dairy products, four servings of fruits and vegetables, and four servings of enriched or whole grain breads and cereals. The supplemental foods included all remaining foods in the menus, such as fat, sugar, sweets, and additional servings of Basic Four foods. . . .

---

*"Evaluation and Modification of the Basic Four Food Guide", by Janet C. King, Sally H. Cohenour, Carol G. Corruccini and Paul Schneeman. *Journal of Nutrition Education*, 10:27–29, January-March 1978. Used with permission.

The Basic Four foods met or exceeded the current RDAs for only 8 of the 17 evaluated nutrients. In addition to energy, the Basic Four foods supplied 60% or less of the recommendations for five nutrients: vitamin E, vitamin B-6, magnesium, zinc, and iron. The folacin, thiamin, and niacin content equaled two-thirds of the standard. The supplemental foods on the menu increased the supply of vitamin E by about 35%, primarily from fats and oils which are not included in the foundation Basic Four Food Guide. About 20% of the recommendations for thiamin, niacin, folacin, vitamin B-6, magnesium, iron, and zinc were provided by supplemental servings of Basic Four foods. Thus, the total menus supplied about 70% of the RDA for iron and vitamin B-6, about 80% for vitamin E, magnesium, and zinc, and about 90% for thiamin, niacin, and folacin.

This menu analysis showed that even though these menus were cited in nutrition publications as examples of good diets, half of the 16 nutrients we evaluated other than energy did not meet the current recommended allowances, and five nutrients in the Basic Four menu items were below two-thirds of the allowances. We therefore felt modification of the Basic Four Food Guide was necessary in order to ensure acceptable intakes of all currently recommended nutrients other than energy.

Modification of the Guide

Our first step in modification of the Basic Four was to identify groups of foods which are good sources of the five nutrients in the Basic Four menus below two-thirds of the RDA, i.e., vitamin E, vitamin B-6, magnesium, zinc, and iron. . . . The serving sizes used for this ranking were the same as specified by the Basic Four Food Guide except 3 oz of meat, fish, and poultry was used rather than 2 oz, and the portion size of cooked legumes, fruits, and vegetables was increased from one-half cup to three-fourths cup. Examination of weighed food intake records from previous studies done by us indicated that these serving sizes were reasonable for adults.

. . . Based on this analysis, the food groups and number of servings for the adult Basic Four Food Guide was modified as below. One serving of fat and/or oil was added to the guide to ensure an adequate intake of vitamin E.

Modified Basic Four

2 svg. Milk and milk products

4 svg. Protein foods:
2 svg. animal protein
2 svg. legumes and/or nuts

4 svg. Fruits and vegetables:
  1 svg. vitamin C-rich
  1 svg. dark green
  2 svg. other

4 svg. Whole grain cereal products

1 svg. Fat and/or oil

The nutritional content of six menus based on the Modified Basic Four was determined by computer analysis. Menu items were chosen from a wide variety of foods. On the average, over 100% of the RDA was supplied for all the nutrients but iron; the iron content averaged 16 mg, or about 90% of the RDA for women. This is 160% of the RDA for men. The average energy content of the menus was 2200 kcal, or 80% of the RDA for men.

The Modified Basic Four Food Guide seems to provide a better foundation for making food choices for a nutritionally adequate diet than the existing Basic Four. . . . Individuals using the guide as a basis for their own food selections, however, may find less latitude in the choices available to them. Specific types of protein foods and cereal products are indicated, and dark green vegetables are recommended daily, rather than dark green or yellow every other day. Also, the energy supplied by the foods in the guide allows women few, if any, additional foods. We think it is important, however, to provide a guideline for the population which is nutritionally sound rather than to suggest a guideline which takes into consideration food preferences and is not optimal nutritionally. . . .

In conclusion, it seems evident that the Basic Four Food Guide needs modification to better meet the current nutrition recommendations for adults. Since many people are familiar with the Basic Four, we chose to modify that guide rather than develop a totally new guide. Because of the recent interest in nutrition, we feel that many people are ready to accept the fact that four food groups are too simplistic and would use a more complex, more adequate food guide. Extensive nutrition education will be needed at all levels, however, if the food choices of the population are to be improved.

> *Here is another update of the Basic Four, this one focussing on eliminating what nutritionist Patricia Hausman calls its "unfortunate acceptance of foods rich in salt, fat and cholesterol."*

UPDATING THE BASIC FOUR*

Patricia Hausman

For almost 25 years, the last word in nutrition has been USDA's Basic Four food guide. The four food groups – milk, meat, fruit-vegetable, and grain – grace virtually all nutrition education materials, and are the basis for countless nutrition programs.

Nutritionists devised the Basic Four in the mid-fifties to translate a myriad of nutrient recommendations into simple food choices that most people could understand. Much planning and thought went into the food guides, and what emerged was a food classification system that placed foods rich in protein, vitamin A, vitamin D, riboflavin, and calcium in the milk group; products high in protein, B vitamins, and iron in the meat group; foods especially rich in vitamins A and C and certain minerals in the fruit-vegetable group; and grain foods providing B vitamins, iron, carbohydrates, and protein in group four. Sweets, fats, and oils fall into the miscellaneous group.

But the Basic Four has become a paradox: it was designed for good nutrition, but today it condones the major problems in our food supply. Half of all adult Americans have blood cholesterol levels above the value suggested in the National Heart, Lung, and Blood Institute's (NHLBI) handbook for physicians, yet the Basic Four says nothing about the diet high in saturated fat and cholesterol that is so closely linked to this problem. NHLBI also estimates that 60 million Americans have definite or borderline high blood pressure, yet the Basic Four does not address the sodium content of the American diet, which experts say contributes to this startling rate of high blood pressure. At the same time, though few Americans have nutrient deficiencies, the Basic Four focuses on the vitamin, mineral, and protein content of the diet.

Still, the Basic Four does provide a simple approach to nutrient adequacy, and the importance of nutrients should not be dismissed. Modifying the Basic Four's message is really all that is needed to turn its unfortunate acceptance of foods rich in salt, fat, and cholesterol into a health-promoting food guide designed to keep intake of these troublemakers at reasonable levels. . . .

*"Updating the Basic Four," by Patricia Hausman. *Nutrition Action* 6:8–9, 1979. Copyright Center for Science in the Public Interest. Used with permission.

	Anytime	In Moderation	Now and Then

Group I:
Beans, Grains
& Nuts
 	
Four or More
Servings/day
	Barley
	Beans
	Bread & rolls
	  (whole grain)
	Bulghur
	Lentils
	Oatmeal
	Pasta
	Rice
	Whole grain
	  cereal
	  (except granola)
		Granola cereals
		Nuts
		Peanut butter
		Soybeans
		White bread and
		  Cereals	

Group II:
Fruits &
Vegetables
 	
Four or More
Servings/day
	All fruits and
	  vegetables ex-
	  cept those
	  listed on right
	Unsweetened
	  fruit juices
	Unsalted veg-
	  etable juices
	Potatoes, white
	  or sweet
		Avocado
		Fruits canned
		  in syrup
		Salted veg-
		  etable juices
		Sweetened
		  fruit juices
		Vegetables
		  canned
		  with salt
			French fries
			Olives
			Pickles

Group III:
Milk Products
 	
Children: 3 to 4
Servings or
Equivalent
Adult: 2 Servings
(Favor
"anytime"
column for
additional
servings)
	Buttermilk
	Farmer or pot
	  cheese
	Lowfat cottage
	  cheese
	Lowfat milk
	  with 1%
	  milkfat
	Skim milk
	  ricotta
	Skim milk
		Frozen lowfat
		  yogurt
		Ice milk
		Lowfat milk
		  with 2%
		  milkfat
		Lowfat (2%)
		  yogurt,
		  plain
		  or sweetened
		Regular cottage
		  cheese
		  (4% milkfat)
			Hard cheeses:
			  blue, brick,
			  camembert,
			  cheddar, (note:
			  part-skim
			  mozarella and
			  part-skim
			  ricotta are
			  preferable but
			  still rich in fat)
			Ice cream
			Processed cheeses
			Whole milk
			Whole milk yogurt

*Trim all outside fat.

"Anytime" foods contain less than 30 percent of calories from fat and are usually low in salt and sugar. Most of the "now and then" foods contain at least 50 percent of calories from fat — and a large amount of saturated fat. Foods to eat "in moderation" have medium amounts of total fat and low to moderate amounts of saturated fat or large amounts of total fat that is mostly unsaturated. Foods meeting the standards for fat, but containing large amounts of salt or sugar, are usually moved into a more restricted category, as are refined cereal products. For example, pickles have little fat, but are so high in sodium that they fall in the "now and then" category.

Important: To cut down on salt intake, choose varieties of the foods listed here that do not have added salt, such as no-salt cottage cheese, rather than the regular varieties. This guide is not appropriate for individuals needing very low-salt diets.

85

	Anytime	*In Moderation*	*Now and Then*
Group IV: *Poultry, Fish,* *Egg & Meat* *Products*	Poultry: Chicken or turkey (no skin)	Fish: Herring Mackerel Salmon Sardines Shrimp Tuna, oil-packed	Poultry & Fish: Deep fried and breaded fish or poultry
Two Servings: (Favor "anytime" column for additional servings. If a vegetarian diet is desired, nutrients in these foods can be obtained by increasing servings from Groups I & III.)	Fish: Cod Flounder Haddock Halibut Perch Pollock Rockfish Shellfish, except shrimp Sole Tuna, water-packed Egg: Egg whites	Red Meats: Flank steak Ham* Leg of lamb* Loin of lamb* Plate beef * Round steak* Rump roast* Sirloin steak* Veal*	Red Meats: Bacon Corned beef Ground beef Hot dogs Liver Liverwurst Pork: loin Pork: Boston butt Salami Sausage Spareribs Untrimmed meats Egg: Egg yolk or whole egg
Miscellaneous Note: Snack foods should not be used freely, but the middle column suggests some of the better choices.	Fats: (none) Snack Foods: (none)	Fats: Mayonnaise Salad oils Soft (tub) margarines Snack Foods: Angel food cake Animal crackers Fig bars Gingerbread Ginger snaps Graham crackers Popcorn (small amounts of fat and salt) Sherbet	Fats: Butter Cream Cream cheese Lard Sour cream Snack Foods: Chocolate Coconut Commercial pies, pastries and doughnuts Potato chips Soda pop

> *In this editorial from* The Community Nutritionist, *editor Steve Clapp argues that the Basic Four has simply outlived its usefulness — that it now contributes to our nutritional problems instead of helping solve them. Let's chuck it, he says.*

CHUCK THE BASIC FOUR?*

Stephen Clapp

A t USDA's annual Outlook Conference in December, a Penn State research team reported that the Basic Four food groups, a staple of nutrition education for three decades, may be hazardous to health.

Analyzing data from the 1977-78 Nationwide Food Consumption Survey, Annemarie F. Crocetti of Anarem Systems Research and Helen A. Guthrie of Penn State found that only about 3 percent of the U. S. population actually follows the Basic Four recommendations to the letter, and the majority of those who do so consume excessive amounts of fat.

"Americans on the whole do better on consuming micronutrients than on balancing macronutrients," Crocetti told the conference. "Perhaps we should chuck the Basic Four."

The researchers found almost half the U. S. population to be consuming more than 35 percent of total calories from fat. Tested for both micronutrient consumption and macronutrient balance, only about 8 percent of Americans show ideal diets. Another 23 percent would receive top grades except for excessive fat intake.

"The intake of the population was not found to conform to the recommendations based on the four food groups approach, and, further, no simple association was found with the quality of the diets and adherence," the researchers said. "The four food groups approach does not address macronutrient ratios of total caloric intake."

The Penn State study would appear to be the final nail needed to hammer home the coffin lid on the Basic Four. Nutritionists have been complaining about its simplistic, easily-misunderstood message for years, and the Society for Nutrition Education in 1978 urged USDA to replace it.

Despite its obvious flaws, the Basic Four has powerful allies in the food industry and the nutrition establishment. When current eating

---

*"Chuck the Basic Four?", by Stephen Clapp. *The Community Nutritionist* 2:1, January/February 1983. Edited portions used with permission.

patterns were challenged by the Senate Nutrition Committee's Dietary Goals, the American Medical Association responded with a 1979 statement of support for the Basic Four, calling it "a model of moderation in developing dietary habits."

When the U. S. Dietary Guidelines posed another challenge in 1980, the Basic Four received a boost from the National Academy of Sciences' Food and Nutrition Board. Introducing their controversial report "Toward Healthful Diets," Alfred E. Harper and Robert E. Olson praised the Basic Four, arguing that it still provides good advice and counsels moderation in consumption of animal foods high in fat.

Politically-entrenched ideas do not die easily. . . .

> *This speech, by one of the editors of the present volume, was given at a time when questions were being raised about eating guidelines, in terms of whether they were consistent with what we had learned since the Basic Four was designed. Gussow suggests that we should begin by looking at our underlying assumptions.*

WHY WE NEED NUTRITION GUIDELINES*

Joan Dye Gussow, Ed.D.

If we need food selection guidelines, what should they look like? . . .

Among the materials I examined in preparing these remarks were descriptions of a number of food grouping systems from this country and elsewhere. I was attempting to understand the rationale that underlay various food classification systems. What became immediately clear was that food guides *sometimes* reflect the relevant knowledge available at the time and place when they were put together and they *always* reflect a set of cultural values. Though the assumptions which underlie our own system tend to get lost the more familiar "our" system becomes, a moment's reflection makes it clear that no food guide begins with a list of essential nutrients translated into some sort of food selection ideal. If that were the case then food guides would look the same the world over. They begin — in fact — with an already established food pattern. The purpose of food guides is to convert the

---

*"Why We Need Nutrition Guidelines," by Jean Dye Gussow. (Speech to the 3rd Conference on Nutrition & the American Food System, Washington, D.C., October 2–3, 1979. Used with permission.

established dietary pattern of a community (or of a more affluent imitated society) into suggested servings of foods. *These foods are grouped together on the basis of decisions about which of their nutrient contributions are important.* The decision about what to group is much less affected by scientific considerations than it is by agricultural, medical, political, cultural and other considerations. . . .

Thus when the first food guides originated in this country some time after the turn of the century they reflected that part of the scientific understanding of the time which said that animal foods supplied protein, grains supplied energy, fruits and vegetables provided what came to be called protective factors, and "useful" fats provided useful fat-soluble growth factors. After the first RDAs were developed in the 1940's, the various food guides attempted to help both applied nutrition professionals and the average homemakers select a diet adequate in the then known nutrients. But all these guides interpreted this newer knowledge of nutrition in the light of the then existing U. S. food pattern, and food availabilities.

Thus when the four food groups were developed in the 1950's they began not merely with the 1953 RDAs but with 1948 household food consumption survey data and national food supply statistics. They were an attempt to set up a guide for selecting food which would be simple, meet the current RDAs, make use of what we produced, and still allow for the expression of existing patterns of food preference. The Basic Seven had included three fruit and vegetable groups, one for leafy green and yellow vegetables, one for citrus fruits and other sources of vitamin C, and one for potatoes and other vegetables and fruits. At a time when knowledge of and consumption of fresh fruits and vegetables were already declining, the four food group system collapsed all this vegetative complexity into a single group — even though it was readily recognized that inappropriate vegetable and fruit selections could easily be made even by someone familiar with the 7-group system.

On what basis was it assumed that the four food group system was better? Presumably on the grounds that it was simpler. Yet it is interesting to note what new assumptions became embedded when we moved from seven groups to four. Not only does the present food plan give no guidance about important nutritive and compositional differences between various fruits and vegetables, but it creates a system in which half of the food classes identified are animal products. Of course we *say* that two items each are to be selected from the milk and meat groups and we *say* that four items each are to be selected from the fruit and vegetable and the grain groups; but we are dealing with the most visually oriented generation in history, and that is not the message our teaching materials convey. Milk products occupy the same space as meat products which occupy the same space as fruits and vegetables which occupy the same space as grain products. Moreover, while the seven food groups were arranged in a circle "to

89

signify that no one group was more important than any other," the four food groups have been most often arranged with meat and milk first and second (or second and first depending on who produced the visual aid), thus conveying a not so subtle impression that it was those requirements that needed satisfaction first, with other foods filling in the cracks. And 2-2-4-4 aside, who has not seen teaching materials in which children are asked to complete a meal so that it contains *one* item from *each* of the four food groups?

What would be the effect of having a food guide which listed grains first, fruits and vegetables second (both of them in large boxes) and then listed meat and milk last in small boxes? Wouldn't even such a modest change completely alter the *impression* of what it is we are apparently trying to say to the American public about the composition of a desirable diet?

Or suppose we developed a nutrition guide which was sensitive to the inevitably rising price of food. It takes no graduate in economics to recognize that animal products are always going to be more expensive than plant products providing similar nutrients. Unless we assume that food prices are going to go down — which would appear to be a foolish assumption in light of world events — we are very soon going to have to decide whether it is morally appropriate — regardless of other considerations — to continue to use a food guide which puts heavy emphasis on animal sources of nutrients.

With price as a consideration, we might consider a food guide which put emphasis on seasonality in produce — a food guide which we would modify according to the part of the country in which it was used. A guide for the Northeastern U. S. in winter might be heavy on storage vegetables (if anyone remembers what those are!) in order to emphasize the importance of reducing transportation and refrigeration costs.

In fact, before we can develop a truly useful food guide for the last fifth of the 20th century, it will be necessary for us to make some guesses about the future — we shall have to decide whether or not the trend toward more centralized food production and processing and more and more "convenience" in food will continue. . . .

We cannot decide on guidelines unless we decide whether or not people will be willing to cook in the future. If home economics classes continue to teach people how to make brownies instead of how to stir fry rice with vegetables, then it is clear that we shall have problems with any food guide that assumes knowledge of cooking. Similarly, if food preparation is viewed as life-denying and sexist by a social movement which presumes to seek full humanness for both the minority (male) and the majority (female) sex, then we may need nutrition guidelines which will minimize food preparation. This might seem to imply that we need pre-prepared convenience foods. I would like to urge, on the contrary, that it might as well put a new healthful emphasis on using raw or lightly cooked foods. Once again, this kind of food

90

guide we are led to develop will reflect our assumptions about what
the citizens of the U. S. are likely to be willing to do.

What other sorts of values could be expressed in our dietary
guidelines? Some of us are very concerned that people have lost touch
with food production — that they no longer recognize their utter dependence on chlorophyll as the primary solar collector. One way of
overcoming this might be to make a food group system which grouped
foods by their source (a system which, incidentally, also groups them
by their nutrients for astonishingly logical botanical reasons). . . .

If one were really concerned with educational effectiveness, one
might want to design a food guide around a food-related topic that
Americans are already knowledgable about — calories. . . . What is
hard — or one thing that is hard — about the present system is that it
is based on a vague concept called "servings" which may have nothing
whatsoever to do with the amount of any given food substance ordinary people serve. Is an orange a serving of fruit? A banana? Is a steak
a serving of meat? Is a quarter plateful of spinach a serving? What if
the plate is small? Is an ear of sweet corn a serving of a vegetable? Is
a baked potato? Instead of talking about servings, suppose we said to
people "try to get about half of your calories from bread, grains, seeds,
nuts, legumes, cooked and ready-to-eat breakfast cereals and so on;
try to get about ¼ of your calories from fruits and vegetables and
about ¼ of your calories from animal products." We could fill in a little
detail about fruit and vegetable types, give a few warnings about lurking fat, and turn them loose. I wonder if they would do any worse than
they do now. . . .

I do not recommend or reject any one of these assumptions —
though I must admit I have my favorites. Nor do I have any particular
bias toward any particular food guide. . . . Whatever it is we decide, I
think it very important that we understand the assumptions we are
incorporating into it. . . .

> *Here then are several examples of proposed new food guides. While some embed very different assumptions about how we should eat, the first from the Department of Agriculture simply bows to reality and adds a fifth group — for fats, sweets and alcohol — to its famous four.*

THE HASSLE-FREE GUIDE TO A BETTER DIET*

Four Basic Servings Daily

Include one good vitamin C source each day. Also frequently include deep-yellow or dark-green vegetables (for vitamin A) and unpeeled fruits and vegetables and those with edible seeds, such as berries (for fiber).

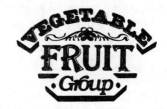

Four Basic Servings Daily

Select only whole-grain and enriched or fortified products. (But include *some* whole-grain bread or cereals for sure!) Check labels.

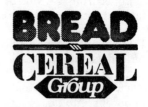

Basic Servings Daily (Based on servings of fluid milk . . .)

Children under 9	2 to 3 servings
Children 9 to 12	3 servings
Teens	4 servings
Adults	2 servings
Pregnant Women	3 servings
Nursing Mothers	4 servings

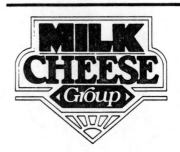

---

*"The Hassle-free Guide to a Better Diet." *Food: a Publication on Food and Nutrition.* U. S. Department of Agriculture, 1979.

Two Basic Servings Daily

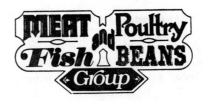

In general, the amount of these foods to use depends on the number of calories you require. It's a good idea to concentrate first on the calorie-plus-nutrients foods provided in the other groups as the basis of your daily diet.

THE HANDY FIVE FOOD GUIDE*

Janice M. Dodds, Ed.D., R.D.

. . . The development of a nutritionally sound food guide is relatively simple when the population to be served is homogeneous with respect to food supply; food preferences; and environmental, economic, and health constraints and objectives. However, the world population is heterogeneous with respect to these considerations; so a guide developed for one group may be meaningless to another. One solution to this problem is the development of a wide variety of food guides, each suitable for use with a specific group. . . .

The purpose of this paper is to present the developmental criteria for the Handy Five Food Guide and some preliminary observations on its usefulness. This guide is intended primarily for use with children or uneducated adults in developing countries. It may also be useful for others who for religious, ecological, or health reasons seek guidance in selecting a nutritionally adequate diet that emphasizes plant foods.

*"The Handy Five Food Guide," by Janice M. Dodds. *Journal of Nutrition Education*, 13:50–52, June 1981. Used with permission.

Developmental Criteria

The Handy Five Food Guide evolved from a discussion by a group of health professionals who were preparing to work with communities in developing countries. We recognized that the people would be eating foods with which we were unfamiliar and that we needed a single guide that would be applicable in several different countries. The criteria for development of the guide considered these circumstances.

The most basic criterion, one which the Handy Five shares with all food guides, is that the plan must satisfy nutritional needs. To the extent possible, the recommended foods should avoid nutrient deficiencies as well as harmful excesses. . . .

A second criterion is that within the constraints of satisfying nutrient requirements, emphasis should be given to foods that nutritionists believe best support health and to foods that are economically available to the target audience. . . .

A third criterion is the *universality* of the food categories so that a variety of specific foods can fit into the categories. The guide then would be adaptable to a wide variety of cultural, religious, economic, and agricultural differences in food preferences or availability.

A fourth consideration that went into development of the Handy Five is that it should recommend foods such that their selection would have a positive impact on the future food supply. The guide should foster the wise use of resources so that food can continue to be a renewable resource. It should encourage practices which preserve resources involved in food production, such as soil, seed, and water. The recommended foods should not depend heavily upon transportation, fuel, containers, storage, and preservation. . . .

A fifth developmental criterion is that the characteristic which determines to which food group a food is assigned be observable rather than abstract, since the guide will be used with children and uneducated adults. . . . Thus, visual characteristics of foods rather than the abstract concept of nutrient composition should form the basis for classification of foods into groups. Anyone can learn to classify a food by recognizing its characteristics and assigning it to the appropriate food group. However, with nutrient-based classification, only persons knowledgeable about food composition and capable of formal reasoning could classify a new or unusual food.

Finally, in order to be a useful educational tool, the guide should be simple and visually interesting so as to be easy to remember. It should serve as a prompter or a cue card so that when one chooses a food, the choice can be checked off against the guide. Of particular importance, there should be only a small number of groups.

The Handy Five

The Handy Five Food Guide is displayed as Figure 1. The foods are classified according to plant parts and animal products. The 5 groups, servings, serving sizes, and some examples of foods in each group are presented in Table 1.

Figure 1. The Handy Five Food Guide

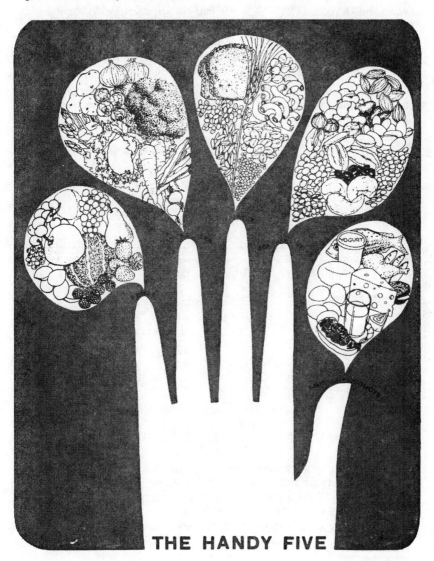

THE HANDY FIVE

Table 1. Handy Five servings and examples

Food Group	Servings	Serving Size	Examples
Flesh around seeds (fruit)	2	½ cup	Orange, apple, tomato, peach, bananas, grapes squash, grapefruit, avocado, payaya, pomegranate
Leaves, stalks, roots, flowers (vegetables)	2	½ cup	Spinach, broccoli, potato, carrot, kale, onions cauliflower
Seeds on grasses (grains)	4	¾ cup	Rice, corn, wheat, barley, millet, oats
Seeds in pods (nuts and legumes)	4	½ cup	Lima beans, peanuts, split peas, walnuts, sunflower seeds, garbanzo beans, black beans, kidney beans
Animal products	2	1 cup (milk)	Milk, cheese, yogurt, eggs
(dairy, eggs, meat)		3 ounces (meat)	Beef, pork, chicken, fish

Table 2. Comparison of number of servings recommended by various food guides

Food Categories	Recommended Servings		
	Four Food Groups	King Modification	Handy Five
Fruits and vegetables	4	4	2 + 2
Grains	4	4	4
Dairy and animal protein	2 + 2	2 + 2	2
Legumes and nuts	—	2	4

If a person eats 2 meals a day, 1 serving from each group with extra large servings from the grain and legume groups will meet most people's needs. With 3 meals a day or 3 meals plus snacks as an eating pattern, a person should include grains and legumes in each meal or snack and distribute servings from the other groups across those meals. Because the amount of food from animal products would be a small proportion of the total food intake, the guide does not distinguish between high-fat and low-fat animal products. People usually use some oil in preparing these foods; so to be accurate, 1 tablespoon of vegetable oil should be indicated as part of the recommended food plan. One and preferably 2 servings of the animal products need to be a dairy food to ensure adequate calcium intake.

Meeting the Criteria

The nutritional adequacy of the Handy Five guide has not been evaluated formally, but this evaluation could be done by analyzing the nutrient content of daily menus prepared for the guide, such as has been done for the Four Food Groups by King et al. . . .

The Handy Five emphasizes foods that suppport good health in harmony with the U. S. Dietary Guidelines. It encourages variety through numerous suggested foods and by specific mention of a legumes-and-nuts food group; it discourages excessive intake of fat through the recommendation of only 2 servings of foods possibly high in fat, saturated fat, and cholesterol. The Handy Five emphasizes complex carbohydrates and fiber because 4 of the 5 groups are plant products; it decreases emphasis on sodium through illustrations of fresh foods rather than processed foods. . . .

The universality of the Handy Five food groups has been demonstrated by the experiences of the health team members who have used the guide in Indonesia, Korea, Egypt, the Philippines, Kenya, and India. In the latter country the author found the guide to be versatile in responding to a wide range of food patterns found in 13 villages across the state of Maharashtra.

The Handy Five particularly addresses concerns for the future food supply. If there is to be enough food, all indications are that the society will need to grow it. The Handy Five emphasizes foods low on the food chain, locally grown, and fresh rather than processed. These characteristics conserve nonrenewable resources and support practices that will preserve land and water resources.

Using the visual characteristics of plant parts and animal products to classify foods, the Handy Five guide fits with the concrete reasoning abilities of the majority of adults and can be used effectively with children, who will initially memorize the groups and their members. But as the children develop their reasoning abilities, the reasons for the classifications will become apparent. The Handy Five helps to educate people about how food grows. At the point of purchase, many of our modern foods are several times removed from their original sources and observable characteristics. A food guide that pictures food as it grows may overcome the notion among children in industrialized countries that food grows in boxes and plastic containers on grocery store shelves. Dry breakfast cereals, for example, have lost much that identifies them observably with the grains on grasses from which they came. . . .

In summary, the Handy Five is a nutritionally sound food guide which emphasizes health promotion, can be adapted easily to a variety of food patterns, reinforces understanding of the ecological nature of the food system, is memorable, and uses observable characteristics for food classification needs. The simplicity of the image and thus the versatility of activities built around the guide make it a creative element for school curricula and for informal education in health centers and social agencies and allow it to serve as an approach for public education.

CONSIDERATIONS FOR A NEW FOOD GUIDE*

Jean A. T. Pennington, Ph.D. R.D.

. . . This guide has the shape of a reverse pyramid (Figure 1). There are 4 main food groups distributed among 4 levels of recommended consumption. Group 1, vegetables and fruits, and Group II, grain products, share the first level. Group III encompasses vegetable, dairy, and meat sources of protein and traverses 3 levels: legumes on the first; skim and lowfat dairy items, lean meat, fish, and poultry on the second; and whole-fat dairy items, nuts, seeds, peanuts, eggs, fatty meats, game, luncheon meats, and sausage on the third level. Group IV consists of luxury foods: desserts, fats, sweets, and alcoholic beverages.

The visual presentation of the guide demonstrates the food selection emphasis, which is to eat liberally from the first level; moderately from the second level; very moderately from the third level; and sparingly from the fourth level. As we look from the top of the reverse pyramid to the apex at the bottom, foods lower down tend to increase in fat content and usually in cost. At the top of the reverse pyramid are foods of plant derivation. At the second level are animal-derived foods which are fairly low in fat. On the third level are the higher-fat animal and plant foods. The fourth level includes both foods that are very high in fat and others that are low in nutrient density. Emphasizing foods near the top of the reverse pyramid encourages lower-cost foods of plant origin and may discourage excessive intake of total fat, saturated fat, cholesterol, sugar, and alcohol. The concept of nutrient density is also expressed within consumption levels and groups.

*"Considerations for a New Food Guide," by Jean A. T. Pennington. *Journal of Nutrition Education*, 13:53–55, June, 1981. Used with permission.

Thus, leafy vegetables appear above other vegetables and fruits; whole grains above refined ones; and low-fat dairy items, meats, fish, and poultry above higher-fat (and lower nutrient-density) animal and plant foods. . . .

Luxury foods are in this food guide because they add flavor to meals and pleasure to eating. However, the quantities are limited. . . .

Figure 1. A suggested food guide

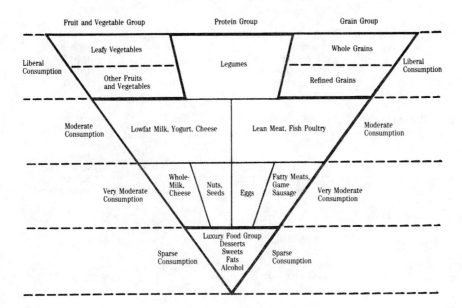

Table 1. Portion sizes and suggested servings per day from the inverse pyramid food guide

Food Group	Example of Portion Sizes	Suggested Servings Per Day	
		Teens and Adults	Children
Vegetables and fruits	¼ – 1 c raw, ½ c cooked leafy greens ¼ – ½ c dried fruit ½ c fruit or vegetable juice ¾ – 1 c other fruits and vegetables	6 or more with at least 1 from leafy greens	4 or more with at least 1 from leafy greens
Grains and grain products	1 slice bread, 1 waffle, 1 tortilla ½ c cooked cereal ½ c rice, noodles, grits ¾ – 1 c ready to eat cereal	6 or more with at least 3 from whole grains	4 or more with at least 2 from whole grains
Protein foods*	1 c milk, yogurt 1 oz cheese, meat, fish, poultry 1 egg ½ c cooked legumes 2 tbsp peanut butter 2 oz seeds, nuts	6 to 15 with at least 2 from dairy foods and at least 4 from others	6 to 15 with at least 3 from dairy foods and at least 3 from others
Luxury foods	Desserts: ½ c pudding, ice cream 2 cookies small slice cake Fats: 1 tbsp butter, oil Sweets: 1 tbsp sugar, honey Alcohol: 1 oz liquor 4 oz wine 12 oz beer	*Children, Teens, and Adults* Desserts: 1 or less Fats: 4 or less Sweets: 4 or less *Adults Only* Alcohol – 1 or less	

*Small portion sizes are specified in order to encourage a wide variety.

> *The last selection in this chapter offers a wholly different way of classifying foods, based on conservation of resources. This excerpt is from the introduction to a cookbook. Its author's previous book,* The Famine Business, *explained some of the reasons why food conservation was appropriate.*

WHAT KIND OF FOOD?*

Colin Tudge

First question, then: What must we grow? Human protein needs have been grotesquely exaggerated, . . . but in designing agriculture it is as well to begin with protein because that is the hardest thing to get right. It would be all too easy to produce too little and so put people in nutritional peril, or too much, and so waste resources. So what is the easiest or most efficient way to produce protein?

The most prolific sources of protein, by a wide margin, are green leaves — a statement that must appear as a misprint to anyone brought up on the nutritional rubrics of the 1950s and 1960s. Yet it is obvious that this should be so, for the protein that finally finishes up in seeds, in meat, or in human flesh was, for the most part, originally manufactured in green leaves, including those of grass. . . .

But leaf protein is too dilute. Cows can get all the protein they need from grass — far more than they need in fact — but only because their enormous barrellike bodies are filled with an astonishingly large stomach called the rumen, which can hold vast amounts of it. . . . Human beings, however, do not seem to have the physical capacity to subsist on leaves.

The potato is the next most productive source; 400 pounds of protein per acre would be reasonable. The protein in potatoes is not too dilute; adult human beings can eat enough to satisfy their protein needs and whole societies, notably the Irish of the early nineteenth century, did subsist almost exclusively upon potatoes. So the potato, rather than the green leaf, can be regarded as the outstanding staple crop.

The cereals, which in practice are the world's leading staples, are the third most abundant protein source. An acre of wheat might yield 250 pounds of protein. Cereals perhaps have the edge over potatoes in that they are easier to store; in general, the two complement each other. Cereals, like potatoes, are adequate sources of protein for adult human beings. . . .

---

*"What Kind of Food?", by Colin Tudge. *Future Food: Politics, Philosophy and Recipes for the 21st Century.* Reprinted by permission of A. D. Peters & Co., Ltd. Copyright 1980, pages 9–12.

The third of the world's great staples are the pulses, the large edible seeds of the Leguminosae: beans, grams, lentils, chickpeas and peas. Yield of protein per acre is of the same order as with cereals but the concentration of protein per seed is generally higher. For this and other reasons — agricultural, nutritional, and gastronomic — the pulses are an admirable foil for the potato and the grains.

These three classes of food — potato, cereal, pulse — should form the basis of every country's agricultural effort and hence of everybody's diet. . . . Once they are taken care of there is little else to do except provide some micronutrients — vitamins, minerals, and essential fats — and exciting flavors; after all, an exclusive diet of cereals, pulses and potatoes would be tedious. But the staples are the bedrock. They are Food of the First Kind.

The foods whose function is merely to abet and enhance the staples are Food of the Second Kind; and the most notable feature of rational agriculture and the gastronomy it allows, is that meat is demoted to this category. I do not suggest we should all be vegetarians; for nutritional as well as gastronomic reasons I would not like to live in or bring up children in a vegan society, and livestock does have clear and important roles in farming. But the Western world's present concentration on livestock is far out of proportion.

Animals produce far less protein than the major plant crops. The most generous farm animal, the dairy cow, yields about 100 pounds of milk protein per acre. The dairy plus beef enterprise, in which the calves are raised alongside their dams, provides about 80 pounds. Broiler chickens give about 70 pounds of protein in return for an acre's worth of feed, laying hens about 60, pigs about 40, and sheep and beef, the jewel in the crown of Western agriculture, about 20 pounds of protein per acre. The developed world, which contains only one-third of the world's people, uses half the world's supply of cereals and feeds 70 percent of its share to livestock — plus, of course, vast amounts of grass. The Third World, with 70 percent of the world's people, feeds only 10 percent of its share of the world's cereals to animals. The Third World could do with more livestock, in the right contexts; but the rich world's prodigality borders on the absurd. There is plenty for animals to do in rational agriculture, however, and the future world can produce, and should eat, meat and other animal products. We should eat less than we eat today, but it will be more flavorsome.

Vegetables are also Food of the Second Kind. As with meat, their nutritional role is as abettors; providing micronutrient vitamins and minerals, dietary fiber and, perhaps above all, flavor. It is probably bad for people to eat too much meat, but it is hard to see that anybody, in practice, could eat too many vegetables provided they ate as varied a selection as possible. . . .

Food of the Third Kind is a mixed bag; almost everything that breathes is potentially edible, and wild fungi, wild leaves, flowers,

102

shellfish, nuts and berries as well as the vast pharmacopoeia of spices can each provide unique and exciting flavor.

All countries should move toward self-reliance in food; . . . partly because one important way to save energy would be to stop shifting food around the world. But self-reliance merely means producing one's own basic foods, so that the people do not starve, even in a blockade. It does not mean an end to all trade, and the tropical spices in particular — which require little land, are cheap to transport, and yet are valuable — should be used and made available worldwide, with the profit going to the producer countries. Agricultural self-reliance has usually been associated with "siege economy" and with extreme austerity, as in Britain in World War II; yet if properly conceived, in peacetime, it implies no hardship. Tomorrow's food should be spicy, and where there's spice there's flavor. . . .

Rational agriculture is at least worth thinking about. The diet it would provide would be heavily biased toward the staples, garnished by masses of vegetables and soupçons of meat, and highlighted with spice and whatever else was to hand. . . . Such a diet would be a considerable nutritional advance on our present one.

Afterword

Well, now! Did you ever think there were so many decisions involved in creating a food guide? Or so many different ways to think about such a simple tool? The reason for the prickliness of the topic is, of course, that we are once more dealing with issues that cannot be resolved by science, but depend on human judgment.

Any food guide we use reflects many assumptions of its designers — about the food supply, about what people prefer to eat, about how people like to learn — but these are not usually stated explicitly, so it is sometimes unclear what people are really arguing about. For example, not until the Dietary Goals (see Chapter 3) proposed that we ought to lower our intake of red meat and full-fat dairy products did it become widely evident that the four-food-group system was not neutral, that it had actually encouraged the heavy consumption of animal products.

When thinking about food groups, what issues do you need to attend to? One interesting question that emerges from these readings has to do with whether certain kinds of food grouping systems are "better" than others. In theory, if we want to settle arguments over which system we should use, we ought to be able to ask which one is better at achieving its goal.

103

In the field of measurement, when an instrument is doing what it intends to do, i.e., achieving its goal, we say it is a "valid" instrument. In a test, validity refers to whether the test is finding out what its designer wants to find out.

In the case of food guides, the validity question has generally been understood to be: "Will people who use the designated number of servings from the designated food groups meet their nutritional needs?" To assess this, researchers have usually done what King and her colleagues did in the paper we reproduced here. That is, they took diets recommended in textbooks as meeting the four-food-group guideline and analyzed them for nutritional adequacy.

But such a procedure is very difficult to carry out in a "valid" manner. One critical problem has to do with who does the selecting. If the diets have been selected by a nutritionist, doesn't it seem likely that she would make wise choices even if she didn't have the guide? So how do you know the guide actually helped?

There is an even more basic problem built into the validity issue. If a good grouping system is intended to be a tool for helping *consumers* select wisely, its validity actually ought to be evaluated in relation to a very different question: "Does this instrument help some specified percentage (a majority, for instance) of consumers who use it to select foods that will meet their nutrient needs?"

It is, of course, very hard to learn why consumers out there in the marketplace make the choices they do, or whether the food system you taught them is having any effect on their choices. You can ask them, but they may not really know themselves. And when you do ask them, as Clapp reports, only about 3% of the population turns out to follow the Basic Four recommendations — and their diets are much too high in fat. Therefore, no food grouping system in this country has actually been shown to be valid!

Although Hayes, Trulson and Stare wonder whether the Basic Seven plan "cannot be made more simple without losing its validity," they provide no evidence that it is valid, nor do they ever ask how many food groups of which sorts a plan would need to have in order to help the public choose a healthful diet.

Consider then, that we do not know whether a four-food group or a seven-food group (or any food guide) actually is valid, and that we moved from 11 to 7 to 4 groups at least partly because we were led to believe that "too many groups" were hard to remember and hence too difficult to use. But back in the 1970s the suggestion that we abandon the Basic Four was often accompanied by a proposal that we turn to some sort of nutrient based system. What happened to simplicity?

The simplest nutrient-based system would be *much* more complex to use than 4 (or even 7 or 11) food groups; there were at last count well over 50 nutrients we would need to pay some attention to! All of this has fueled the argument that we moved from 7 to 4 not for simplicity but for product promotion — but we have no real evidence to prove that there was anything so logical behind the proposal.

Hayes, Trulson and Stare raise some other problems common to most food grouping systems: Suppose someone made the worst possible choices in each group? What is meant by a serving? How large or small should these servings be? All these problems, as they point out, "are inherent in any simple teaching device."

What the public views as a "serving" of various foods has been shown to vary widely from what is usually recommended as "standard." (S. M. Krebs-Smith and Helen Smikiklas-Wright. Typical serving sizes: Implications for food guidance. *Journal of the American Dietetic Association.* 85:1139–1141, September 1985.) Gussow noted that establishing a workable "serving" represented a major problem for food guide designers, and suggested that calorie content might be a more familiar unit to a weight-watching public.

Hayes, Trulson, and Stare suggest that someone choosing from the Basic Seven might "habitually select green and yellow vegetables of such low vitamin A content" as to fail to meet his or her nutrient needs. But such a problem is clearly much more serious in their proposed four-group system, which (like ours) lumps into a single group all fruits and vegetables, some containing no vitamin A at all.

While there is little evidence to support the claim of food guide critics that we were promoted into adopting the four-food-group system by the meat and dairy industry, there can be no dispute about the fact that our national view of what constituted a "proper" meal (meat, potatoes, vegetable, bread, beverage) was, over time, shaped by the four-food-group concept, and that concept was in turn shaped by a desire to make full use of the commodities our nation produced. Many countries have a basic starchy staple as the centerpiece of their diets — and of their food guides. Only rich countries can afford to have meat and milk as the mainstay of their meals.

It is also true that many of the teaching devices that have been used to teach small children the Basic Four were guilty of overemphasizing the meat and milk groups. Even Hayes and her colleagues — at the dawn of the system — urged that "a unique way of teaching nutrition for school children might be to serve their lunch on plates or trays partitioned into four segments, each segment bearing a picture of a basic food group." All such approaches, as Gussow points out, create the idea that at any given meal *one* selection from each group is OK — the message being not 2, 2, 4, 4, or even 4, 4, 2, 2, but 1, 1, 1, 1.

A difficult problem for any food guide is the increasing availability of what Mayer calls "'fabricated foods' like cocktail cheese puffs, imitation cream, vegetable-protein 'bacon' chips or the complex convenience foods like TV dinners. . . ." As he points out, no food guide can provide guidance for dealing with such foods. The old faithful indicator nutrients which we mentioned in the last chapter no longer indicate anything, since they can be added by manufacturers to products which have no other nutritional value.

Also, incomplete nutrient composition data on most foods, including some processed foods, makes it difficult to take account of nutrients like B-6, zinc, vitamin E, folate and other vitamins and minerals not included in many nutrient data bases and not normally identified on food labels. (It is even more difficult to take account of non-nutrient substances that may be important to health — see Chapter 6 on Nutritional Supplements.)

Fabricated foods are thus not only unlikely to be fully equivalent nutritionally to foods they resemble in form or function, but they are unlikely to fit honestly into existing food groups since their nutrient composition is largely determined by what has been added to them. For example, even though we teach that vegetable foods do not contain B-12, some brands of corn flakes are a better source of vitamin B-12 than they are of thiamine, a nutrient normally found in grains.

Whether the availability of fabricated or fortified foods is good or bad overall is a matter of dispute. As we saw in Chapter 1, Dr. Brin seemed to approve of such products, while Dr. Hall thought they were disastrous. Whichever one is right, lumping these foods into guideline food groups containing traditional foods would make it possible for consumers to inadvertently select a diet made up entirely of foods whose nutrient composition is markedly deficient, and whose nutrients are derived largely from fortification. Few nutritionists would judge such a diet safe or adequate.

Both of these kinds of objections — that the four food groups overemphasize animal products and that they allow for too many fabricated foods — are dealt with to some extent by the modifications suggested by King and Hausman. All of these plans emphasize whole "natural" foods, and Hausman de-emphasizes animal products. But another kind of objection has been raised which applies to any system based on grouping foods solely on the basis of the nutrients they contain. Can such a system be a good teaching tool?

In this chapter, Ullrich argues that even nutritionists don't use the four-food-group system, and other critics have questioned whether children can really grasp a system that groups foods together by the "nutrients" they contain.

Michela and Contento looked to see whether children classified foods into anything like the Basic Four and found that they did not. Children may have the "*capacity* to learn abstractly about nutrients and existing food grouping systems," they say, but as their own research makes clear, children's "naturally occurring" conceptualizations are overwhelmingly functional, i.e., "drinks" or "foods served with meals." Their finding suggests that more logical classifications based on visible qualities — like Dodds' system which groups plants by concrete characteristics and puts all animal products into a single group — may be easier for children to learn.

Dodds' article makes clear that all food guides are based on a number of underlying assumptions. Most of the suggestions for modification of our present food guide never ask whether the common underlying assumptions are correct. One of these underlying assumptions, as Gussow notes, is that we should consume as much as possible of what our country produces. A food guide like that of Dodds, or the approach to food groupings Tudge suggests, have quite different underlying assumptions — namely that we should pay attention to food economy, rational land use, relocalization of the diet, or the botanical characteristics of food items.

Such suggestions should help us to think more carefully about what we want and need in a food guide that will serve us into the 21st century. In the end, it is people's judgments about what values dietary planning ought to take into account that will help determine the sort of food guide we have in the future.

But do we need a food guide at all? Probably we do. Some way (or ways) of grouping foods is probably necessary just to help people make sense out of the multiplicity of foods available to them in this society. Other countries have food guides, many of them simpler than those we have had. Hayes and her colleagues remark, in defense of a four-group system, that no other country has found it necessary to have as many as seven groups. But many countries also have much simpler food patterns than ours.

What makes designing a food guide so difficult in this country is that we have an abundant and varied food supply, many ethnic groups, a range of "traditional" food patterns, an aggressive food industry, and a remarkable zest for novelty. In the face of such barriers to commonality, it is probably inevitable that any sort of food guide will cause controversy.

Perhaps we have passed the time when a single food guide will do. Perhaps we need different food guides for different seasons, different parts of the country, and for different groups of people choosing to eat vegetarian or other special diets. When you get to Chapter 6 on Nutritional Supplements, where we suggest

107

you check your own diet against a food guide, you will have to decide for yourself whether any of those we have presented in this chapter fits into your own assumptions about yourself and the world.

3 Dietary Goals and Guidelines: A Progressive Jump or Jumping the Gun?

I f the RDAs tell us what nutrients we need, and the Food
Guides tell us where we can find those nutrients in foods, what
on earth do we need Dietary Guidelines for? In this chapter we
take up a topic that has been hotly debated in public during the
last few years.

The U.S. has never had a food policy — at least not an intentional one. As was suggested in the previous chapter, however, the
effect of the Four Food Groups was to promote, or at any rate to
validate, a dietary pattern relatively rich in animal products, a situation that made livestock and dairy producers happy. In 1977, 30
years after the Four Food Groups was first adopted, a Senate
Select Committee chaired by then South Dakota Senator George
McGovern brought out a small report entitled "Dietary Goals for
Americans." The booklet was based on research done by the committee staff and on many months of hearings on the relationship
between the health of U.S. citizens and the nation's dietary pattern.

The report concluded that the American diet was much too
high in fat, especially saturated fat, and in cholesterol, sugar and
salt. To help the public decrease its intake of these substances to
specific targeted levels, the report recommended lowering average
consumption of specific foods, most notably red meat, eggs, and
processed foods containing high levels of salt and refined sugars.

The report was a bombshell. As you will see from some of the
excerpts included here, many people, among them the producers
of red meat and eggs, were outraged. In the battle that ensued,
nutritionists took both sides and quarreled over many details, but
the underlying argument was over something very simple: Did we
have enough evidence linking our dietary pattern to cancer, cardiovascular disease, hypertension and the other major "killer diseases" to justify recommending that ordinary healthy people
should eat differently? The Senate Select Committee, and subsequently a number of other groups, including some nutritionists
and some food producers, said "yes." A number of nutrition scientists, physicians and some other food producers said "no."

Over the years so many positions have been taken in this debate that the contestants are hard to keep straight without a program. Therefore, our second selection is a chronology to help you
keep score. Although there are much fought-over differences between the reports that have followed the Dietary Goals, their basic
recommendations (and the major arguments supporting and
objecting to them) are similar enough to refer to collectively as
"Goals and Guidelines." We hope you can keep your head and enjoy the battle.

111

- Dr. Wilbur Olin Atwater, called the father of American nutrition, announced in 1887:

  *. . . our food production is one-sided. It includes a relative excess of the fat of meat, of starch and of sugar.** *

- A. S. Truswell:

  *Since the modern messages have major negative items, anyone embarking on nutrition education is likely to meet lack of interest from politicians, anxiety or delay by civil servants, apathy from the medical profession, a tough counter-attack by the producers and processors of the food(s) you think people should eat less of, and confusion or indifference from the general public.*** *

- John R. Block, Secretary of the U.S. Department of Agriculture under President Ronald Reagan (1981 – 1986):

  *I know that they are not the same, but hogs are just like people. You can provide protein and grain to a hog and he will balance his ration. He will eat about the right amount of protein to go along with the grain. He will not overeat on the protein or the grain. People are surely as smart as hogs. Really, I think people deserve that prerogative. I am not so sure that government needs to get so deeply into telling people what they should or should not eat.**** *

- Richard Eamer, Chairman and Chief Executive Officer of National Medical Enterprises, a hospital management company:

  We have no food policy. You can live on Mars bars and Coca-Cola if you want. But you can't go to the drugstore and get any drug you want. That's because we have a drug policy.

  *But the funny thing is: It's probably a hell of a lot more important to have a food policy than a drug policy.***** *

---

*Tom Monte. "The U.S. finally takes a stand on diet." *Nutrition Action.* 6:3 – 6, September 1979.
**H. M. Sinclair and G. R. Howat, editors. (1980). *World Nutrition and Nutrition Education.* Oxford: Oxford University Press. Pages 44 – 50.
***Michael F. Jacobson. (1985). *The Complete Eater's Digest and Nutrition Scoreboard.* Garden City, New York: Anchor Press/Doubleday. Page 17.
****N. R. Kleinfield. "Total health care approach: N.M.E. stirs competitors to diversify." *New York Times.* July 19, 1983.

> *In the teeth of the controversy generated by the Dietary Goals, the General Accounting Office released a report outlining the limitations consumers faced in knowing what they were eating and whether it was good for them. Vitamin and mineral deficiencies were no longer our major problem, the report observed, and the public needed guidance about other substances in foods.*

WHAT FOODS SHOULD AMERICANS EAT? BETTER INFORMATION NEEDED ON NUTRITIONAL QUALITY OF FOODS*

General Accounting Office

. . . . The recommended dietary allowances (RDAs) serve as a basis for expressing human nutritional needs. . . .

No RDAs have been established on several of society's most controversial food components — fat, cholesterol, sugar, salt, alcohol, and fiber. . . . The lack of such authoritative guidance often creates a dilemma for consumers concerned with diseases statistically associated with these food components. For example, nutrition literature may recommend liver, milk, and eggs as good sources of protein, vitamins A and B, and iron. Other nutrition literature may recommend avoiding these same foods to prevent atherosclerosis because they are high in fat and/or cholesterol. Authoritative guidance on safe levels of intake for these controversial dietary substances would help consumer nutrition decisions. . . .

Even though no RDAs have been set for these controversial substances, the Food and Nutrition Board's eighth RDA edition does cite information which correlates food components to certain diseases. For example it states that (1) diets high in sticky forms of refined and processed sugar are linked to dental cavities (2) saturated fats are linked to coronary heart diseases (the American Heart Association recommends a goal of less than 10 percent of total calories from saturated fat), and (3) cholesterol intake is linked to heart disease. . . .

---

*"What Foods Should Americans Eat? Better Information Needed on Nutritional Quality of Foods." *General Accounting Office, Report CED-80-68*, April 30, 1980, pp. 15–16. Comptroller General of the United States.

SUMMARY OF DIETARY RECOMMENDATIONS MADE FOR HEALTHY AMERICANS BY 10 FEDERAL, PROFESSIONAL, AND HEALTH ORGANIZATIONS*

Title and organization	Nutrient adequacy	Weight control
Dietary Goals for the United States, 2d edition U.S. Senate Select Committee on Nutrition and Human Needs, 1977	([1])	To avoid overweight, consume only as much energy as expended.
Diet and Coronary Heart Disease: General Dietary Recommendations American Heart Association, 1978	([1])	Balance calories to maintain ideal weight.
Healthy People — Surgeon General's Report on Health Promotion and Disease Prevention U.S. Department of Health, Education, and Welfare, 1979	Balance and vary food choices every day.	Exercise and balance calories to maintain desirable weight.
Concepts of Nutrition and Health Council on Scientific Affairs American Medical Association, 1979	Vary diet to increase nutrient adequacy.	Maintain desirable weight through dietary control and exercise.
Recommended Dietary Allowances Committee on Dietary Allowances Food and Nutrition Board National Research Council National Academy of Sciences, 1980	Nutrient recommendations are to be met by a variety of foods.	Balance energy intake with output to maintain desirable weight.
Nutrition and Your Health: Dietary Guidelines for Americans U.S. Department of Agriculture and Department of Health and Human Services, 1980	Eat a variety of foods.	Maintain ideal weight. If obese, lose weight gradually; increase physical activity.
Toward Healthful Diets Food and Nutrition Board National Research Council National Academy of Sciences, 1980	Select wide variety of foods from the major food groups	Adjust energy intake to maintain appropriate weight for height
Diet, Nutrition, and Cancer Committee on Diet, Nutrition, and Cancer National Research Council National Academy of Sciences, 1982	([1])	([1])
Nutrition and Cancer: Cause and Prevention — A Special Report American Cancer Society, 1984	([1])	Avoid obesity.
Cancer Prevention National Cancer Institute National Institutes of Health U.S. Department of Health and Human Services, 1984	Vary diet Eat variety of foods every day.	Prevent being overweight; increase physical activity.

114 *"Dietary Recommendations for Healthy Americans Summarized," by Patricia M. Behlen and Frances J. Cronin. *Family Economics Review*, No. 3, 1985, pp. 17–24. U.S. Department of Agriculture.

DIETARY GOALS AND GUIDELINES

Patricia M. Behlen and Frances J. Cronin

Fat			Cholesterol
Total	*Saturated*	*Polyunsaturated*	
Reduce to 27-33 pct of total energy.	Reduce to 8-12 pct of total energy.	Intake should be 8-12 pct of total energy intake.	Reduce to 250-350 mg/day.
Reduce to 30-35 pct of total calories.	Reduce to less than 10 pct of total calories.	Up to 10 pct of total calories.	Reduce to 300 mg/day for adults.
Reduce excess intake.	Consume less.	(1)	Consume less.
Moderate intake regardless of source.	Proportion of saturated and polyunsaturated fat is not of universal importance.		Level in the diet is not of universal importance.
Reduce to not more than 35 pct of dietary energy, particularly in diets below 2000 calories.	Reduce.	Upper limit intake of 10 pct of dietary energy.	(1)
Avoid too much.	Avoid too much.	(1)	Avoid too much.
Reduce intake if overweight, or if energy needs are low.	Recommendations not warranted for the public.	Recommendations not warranted for the public.	Recommendations not warranted for the public.
Reduce intake to 30 pct of total caloric intake.	Reduce intake.	Reduce intake.	(1)
Cut down intake.	(1)	(1)	(1)
Keep intake of all fats low — both saturated and unsaturated.	Keep intake of all fats low — both saturated and unsaturated.	Keep intake of all fats low — both saturated and unsaturated.	(1)

115

[1] No specific dietary advice is stated in the published report. If a group specifically stated that recommendations are inappropriate or unwarranted, this is noted.

Title and organization	Carbohydrates	
	Starch	Fiber
Dietary Goals for the United States, 2d edition U.S. Senate Select Committee on Nutrition and Human Needs, 1977	Increase complex carbohydrates and naturally occurring sugar to 45-51 pct of total energy.	Increase.
Diet and Coronary Heart Disease: General Dietary Recommendations American Heart Association, 1978	Increase carbohy-drates, particularly complex.	Increase carbo-hydrates, partic-ularly complex.
Healthy People — Surgeon General's Report on Health Promotion and Disease Prevention U.S. Department of Health, Education, and Welfare, 1979	Consume more complex carbohydrates.	Consume more complex carbohydrates
Concepts of Nutrition and Health Council on Scientific Affairs American Medical Association, 1979	([1])	([1])
Recommended Dietary Allowances Committee on Dietary Allowances Food and Nutrition Board National Research Council National Academy of Sciences, 1980	Maintain or increase consumption of complex carbohy-drates.	Moderately in-crease intake.
Nutrition and Your Health: Dietary Guidelines for Americans U.S. Department of Agriculture and Department of Health and Human Services, 1980	Eat foods with adequate starch.	Eat foods with adequate fiber.
Toward Healthful Diets Food and Nutrition Board National Research Council National Academy of Sciences, 1980	([1])	([1])
Diet, Nutrition, and Cancer Committee on Diet, Nutrition, and Cancer National Research Council National Academy of Sciences, 1982	([1])	([1])
Nutrition and Cancer: Cause and Prevention — A Special Report American Cancer Society, 1984	([1])	Eat more high fiber foods.
Cancer Prevention National Cancer Institute National Institutes of Health U.S. Department of Health and Human Services, 1984	([1])	Eat foods with fiber.

Carbohydrates Refined sugar	Sodium	Alcohol
Reduce to 8-12 pct of total energy.	Decrease salt intake to 4-6 g/day (1600-2400 mg/day sodium).	Keep intake moderate.
([1])	Avoid excess sodium.	Keep intake moderate.
Consume less.	Consume less salt.	([1])
([1])	Moderate intake of salt to less than 12 g/day (4800 mg/day sodium).	
Reduce intake.	Safe and adequate range of sodium is about 1100-3300 mg/day.	For many individuals. reduced intake will assist energy balance.
Avoid too much.	Avoid too much	If you drink, do so in moderation.
Reduce intake if energy requirement is low.	Use salt in moderation: 3-8 g/day (1200-3200 mg/day sodium).	Reduce intake if energy requirement is low.
([1])	([1])	If consumed, do so in moderation.
([1])	([1])	Keep consumption moderate, if you drink.
([1])	([1])	If you drink, do so in moderation.

[1]No specific dietary advice is stated in the published report. If a group specifically stated that recommendations are inappropriate or unwarranted, this is noted.

*In a series of statements made in successive years after the
Dietary Goals had been released by the McGovern Committee,
D. Mark Hegsted, a nutrition scientist with a public health
viewpoint, presented arguments in favor of the Dietary Goals.
Is the science base for Dietary Goals, he asked, really less
adequate than that used to establish Recommended Dietary
Allowances?*

DIETARY GOALS — A PROGRESSIVE VIEW*

D. M. Hegsted, Ph.D.

The Dietary Goals for the United States published by the Senate
Select Committee on Nutrition and Human Needs recommend that
Americans should eat less food and specifically that they should eat
less fat, particularly saturated fat, less cholesterol, less sugar, and less
salt, and that they should increase their consumption of fruits, vegetables, grain products, and unsaturated oils. It is not surprising that
various segments of the food-producing and manufacturing community
find fault with these guidelines. Of more significance, perhaps, are the
adverse comments of some of the current leaders of the nutrition
community. . . .

These opponents find the report either premature or unjustified
on the basis of current knowledge. We should be very clear what is
being said, . . . either . . . that the intake of fat, cholesterol, salt, and
sugar has no nutritional significance and, therefore, does not deserve
attention by serious nutritionists or the public, or that, having reviewed all of the evidence, the current American diet estimated to
provide about 40% of the calories as fat, about 20% of the calories as
sugar, 500 to 700 mg of cholesterol per day, and 8 to 10 g of salt is
the best diet that can be recommended for Americans. We should note
that these are estimates of average intake so that half of the population is consuming larger amounts. Frankly, I find it inconceivable that
anyone familiar with the literature can arrive at either conclusion.

The Dietary Goals have been criticized that they were not a complete prescription for health — that there was inadequate discussion of
obesity, fluoridation, alcohol, exercise, etc. The legitimacy of this argument depends entirely upon one's point of view. It is perfectly clear to
everyone, however, that the Goals were not intended and do not pretend to be a substitute for other well established information and

*"Dietary Goals — A Progressive View," by D. M. Hegsted, Ph.D. *American Journal of
Clinical Nutrition*, 31:1504 – 1509, September 1978. American Society for Clinical
Nutrition. Used with permission.

other legitimate goals. What they were intended to do was to call forceful attention to issues that the nutrition and biochemical community have so far failed to deal with in adequate fashion. . . .

Rather invidious comparisons have been drawn between the RDA and the Dietary Goals with the implication that whereas the RDA are obviously justified, the Dietary Goals are not. The change in the Goals on salt intake in the second edition is said to demonstrate that the recommendations are premature. We should compare what has happened to the RDA. In the 1948 edition the recommended intake of riboflavin and vitamin C were much higher than they are currently and the recommended intake of iron was the same for men and women. The last edition dropped the recommendation of vitamin C for men from 60 to 45 mg. Does this mean we never knew anything about desirable vitamin C intakes and possibly still do not? It has always been understood that dietary recommendations should be continuously reviewed and will inevitably change. Otherwise, research is useless.

It should also be emphasized that the RDA have always been derived from informed judgment based upon all possible sources of information — epidemiology, metabolic studies with human subjects, and studies with experimental animals being the primary sources of information. If this procedure is valid for establishing "best estimates of nutrient need," it is equally valid for establishing best estimates of desirable intakes of fat, sugar, salt, or any other dietary constituent.

A major criticism of the Dietary Goals has been that there is no proof that adoption of the dietary pattern recommended will benefit the public. . . . It is a somewhat strange argument for nutritionists to make. Where is the proof that an intake of 45 mg of vitamin C is better or worse than an intake of 60 or 70 mg? . . . It is obvious that recommendations do have to be made before all of the desired evidence is available and this has always been accepted.

We should note that the RDA have always been set (at least in theory) at relatively high levels to minimize "risk" of deficiency. . . . If the RDA is correctly estimated, it follows that very few individuals would benefit from an intake that high. Similarly, it is perfectly clear that some individuals are more adversely affected by diets high in fat, cholesterol, salt, and sugar than others. A few will have little or nothing to gain from a lower intake in the same way that an individual with a vitamin A requirement of 2500 IU per day will have nothing to gain from an intake of 5000 IU. This, however, cannot mean that no advice about intake can be given to the public, particularly when a very large proportion of Americans are at risk from excessive intakes. . . .

Much has been made of the fact that iron deficiency is a problem in the United States and that decreased consumption of meat might exacerbate this problem. . . . There is a curious inconsistency in the way [some critics] consider the major chronic diseases and iron deficiency. They argue that dietary recommendation for coronary artery disease, diabetes, etc. should be reserved as *therapy* after susceptibles have been identified while *prevention* of iron deficiency is a high priority item. Most nutritionists, I think, agree that iron deficiency ought to be prevented. Yet this is a disease that is easily identified, easily treated and, as far as we know, has no residual effects. Furthermore, the actual impairment in health of the modest degrees of iron deficiency which occur have been difficult to document. In contrast, coronary heart disease (CHD), stroke, diabetes, hypertension, etc. are devastating diseases and dietary or other forms of treatment are relatively ineffective. Any major health gains to be made in the United States must be aimed at prevention or amelioration of these diseases. . . .

There are obviously two philosophies that may be used in establishing dietary recommendations, either of which can be defended. One is to establish desirable *goals* regardless of whether they can be achieved or not. The RDA have often been defined as "goals which we should strive to meet" even though the consequences of not achieving the specific goal cannot be precisely defined. The other approach is to develop a specific "cut-off point," below or above which, "health cannot be assumed." These different approaches may yield somewhat different recommendations but some goals or guidelines are necessary. Above all, we cannot assume that dietary habits are immutable. This is denied by everything that has happened in the United States during the past 30 to 40 years and what is happening all around the world.

In discussing "The Code of the Scientist and its Relationship to Ethics", André Cournand emphasizes that "We must find a means of establishing control over the processes of emergence so as to favor man's survival," and that "Unchecked, this blind emergence overpowers its antithesis, which . . . I shall refer to as humanizing emergence." Our current dietary habits represent an example of "blind emergence." They can certainly not be said to have been planned for any nutritional purpose. Although the recommendation to "eat more meat, more milk, more eggs — more of everything – but don't get fat" has characterized our nutritional strategy for the past 50 years, and nutritionists, therefore, bear some responsibility, these recommendations were not based upon any knowledge of the ultimate effects of such a diet. Such knowledge is now available.

The total evidence related to coronary disease, stroke, diabetes, cancer, hypertension, obesity, etc. — the major health problems of Americans — indicates that a more moderate diet will lessen the impact of these diseases. There are no reasons to believe that such a diet will impose nutritional risks. Nutritional deficiencies are not the important nutritional problems of our population and a more moderate diet will not create nutritional deficiencies. If the proper dietary recommendations are not those specified in the Dietary Goals, they are certainly something very similar.

It is the responsibility of the nutrition community to provide some leadership. It must answer the questions put to it — How much sugar, how much salt, how much cholesterol, how much fat, and what kind of fat, etc. are *desirable* in the American diet? To simply argue that we are ignorant, that we have not learned anything useful, and that we have no advice to offer, is self-defeating and irresponsible.

FINDING A COMMON LANGUAGE TO EDUCATE AND PLAN*

D. M. Hegsted, Ph.D.

. . . One of the arguments against the goals is that the levels specified are unrealistic. The goals specify about 30% of the energy as fat, about one-third of which should come from saturates and one-third from polyunsaturates; about 300 mg of cholesterol daily; about 15% of the energy as sugar and about 3 g of salt daily. We should not be unduly distracted by these figures. The goals represent some kind of compromise between what is desirable and what might be achievable. Completely unrealistic goals do discourage acceptance yet one can argue that the goals are something to aim at. Many of us may have a goal of being a millionaire but we will not be completely unhappy if we do not quite reach the goal. . . .

The major point . . . is that it can be expected that improvements in health will occur if the national diet is moved in this direction. It is not that we will suddenly blossom with great health when we reach a magical number and nothing is achieved before the goals are reached.

A second objection is that we have not proven what the benefits are. We need field trials, more research, etc. to demonstrate the benefits. I say to you and those critics that we do not have that option and for several reasons.

To assume that we have spent multimillions on research during the past several decades and still know nothing is ridiculous. The public and the Congress are tired, and rightly so, of researchers who never know enough to reach a decision. Many, perhaps most, of the important public decisions are made with much less evidence than we have. Consider a Supreme Court decision of 4 to 5, a statistically insignificant difference, that becomes the law of the land or a Congressional vote with a majority of one or two. Once the question is raised they cannot simply duck the issue; they have to consider the evidence and arrive at a conclusion. We are now in that position. We know that living in the United States carries a risk of about 7 or 8 out of 10 of dying of a heart attack or of cancer or of developing diabetes. The

"Finding A Common Language to Educate and Plan," speech by D. Mark Hegsted, Ph.D. Edited portions used with permission.

question is "What are the possibilities of modifying this risk and what risks are associated with dietary modification?"

We tend to avoid the decision by asking the wrong question. We talk about the American diet as though it were something fixed when we know that it has, is, and will change. The diet we eat is not something that was planned. If it was planned, the plan was certainly not based upon any evidence of need or knowledge of the result. No field trial was done. Our diet is a happenstance of affluence, the productivity of American farmers, and the influence of the food industry. The question that really should be asked of nutritionists is "Given two diets, one of which contains 40–45% of the energy as fat, most of which is saturated, contains 700–1000 mg of cholesterol, 20–25% of the energy as sugar; 10–15 g of salt, etc. and another that approximates the dietary goals, which is the most likely to be beneficial or which would you recommend?"

. . . The question should be put in such a way that we do not have the luxury of avoiding a decision.

The major question, then, is what are the likely benefits and risks associated with dietary recommendations? Every physician makes this kind of judgment daily. His job is to do the best he can with the available knowledge. He is not asked to guarantee results but he cannot tell the patient to go home and come back in a few years after his research is complete. The public health, to a major degree, must be treated the same way. The public deserves the best advice available at any particular time.

The argument that we need more research is, of course, valid. There simply is not any other avenue open to us. There may be better solutions available at some time. It is simply not clear, however, whether we have the capability of solving some of these complex problems in any reasonable period of time. If one considers cancer and diet, for example, where the incubation period may be 10, 20, 30 or more years and it is certain that multiple etiologic factors are involved, it is unlikely that we will have all of the knowledge we need to define what needs to be defined in any reasonable time. If we could simply stop the world and get off and view it from afar for the next 50 years, things would be simpler. But diet is changing and decisions must be made.

There is also legitimate concern about bureaucratic control. We find ourselves in an age when everyone asks for less governmental interference yet continues to heap additional responsibilities on government. I do not want Washington or anyone else telling me what I must eat. We have a right to make fools of ourselves, within some limits, and that right must be preserved. We also have an obligation to present the current state of knowledge to the public. Innumerable decisions are made daily which influence the food supply and the consumption patterns of the American public. Those decisions should be made in the light of and aimed at the improvement of public health — not the reverse. . . .

122

FOOD AND NUTRITION POLICY: PROBABILITY AND PRACTICALITY*

D. Mark Hegsted, Ph.D.

. . . Some of the activist-consumer representatives have not been very helpful. By over-emphasizing and overstating the risks associated with the American diet, demanding excessive controls, suggesting that we are all being deliberately poisoned, and such, they have often polarized the situation to the point that the voices of moderation become lost in the argument.

The issue is *not* natural vs. processed foods. We don't really know how to make that distinction — some people consider such items as pasteurized milk and frozen vegetables as processed foods. The issue is: How to apply the best nutritional knowledge. Certainly, there is abundant evidence that a diet of natural foods in itself does not assure adequate nutrition. It is also true that the food industries are able to apply better control in their production than many cooks at home; processed foods will often have greater nutritional value than those prepared from scratch at home. On the other hand, we also know that nutritional knowledge is not complete. A diet composed entirely of highly processed foods does pose some risks, some of which we cannot define. To some degree, we are forced to rely on experience, and our long-term experience is based primarily on less refined foods than many now available. We cannot assume that throwing a vitamin-mineral supplement into a food fulfills essential nutrient requirements. The message again, I think, must be one of moderation and common sense, but with some degree of conservatism, which will not please all manufacturers.

. . . The challenge to the food industry is to produce products with the kinds of nutritional properties that are desirable and which also combine other characteristics of flavor, consistency, convenience, and price that do make them acceptable. The food industry has adequately demonstrated in the past couple of decades that the definition of "acceptable" does change — or that it can be changed. . . .

*D. Mark Hegsted, Ph.D.: "Food and Nutrition Policy: Probability and Practicality." Reprinted from *Journal of the American Dietetic Association*, Vol. 74:534, 1979.

> *When the debate over the Dietary Goals was raging hot and heavy, one of the authors of this volume was asked to debate one of the Goals' most influential and articulate critics. The excerpt that follows is from her remarks prepared for that encounter.*

DO WE KNOW ENOUGH TO EAT?*

Joan Gussow, Ed.D.

Let's begin by talking about the impact of the Goals on the food industry. It has long been clear to me that if ordinary citizens began for some inexplicable reason to listen to nutritionists and turned to eating relatively simple, minimally processed, low calorie diets, much of the food industry would be in serious financial trouble. For much of the profit of the food industry is derived from the sale of complex highly processed products rich in salt, fat, and sugar and other refined carbohydrates. I have long been aware of this problem. The death of Pringle's would idle a lot of expensive machinery and a large number of Pringle workers — and that is a very real problem. But it is not *my* problem; and it is not yours. Our job is to tell the nutritional truth to the best of our abilities, and to ask the economists to tell us how to make the system work like it is supposed to.

The Dietary Goals recommend, among other things, that we eat less fatty meat, butter and eggs and more fruits, vegetables, grains and fish. Thus it is hardly surprising that among the groups which have come out in support of the goals are the United Fresh Fruit and Vegetable Association, the National Fisheries Institute, the National Association of Wheat Growers, and *Milling and Baking News*. Neither is it unexpected that the goals should be opposed by the egg producers, the Dairy Associations, the American National Cattlemen's Association, the National Livestock Feeder's Association and the National Livestock and Meat Board. . . .

(Their opposition is really quite predictable.) So, of course, is the opposition of the other trade groups whose members would presumably also be harmed by widespread adoption of the goals. But such consumption shifts are a part of the workings of the free-enterprise system — harness makers were devastated by the invention of the automobile. The story we tell ourselves is that this is progress.

---

*"Do We Know Enough to Eat?," by Joan Dye Gussow. *Speech to the Food and Nutrition Council of Greater New York and the New York State Nutrition Council*, January 31, 1978. Used with permission.

I believe, however, that we ought not to let workers suffer merely because our wisdom increases. While nutritionists should not be *blamed* for economic dislocations, we ought not to be indifferent to the problems of the cattle raisers and the egg producers — since our concern must always be with food and those capable of producing it. We, as professionals, ought to be calling attention to the reality of the economic problem and demanding that our economists tell us how to make the system produce both health and economic well being instead of producing, as it does, "a shortage of whatever does in fact make people whole, well, and happy," what economist Herman Daly calls "existential scarcity."

What I am saying, in short, is that we must concern ourselves with the economic problems that a change in diet might bring, but that we must not let that concern keep us from recommending whatever changes are *nutritionally* rational. . . .

In any case, one of the things I have been trying to understand in the great debate over the Dietary Goals is why the Four Food Groups are acceptable and the Dietary Goals are radical. And I have concluded that it is because *anything* goes under the Four Food Groups. It is an acceptable guide because it is totally ineffectual — and probably actually misleading about the dietary pattern that might promote optimal health. You can put together a perfectly appalling diet, grossly high in fat, sugar, salt, calories and still tuck it comfortably under the skirt of the Four Food Groups. Even pink, yellow, green and purple breakfast confections composed of 50% or more sugar can be comfortably fitted into the grain group, so long as they are advertised as cereals.

When I first saw the Dietary Goals, I recognized it as a radical document. Yet its food recommendations are what we have all been giving out for years (eat less fatty meat, more chicken and fish, less sugar and fat, more fresh fruits and vegetables and whole grains). Why then is it radical? It seems radical because it is an attempt to tell what its authors have concluded is the truth without reference to which power blocs might be offended. What an astonishing definition of radical! . . .

. . . Our choice is not one between doing nothing because we do not yet have enough information, and taking an action which will suddenly move us away from a well-established dietary pattern. To do nothing, as I point out to my classes each year, is to do something. Not to act, is to act. Not to object to the present direction of the diet — for the diet is not fixed, it is rapidly changing — not to object to that is to acquiesce in it.

We are told that by urging a dietary change we run the risk of producing ill-health. Where were all these concerned scientists over the last decades when, propelled by the demands of commerce alone, the American people undertook a drastic dietary change?

Major dietary changes have occurred in the U. S. over the last half-century, without regard to whether a knowledge base existed or not. These changes have taken place in the service of free-enterprise and, **125** lately, with the help of staggeringly large expenditures in the mass media. The response from those who now argue that we don't know enough to change diets has been deafening silence. Therefore, the message appears to be that without direct and irrefutable evidence that a change in the food supply causes harm, anyone may promote *anything* — anything, that is, except a food pattern that is likely to be healthier than the existing one.

Another point to be made is that the diet recommended by the Dietary Goals is neither novel, exotic or radical, unless radical is taken in relation to its real meaning — "relating to roots." For nutritionists have been urging such a dietary pattern on Americans for more years than I had imagined.

In 1927, almost 60 years ago, Dr. Grace McLeod of Teachers College, in an address to the National Canner's Convention demonstrated how the diets of that era would be improved if a larger proportion of the budget were spent for fruits and vegetables and whole grains, and a smaller proportion for meat. A quarter of a century later, in 1950, Columbia's distnguished Dr. Henry T. Sherman (in his *Nutritional Improvement of Life*) compared the diet of "an individual adult nutritionist" (presumably himself) with that of the general public and concluded that his diet was much higher in mature legumes and nuts, in total fruits and vegetables and in milk and its products — while he consumed at least 50% less than the population average of eggs, meats, fat and sugar. The public, he concluded, would be better off eating like he did. . . .

So please, as the argument progresses, keep hold of your common sense. Do not lose sight of the fact that we are talking about Dietary Goals that consist almost entirely of what we have been teaching for 50 years — that this is not some sort of exotic document that the Senate Committee has produced which urges onto us a diet of tofu and carrot sticks. . . .

So much for the advocates. Here come the spokesmen for the opposition. Robert Olson is a nutrition scientist who has battled fiercely against the goals. Here, in an article published in the Journal of the American Dietetic Association, *are some of his reasons.*

ARE PROFESSIONALS JUMPING THE GUN IN THE FIGHT AGAINST CHRONIC DISEASES?*

Robert E. Olson, M.D., Ph.D.

At present, there is an intense interest in the subject of nutrition in this country — by our people, by consumer advocate groups, by health food interests, by voluntary health agencies, and by the government through its National Institutes of Health and the various Congressional committees. This interest provides unprecedented opportunities for health education in the field of nutrition, and it behooves all of us, as professionals in the field, to take advantage of this receptive market but not to abuse it by promising a health panacea through inappropriate dietary intervention. Obviously, a receptive audience also provides opportunities for quacks and charlatans to sell inflated values for health foods, nostrums, and even dangerous drugs, such as laetrile.

In a way, the American public has become a battleground for the selling of nutritional ideas based on both fact and fraud. On one hand, qualified scientific bodies are shaking their heads and stressing the need for more research to develop a solid base of scientific knowledge to make better dietary recommendations. On the other hand, the health quacks are promising cures for all chronic diseases through the ingestion of nuts, fruits, fad diets, and attractively packaged powders. One might ask: What has led to this nutrition mania? *And:* What can health professionals do about it? . . .

Mythology of Foods

. . . The present craze about nutrition . . . fits very well into the psychology of the Vietnam alumni in that they are concentrating on one aspect of self-preservation, one important avenue of which is good

---

*Robert E. Olson: "Are Professionals Jumping the Gun in the Fight Against Chronic Diseases?" Copyright The American Dietetic Association. Reprinted by permission from *Journal of the American Dietetic Association, Vol. 74: 543, 1979.

health and good health care. Because there is a general distrust of scientific institutions and disenchantment with professional approaches to these problems, mythology has been substituted for science. . . .

The interesting thing about the etiology of the chronic degenerative diseases is that dietary determinants do contribute to the progression or retardation of these diseases. It is easy for "believers" to take this basic concept of dietary determinants in chronic diseases and fuse it with the "mythology of foods" to reach conclusions beyond the proper scientific limits. Their conclusion is that, because there are some dietary determinants for coronary disease, hypertension, cancer, diabetes, and cirrhosis of the liver, it should be possible to prevent these diseases by manipulation of the ratios of macronutrients in our diet. The question I would like to put to us, as health professionals in the field of nutrition, is: Are we promoting these ideas on the basis of hope, fear, and charity, or are we critically evaluating the data base underlying these proposals in an attempt to carry out sound nutrition education?

National Nutrition Policy

Since 1941, the national nutrition policy in the United States has been to create and distribute a supply of foods which will meet the nutritional requirements of our population. . . .

Although the nutrition policy for this country, embodied in the RDAs, has not formally been endorsed by any branch of the government, tacit acceptance has come from the widespread use of RDAs by both governmental and non-governmental agencies. . . .

With the current scientific data available, can any authoritative body in the field of clinical nutrition move further in making sound recommendations regarding an optimal diet for the U.S. population? Is it likely that changes in the macronutrient and mineral composition of the American diet will modify the mortality from the major chronic diseases? One problem which complicates the dietary regulation of these diseases is their intricate and multiple etiology.

In Figure 2, the genetic vs. nutritional determinants for thirteen diseases are shown. For each, a bar is positioned to indicate the extent to which nutrition can influence the course of the illness. . . .

The killer chronic diseases are intermediate on the scale of genetic and nutritional determinants and hence, will never be totally controllable by dietary intervention.

. . . Let me contrast the decision of a physician to treat a patient whose disease is incompletely understood "on the basis of current research findings" with the decision of a public health official to make a recommendation to prevent the same disease in the general population. In the first instance, the physician has studied his patient. He

128

knows something about his/her history, physical examination, laboratory findings, and past course of his/her disease. He has evaluated the relevant risk factors and takes action with much more knowledge about the object of his decision-making than does the public health official who has no direct contact with any subject and only a statistical view of the disease problem. For what percentage of susceptible subjects in a given population is a public health official justified in imposing a regimen on all? Is such action *ever* justified in the absence of a positive clinical trial showing clear benefits from the regimen in the form of reduced morbidity and mortality?

Figure 2. Reciprocal genetic and environmental determinants of thirteen diseases as shown on a linear scale. Extent to which nutritional intervention can modify the disease is indicated by the degree of displacement of each bar to the right of the line.

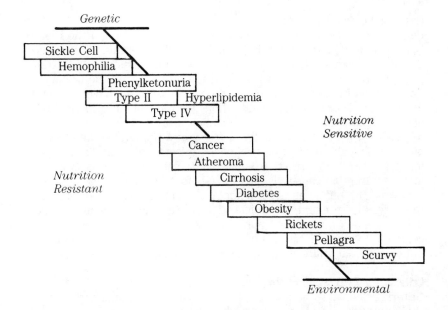

Dietary Recommendations to the Public "beyond the RDAs"

. . . The issue here is not the doctrine of prevention, but the scientific soundness of a given preventive program. The soundness of "Dietary Goals" as a preventive program remains in doubt. No preaching about a diet alleged to combat the six major killer diseases in the U.S. will substitute for a sound program of preventive medicine, including periodic vists of healthy individuals to their physicians, the evaluation of

129

individual risk factors, and the individualization of medical care. Furthermore, to exclude the medical profession and the allied health professionals from a basic plan, dietary or otherwise, to prevent our major chronic degenerative diseases is sheer folly and is doomed to failure.

Critique of the "Dietary Goals"

In principle, I believe in selective dietary goals beyond those implicit in the RDAs. However, I doubt that any single dietary recommendation will be appropriate for all segments of our population, i.e., infants, children, young men, pregnant and lactating women, non-pregnant women before menopause, women after the menopause, and persons beyond the age of seventy. The frontier in public health nutrition is moving, and we must be prepared both to make and to criticize recommendations which arise from an expanding data base. . . .

Need for Clinical Evidence

Perhaps the most cogent argument against the adoption of the Dietary Goals in the hope of preventing the chronic degenerative diseases is that the efficacy of this regimen has not been demonstrated in extensive clinical trials. Even Hegsted, a strong proponent of the Dietary Goals, noted in his introduction to the report that "we have not demonstrated that the dietary modifications we recommend will yield the dividend expected . . . but . . . we cannot afford to temporize."

Many of us, on the other hand, feel that a properly conducted and positive clinical intervention trial of the effect of diet (and/or drugs) on morbidity and mortality from coronary artery disease, as well as mortality from all causes, is necessary before one can advise physicians and the public at large to adopt a regimen designed to prevent this disease. For example, clinical trials of the value of small pox and polio vaccination were strikingly positive, and only after they were completed was public health action initiated which has now resulted in the essential eradication of these two diseases. . . .

Criteria for Evaluation of Programs

Criteria I believe to be important in evaluating recommendations to the public about diet and chronic disease are the following:

a. Epidemiologic studies are not, of themselves, sufficient evidence to assume cause-and-effect relationships between associated health variables. For example, when Robert Koch discovered the tubercle bacillus, the general view of epidemiologists of his time was that tuberculosis was a disease of malnutrition. He had to demonstrate in the laboratory, by application of his four postulates, that the tubercle bacillus was, in fact, the agent of the disease. Contrariwise, when Joseph Goldberger began to investigate pellagra in southern

United States, the prevailing view, based on the epidemiology available at the time, was that pellagra was an infectious disease. By
careful epidemiologic and clinical studies, Goldberger showed it to
be a disease of malnutrition.

b. In diseases of multiple etiology in which genetic factors are apparent, it is necessary to understand the extent to which dietary intervention can be successful under the best conditions.

c. Clinical intervention trials using the recommended dietary regimen
in the population at risk should be positive before public health
education is contemplated. In the case of scurvy, dietary intervention with citrus fruits cured the disease, and lime supplements to
the diet of healthy sailors prevented its appearance. In the case of
pellagra, feeding either animal protein or nicotinic acid prevented
and/or cured the disease. It would seem important to demand similar evidence of the efficacy of dietary change in given chronic disease before recommending sweeping changes in the U.S. diet.

d. Strong support from the medical and paramedical professions for a
contemplated dietary change to control disease should be obtained
before initiating a given public health nutrition program. . . .

*Why have Dietary Goals at all? Here, another well-known
nutrition scientist argues that we are promoting a nationwide cure before it is clear that we have a disease.*

DIETARY GOALS — A SKEPTICAL VIEW*

A. E. Harper, PhD.

The Senate Select Committee on Nutrition and Human Needs has
proposed "dietary goals" for the United States . . . because *1*) heart
disease, stroke, cancer, and various other chronic diseases are "killer
diseases" that are "epidemic in our population," *2*) "six of the ten
leading causes of death in the U.S. have been linked to our diet," and
3) this "epidemic" is associated with changes that have occurred over
the past half century in the composition of the U.S. diet which "represent as great a threat to public health as smoking." The implication of
these statements is that the dietary goals have been proposed as a

*"Dietary Goals — A Skeptical View" by A. E. Harper, Ph.D. Copyright *American Jour-
nal of Clinical Nutrition*, 31:310–321, February 1978. American Society for Clinical
Nutrition. Used with permission.

prescription for the prevention of an epidemic of killer diseases caused by changes in the U.S. diet and that the benefit to be expected is control of the epidemic.

The Council for Responsible Nutrition, a trade association of food supplement manufacturers, drafted a resolution endorsing the dietary goals. Several well-known nutritionists . . . have signed this endorsement. . . . They presumably accept the view that dietary modification is an important measure for reducing the incidence of chronic diseases that are not primarily nutritional. The goals have also been endorsed by a number of consumer advocate organizations and industry groups. . . .

Those from the fruit, vegetable, cereal, fisheries, and nutritional supplement industries who endorsed the goals represent industries that would benefit if the recommendations to reduce substantially the consumption of whole milk, meat and eggs were to be adopted.

The dietary goals may appear superficially to be innocuous but if the goals and the rationale for them were to be adopted by Federal agencies and were to serve as the basis for food, nutrition, health care, and education programs, as those endorsing them have requested, this would have far reaching implications. The approach in nutrition education would be completely altered. Programs would be directed toward providing guidelines for nutritional treatment of diseases that are not primarily nutritional rather than guidelines for a wholesome and nutritionally adequate diet. Health programs that prescribed adoption of the dietary goals for prevention and treatment of chronic diseases would be, in essence, the practice of medicine with uniform nutritional treatment for all, irrespective of the nature of their health problem or whether they were ill or well.

Also, the report of the Senate Select Committee represents a sweeping indictment of the U.S. food supply. The changes that would be required in the composition of most diets in order to meet the dietary goals would necessitate substantial changes in the food habits of consumers. This, in turn, would require drastic modification of the U.S. food supply. The basis for the goals, should, therefore, be extremely sound and the U.S. public should be assured of substantial benefits from their adoption.

The resolution endorsing the goals states "We live in the present and cannot afford to await the ultimate proof before correcting trends we believe to be detrimental". . . .

Incidence of Chronic Diseases and Life Expectancy

How valid is the rationale for the dietary goals, i.e., the claim that the U.S. is suffering from an "epidemic" of "killer diseases" associated with changes in the national diet over the past half century? While our diet

132

has been undergoing these assumed undesirable changes, life expectancy has increased by 20 years. It has increased since 1950, although more slowly than previously. Nutritional deficiency diseases have all but disappeared and most infectious diseases have been effectively controlled. Infant and child mortality, in particular, have thereby been reduced far below what they were at the turn of the century. This and control of infectious diseases among all age groups has resulted in an aging population. . . . It is not surprising, then, that the incidence of chronic diseases should increase and that heart disease and cancer should be major causes of death.

Despite the aging of the population, however, U.S. health statistics . . . show that, when the incidence of heart disease and stroke are adjusted for age, the rates of occurrence of these diseases have been decreasing. . . . It is obviously fallacious and misleading to call this situation an "epidemic" of "killer diseases" attributable to deterioration of the food supply or to indict the U.S. diet as "pathogenic." Such statements are political, not scientific. They create unjustifiable fear of food and fear for health. . . .

Diet and Health in This Century

With life expectancy having increased by 20 years since 1900; with the age-related incidence of heart disease decreasing since 1950 and that of stroke since 1930; with the average amount of time lost from work, in the U.S., including work loss from accidents, being only between 5 and 6 days per year; and with nutrition survey reports indicating that at least 85% of people surveyed show no evidence of nutritional deficits and that the major deficit is mild iron deficiency; there can be no doubt but that the food supply is sound if it is used appropriately, as it obviously is by most people. The fact that the major health problems of the U.S. are chronic diseases associated with aging is, in itself, evidence of this. The countries with health statistics equivalent to or better than ours in 1975 were those of western Europe and northern North America where diets resemble those of the U.S. When our knowledge of diet and health is viewed in proper perspective, a far stronger case can be made for concluding that the changes in our food supply during this century have been associated with improved health rather than with deteriorating health.

Nevertheless, evidence that we are basically a healthy people is no reason for complacency about health and nutrition problems. However, we must recognize that relationships between diet and most current health problems are complex and poorly understood. These problems will not be solved by drawing unwarranted conclusions from insufficient and inappropriate research results, nor will they be solved by accepting simplistic proposals as if they were panaceas. They will be

133

solved only by careful, imaginative, well-designed research that provides valid answers to difficult questions, particularly to the question of what role nutrition has in aging and in the development of chronic diseases. . . .

Oversights in the Dietary Goals

It is difficult, after reading the dietary goals document critically, to avoid the conclusion that the dietary goals were preconceived and then evidence was marshalled to support them. *1*) Anemia attributable to iron deficiency, which is considered to be the major nutritional problem of the U.S., is not mentioned and a recommendation is made for reducing the consumption of meat, a major source of iron in the food supply. *2*) Major emphasis for the control of dental caries is placed exclusively on lowering sugar consumption rather than on a measure that has proven effective, fluoridation of the water supply. *3*) The recommendation for reducing salt consumption is a recommendation for treating the entire nation for hypertension even though many may have a high need for salt. . . . *4*) The nutrient content of plant products is not compared with that of animal products but with that of purified sugars and fats. *5*) Processed foods are denigrated for their contribution to the sugar content of the diet, yet sugar consumption has remained constant for 50 years. *6*) The report states that views on the role of diet in the development of heart disease and other chronic diseases are controversial but does not hesitate to conclude that the proposed dietary changes will be beneficial. *7*) Obesity is cited as an important nutritional problem but the only recommendation for controlling it — to alter the composition of the diet — is a discredited one.

The dietary goals report is not scientifically sound: it is a political and moralistic document. It will appeal to those who accept pseudo-scientific reasoning about the wisdom of returning to the diet of last century and to that of the peasant of poor countries. Back to nature movements have occurred regularly throughout history when the problems to be solved were complex and solutions for them were not readily attainable. Treatment with some natural product assumed to have magical properties has often been the substitute for appropriate knowledge. We had the medieval doctrine of signatures. The thistle with prickly leaves was appropriate as a treatment for internal prickling. Port wine, which was red, was appropriate treatment for pale blood. And occasionally one of these chance remedies proved effective, for example, digitalis for heart disease. But why, when we have the ability to apply the scientific method to solve our problems, should we fall back on preconceived conclusions because the answers we would like to have cannot be obtained as quickly as we want them through sound, basic research? . . .

134

On Panaceas and Common Sense

The rationale for the proposed dietary goals for the treatment of chronic diseases bears a striking resemblance to that of the nutrition healers who recommend large doses of vitamins to prevent colds, influenza and cancer and large doses of vitamin E to ensure sexual potency and freedom from heart disease and aging. The nutritional healers and the proponents of the dietary goals both say there are no risks involved and important benefits can be expected. This is also the stock in trade of food faddists and nutritional supplement companies. Neither consumers nor nutrition professionals stand to gain from this approach to health problems. It has great potential for undermining both the science of nutrition and nutrition education. It raises false hopes among consumers on inadequate grounds. It is a promise to deliver a panacea that cannot be delivered.

The necromancers of old promised to provide the elixir of life but their credibility was eventually undermined by the rise of science. The international experts who proposed protein supplements and amino acid fortification for the prevention and cure of world-wide malnutrition lost credibility when that simplistic solution for a complex problem was proven invalid. There is no need for nutritionists to fall into this trap again by joining those who would promote a simplistic nutritional cure for all the ailments of old age. In fact, it would not be important to discuss the dietary goals at all were it not for the possibility that they might be adopted and thereby influence Federal nutrition policy to the detriment of both the consumer and the professional nutritionist. . . .

A Federally-supported nutrition education program based on established knowledge that would help to teach people what sound nutrition practices are *and more particularly what can, and what cannot, be expected from following such practices,* would be of infinitely more value to the general public than a set of recommendations for nutritional treatment of chronic diseases based on fear of food and fear for health and proposed on the basis of highly selected information under the guise of dietary goals.

We do need Dietary Goals, says Dr. Leveille, formerly of Michigan State and more recently of Nabisco Brands, Inc. But the ones proposed are the wrong ones. The American diet may be the best in the world.

ESTABLISHING AND IMPLEMENTING DIETARY GOALS*

by Gilbert A. Leveille

The need for dietary goals is obvious. It is clear that the consuming public has a definite need for guidance in making appropriate food selections that will ensure, insofar as possible, the consumption of a diet providing the essential nutrients and ensuring maximal health. The selection of such a diet is not a simple matter and must be based on current scientific information. The public cannot be expected to be conversant with the scientific information and, therefore, this information must be translated into food terms which the consuming public can understand and use. The need for such goals should be inherent in any national food and nutrition policy. . . .

. . . The Senate Select Committee on Nutrition and Human Needs published a set of dietary goals. This effort is laudable, but unfortunately the goals leave a great deal to be desired. In many respects these goals are not based on the contemporary science and if implemented would not be in the public interest. . . . These goals are not based on the whole of the scientific evidence available; they fail to recognize significant problems which exist in our society; and unfortunately, fail to recognize the possible negative impacts which their implementation might have.

Ideally, dietary goals should take into account those positive aspects of our current national diets and should assist in sustaining them. Further, they should correct the poor eating habits which can be identified. The American diet has been referred to as "pathogenic" by some and as "disastrous" by others, implying that our diet has "deteriorated" in the past 50 to 75 years. I submit that such a conclusion is erroneous and misleading. The American diet today is better than ever before and is one of the best, if not *the* best, in the world today. There is much supporting evidence for this statement. One need merely consider the stature of the current generation of Americans, which is coming closer and closer to the achievement of maximum

*"Establishing and Implementing Dietary Goals" by Gilbert A. Leveille. *Family Economics Review,* Winter-Spring 1978, pp. 7–11. U.S. Department of Agriculture.

genetic potential. We have virtually eliminated morbidity and mortality from acute nutritional deficiencies. A prime example is pellagra resulting from niacin deficiency, which claimed thousands of lives only a few short decades ago but which is virtually unheard of today. The same could be said for rickets, which was overcome by the fortification of milk with vitamin D, and of goiter, which was eradicated by the iodization of salt. We have seen a remarkable increase in the life expectancy of the American population. We have seen many improvements in the quality of our food supply as measured by its safety, wholesomeness, and variety; it is unparalleled in the world today.

Taking all of these factors into account, it seems abundantly clear to me that we can put to rest serious concerns about the quality of our diet and any consideration of returning to the diet of days gone by. Any notion that a return to the diet of the past would improve the well-being of Americans is nostalgic nonsense. Rather, we should identify existing nutritional problems and attempt to develop solutions to them. This, it seems to me, is the appropriate challenge of today and the challenge of developing appropriate goals for the American population.

The goals developed by the Senate Select Committee imply that we have been a Nation without dietary goals. This is not completely true. Admittedly we have not had a national food and nutrition policy to give visibility to dietary goals, but assuredly we have had guidelines which have served effectively to direct many food and nutrition programs in this country. The guidelines of which I speak are the Recommended Dietary Allowances (RDA's). . . .

. . . Any dietary guideline must have, as a fundamental basis, the objective of meeting essential nutrient needs and, secondarily, must deal with other recommendations that would contribute to insuring the public health. If such guidelines are to deal with the prevention of specific diseases, there should be a sound scientific basis for their establishment and they should not put any segment of the population at nutritional risk. Unfortunately, the Senate Select Committee's dietary goals have not provided this assurance, and they are not based on the whole of available scientific evidence.

The dietary goals published by the Senate Select Committee assume (1) that the diseases of primary concern, namely cardiovascular disease and cancer, are of epidemic proportions in the United States, and (2) that appropriate dietary modifications can delay or prevent these diseases. I would like to spend a brief time reviewing these two fundamental assumptions. There is little question that the proportion of the U.S. population dying from cardiovascular disease and cancer has increased dramatically over the past 50 years. I submit that this is not surprising and is to be expected. Accompanying the increase in mortality from cardiovascular disease and cancer has been a significant reduction in mortality from infectious diseases. Advances in medical science have greatly reduced mortality from such causes as

137

tuberculosis and pneumonia. The old adage that "death and taxes are assured" remains to be disproved. Consequently, one would expect that the elimination of death from infectious diseases would simply involve some other cause of death becoming primary. . . .

It seems that the recommendations for dietary change made by the Select Committee have not been evaluated from the standpoint of other potential, undesirable impacts which they might have if implemented. For example, it is recognized that a significant proportion of the total iron consumption by the U.S. population is derived from meats and meat products. Further, it is recognized that a large proportion of the iron derived from meat is in the form of heme, which has a much higher availability than does nonheme iron. If the recommendations of the Select Committee were followed, the likely effect would be a significant reduction in total iron intake and a decreased availability of that iron which was consumed. If this were to occur, the effect on the problem of anemia, which already appears to be widespread, would be disastrous. Thus, the recommended changes cannot be made without recognizing the need for increased iron fortification or somehow increasing the availability of iron from sources other than meat.

Similarly, the American population derives a significant proportion of its dietary zinc from meat. A reduction in meat intake would result in a significant reduction in zinc consumption. Further, the increased intake of cereal grains would increase the dietary content of phytic acid which is known to bind zinc and reduce its availability. Thus, there is a reasonable probability that implementation of the Select Committee's goals might result in serious zinc deficiency in some segments of the population.

Careful evaluation of the Select Committee's recommendations demonstrates that they are not based on the available scientific information. Further, there are many inconsistencies and outright errors in the development of the goals. The errors of omission and interpretation are sufficiently great to cause serious concern if they were taken seriously and applied to any current feeding programs.

There is a need for sound dietary goals to guide feeding programs and to guide individual consumers in their food choices. There is no question, in my opinion, that the Senate Select Committee's goals are inappropriate and that a totally new effort is required. Such an effort should involve a broad cross-section of expertise from the nutrition, food, and medical communities. It should involve consumers and consumer advocates who are knowledgeable about the application of nutrition and food information by consumers. Only in this way can a realistic set of dietary goals be established which will serve the best interests of the U.S. population. . . .

138

> *Like the Live Stock and Meat Board and the egg producers, the*
> *American Medical Association also objected to the Dietary*
> *Goals. Many people read their objection as saying, "see your*
> *doctor for individualized dietary advice." Judge for yourself.*

STATEMENT OF THE AMERICAN MEDICAL ASSOCIATION*

. . . The evidence for benefits to be derived from the adoption of the dietary goals . . . is insufficient and the potential for harm for the radical long term dietary change in "the American diet" is unknown. Further, the genetic and cultural heterogeneity of the population in the country would, no doubt, resist a rigid policy with respect to dietary goals. While the goals set forth . . . would appear to be laudable in many respects, the American Medical Association believes that at this time it would not be appropriate to adopt such dietary goals.

The dietary goals . . . concerning modification in the amount and type of fat and cholesterol and the restriction of salt intake to no more than 3 grams daily are comparable in many respects to therapeutic diets. Such diets must be formulated to meet the individual needs with appropriate medical dietary counselling on an individual basis. Strict adherence is required to obtain the desired results.

The American Medical Association does not consider it appropriate for the government to adopt national goals that specify such matters as the amount and proportions of total fat, type of fat, sugar, cholesterol, or salt content in the diets of the general public as these national goals advocate.

Rather, we believe that individual programs to prevent or to treat obesity through decreased caloric intake along with programs aimed at improving physical fitness would be the most effective means of improving the health of our American citizens.

As to the recommendations . . . we believe that they should not be adopted . . . the recommendations would encourage the Federal government to undertake a massive, nationwide educational program to gain public acceptance and incorporation of the dietary goals as personal goals. Furthermore, the recommendations carry with them the underlying potential for prohibiting the sale or for discouraging the agricultural production of certain food products which may not in the view of the government be supportive of the dietary goals. . . .

Statement of the American Medical Association (to the Senate Select Committee on Nutrition and Human Needs) April 18, 1977.

139

In 1980, a committee of the National Academy of Sciences'
Food and Nutrition Board published a small booklet intended
to refute the recommendations of the Dietary Goals. Here is a
part of the rationale from Toward Healthful Diets.

TOWARD HEALTHFUL DIETS*

Food and Nutrition Board

Associations between dietary patterns and disease prevalence have
been observed in a variety of epidemiological investigations of coronary heart disease, hypertension, and diabetes. These observations
have raised the question whether it is possible to develop additional
nutritional guidelines for improving health. In fact, general recommendations to alter consumption of dietary fat, cholesterol, complex
carbohydrates, sugar, salt, and fiber have been made to the public by a
number of organizations. Such nutritional guidelines for improved
health deal not with requirements for essential nutrients but with the
pattern of intake of nonessential nutrients or with the intake of essential nutrients in amounts that greatly exceed requirements.

The Board considers it scientifically unsound to make single, all-
inclusive recommendations to the public regarding intakes of energy,
protein, fat, cholesterol, carbohydrate, fiber, and sodium. Needs for
energy and essential nutrients vary with age, sex, physiological state,
hereditary factors, physical activity, and the state of health. The nutritional needs of the young growing infant are distinctly different from
those of the inactive octogenarian; those of the vigorous active young
person differ from those of the sedentary, obese person of middle age.
Variations in requirement due to age, sex, physical activity, and individual variability are taken into account in the formulation of the RDA.
Guidelines for a healthful diet must also take into account these same
variables if they are to be realistic.

The Surgeon General's report on healthy people (DHEW, 1979) has
stated that the population of the United States has never been healthier. It reported that age-corrected mortality rates have been falling
throughout this century, that life expectancy at birth is continuing to
rise, and that the mortality rate for coronary heart disease has declined 20 percent during the last 20 years and is currently falling at a
rate of 2 percent per year. Likewise, death rates from cancers not
associated with excessive cigarette smoking have not been rising, and

*"Quest for Guidelines Toward Healthful Diets; Decision-making in Public Health,"
Toward Healthful Diets, ©1980, pp. 4–5, 17–18. Food and Nutrition Board, National
Academy Press. Used with permission.

some have been falling. Nonetheless, heart disease and cancer continue to be the leading causes of death in the United States, together accounting for about 66 percent of total mortality. Both are diseases of multiple etiology. Some argue that because there are associations between dietary practices and the incidence of these diseases, it should be possible to reduce death rates from them by proper nutritional practices.

Although the Board considers it appropriate to set dietary guidelines beyond those implicit in the RDA, in the hope of correcting metabolic patterns in susceptible individuals in such a way as to prevent or delay the onset of chronic degenerative diseases, it is concerned about the adequacy of the scientific undergirding on which these recommendations are based. The Board recognizes that epidemiology establishes coincidence, but not cause and effect. Epidemiologic findings, however, lay the groundwork for further studies to test given hypotheses. Many such studies are in progress. The Board believes that advice should be given to the public when the strength, extent, consistency, coherence, and plausibility of the evidence from lines of investigation ranging from epidemiology to molecular biology converge to indicate that certain dietary practices or other aspects of lifestyle promote health benefits without incurring undue risks.

The American food supply on the whole is nutritious and provides adequate quantities of nutrients to protect essentially all healthy Americans from deficiency diseases. The excellent state of health of the American people as documented in the Surgeon General's report could not have been achieved unless most people made wise food choices. It is clear, however, that appropriate selections are not made and equitable distribution of nutrients is not currently attained by a portion of the population because of economic, educational, and cultural factors. . . .

Good public health practice depends upon the application of sound principles of preventive medicine to population groups. One of these principles is that primary prevention of disease is preferable to treatment, provided the preventive intervention is effective and safe. Another is that primary prevention is preferable to secondary prevention, i.e., the prevention of the progression of a disease, once established. Immunization of healthy persons against preventable infectious diseases is a classic example of primary prevention and constitutes good public health practice. It is clear that risk-benefit considerations for proposed new interventions constitute an important aspect of decision-making in public health.

Any public official considering a new public health program for disease prevention must evaluate the potential effectiveness of the proposed action before recommending its adoption. If there is uncertainty about its effectiveness, there must be clear evidence that the proposed intervention will not be harmful or detrimental in other

141

ways. In the case of diseases with multiple and poorly understood etiology, such as cancer and cardiovascular disease, the assumption that dietary change will be effective as a preventive measure is controversial. These diseases are not primarily nutritional, although they have nutritional determinants that vary in importance from individual to individual. Authorities who resist recommendations for diet modification express a legitimate concern about promising tangible benefits from controversial recommendations that alter people's lives and habits. Many also have an equally valid concern about diverting attention and resources away from investigation of the underlying causes of these diseases toward unproven action programs. Those experts who advocate a more aggressive approach and seek to change the national diet in the hope of preventing these degenerative diseases assume that the risk of change is minimal and rely heavily on epidemiologic evidence for support of their belief in the probability of benefit. Neither the degree of risk nor the extent of benefit can be assumed in the absence of suitable evidence. . . .

What accounts for the differences in viewpoint expressed in the previous selections? How is it possible that one group of scientists can be convinced we need to recommend a modification of the U.S. diet while another group of equally competent scientists is convinced that such a recommendation is wildly premature? Here, in an excerpt from a speech given to a home economics conference, is one explanation for the conflict.

NUTRITION DILEMMAS — WHAT'S THE TRUTH?*

Katherine Clancy, Ph.D., R.D.

The question is, . . . how did it happen that after all the research and reports and recommendations to the general public to modify their diet [The Dietary Guidelines] there was another scientific body suggesting just the opposite [Toward Healthful Diets]? . . . When one got through the publicity problems and the arguments back and forth and the press conferences what one found were 2 reports that made very similar recommendations regarding overall diet except in the area of cholesterol and fat.

---

*"Nutrition Dilemmas — What's the Truth?," by Katherine Clancy. *Speech to the Nutrition Update Conference for Home Economics/Health Education* (Annapolis, MD), February 11, 1981. Used with permission.

Here was a dilemma — or as one of Webster's definitions has it, "an argument presenting two or more equally conclusive alternatives". I choose that definition, of the several that define "dilemma," because we know that all of those scientists had looked at the same studies, the same data, and all had equally good qualifications as scientists. . . .

The basis for the dilemma is that the different groups were using different models, or paradigms, to guide their deliberations. The FNB report [Toward Healthful Diets], which was written in good part by a physician, followed a medical or clinical model. This model exists within the traditional health care system and consists of the doctor-patient dyad, with much greater emphasis on treatment than prevention, and a research model that engages in clinical studies which test hypotheses in hopefully well-controlled experiments.

This model does not accept epidemiological data as applicable, nor does it admit that large population statistics which denote relationships but not causes are adequate bases for recommendations to the public. Only people who are already designated by various tests as being at risk are seen as reasonable targets for dietary modifications. This latter concept leads logically to the acceptance of the assumption that the average American diet is optimal except when proven otherwise, i.e., by the development of risk indicators.

The model I just delineated exists next to a public-health model which describes the world differently. The field of public health in general deals with community-wide as opposed to individual problems and focuses action toward a broader aggregate population. Epidemiology is one of the major research tools in this model and logical, statistically-significant relationships are used often as the basis for action. Prevention is paramount and suggestions for modifications in lifestyle are recommended if there does not appear to be the possibility for harm.

So — the FNB, using its model, stated that only people with identified risk factors should think about modifying their diets, because there is so much controversial evidence regarding the relationship of diet and heart disease and because large clinical trials where dietary modifications were instituted have not been conclusive. On the other side, the government agencies and private organizations like the American Heart Association recommend to the public at large that they modify their diets based on the assumption that adequate evidence exists to say the prudent person would do so, and that there appears to be no harm in taking such steps (the steps outlined in the Dietary Guidelines).

Now, I hope you've stayed with me this far to see that the scientific facts are the sam for both models. But the models choose to emphasize different assumptions and to accept different research modes. Therein lies a dilemma. The public are interested observers as the scientists duel and debate. . . .

143

Psychologist Philip Slater once wrote that if quantity is the important characteristic of data, then it is more important to be right about details than about wholes because there are more of the former. Mike Jacobson seems to be saying something similar. More studies, he argues, seem not to resolve anything, but to take us ever further from certainty about diet and disease relationships.

HOW THE 'EXPERIMENTAL IMPERATIVE' SUBVERTS A 'PUBLIC HEALTH PERSPECTIVE'*

Michael Jacobson, Ph.D.

Scientists and medical researchers like to think that their years of study and struggle to understand the causes of important diseases will ultimately result in greater control over those diseases. That intellectual optimism is instilled in every pre-med and graduate student. Regrettably, understanding does not always lead to control. In some cases, ironically, the more a disease is studied, the less it can be controlled.

Due to the extraordinary capabilities of many branches of science, medical researchers and the public are attracted by the idea of doing ever more detailed studies to gain a better understanding of the causes of a disease. Because studies *can* be done, they *will* be done. This is the "experimental imperative." Thousands of scientists form a vociferous constituency for pushing experimental science to its limits. Never satisfied with current evidence, scientists place great faith in the next study, which is always expected to be definitive, but somehow never is. Most government regulatory officials are also captive to this way of thinking.

Until recently, the experimental imperative held little sway on public health issues. For example:

- Sailors in the 1800s got their ration of citrus fruit, even though the relationship between the fruit and scurvy — a disease of vitamin deficiencies — was not understood at all. Now, health research bureaucrats would probably be reluctant to defend the ration. "Why give out oranges," they might ask, "when not all sailors develop scurvy? We should devote our efforts to identifying the sensitive sailors, and not waste oranges on the others."
- Seventy-five years ago, sanitation engineers chlorinated the water

*"How the 'Experimental Imperative' Subverts a 'Public Health Perspective.'," by Michael Jacobson. *Nutrition Action* 7:6–7, November 1980. Copyright, Center for Science in the Public Interest. Edited portions used with permission.

supply and cleaned up city streets to prevent the spread of infectious diseases. Action was not postponed until researchers understood exactly how the micro-organisms caused the diseases.

- Most doctors advise patients that smoking can lead to lung cancer, even though statistics demonstrate that only a small fraction of smokers ultimately develops the cancer. The present logic used by some people suggests an alternative approach: cancer-prone (or heart disease-prone) individuals should be identified and told not to smoke, so that the rest of the public could continue to puff away.

Today's major health problems are not always dealt with as sensibly as previous problems. Now, scientists understand the major causes of heart disease, hypertension, and dental caries. But industries whose economic interests are related to causes of those health problems prevent health officials from instituting preventive measures. The industrial forces frequently take advantage of new scientific findings to justify postponing action. They say that broad societal actions should not be taken, because we are not all likely to run the same risk of contracting a particular disease.

Rather, they argue, people at high risk should be identified, and encouraged to take appropriate steps. Never mind that identifying all high-risk individuals is not possible. Never mind that the poor and the less educated are more likely to escape identification and not take preventive measures — such as special medical examinations or dietetic foods — they cannot afford. Never mind that the ultimate cost to society — in dollars and lives — is likely to be enormous when diseases are dealt with on an individual rather than a community-wide basis.

Industry spokespersons often argue that while statistical correlations indicating a cause-effect relationship may be interesting, they do not prove anything. No regulatory actions should be taken until the underlying biochemical or physiological mechanisms are understood, they say. Though such an understanding may be within the grasp of science, to actually do the studies might take years or decades, exposing people to health hazards all the while. . . .

Medical technology may soon be at a point where detailed information about the risks of most major diseases could be provided to individual patients. For those wealthy enough to pay for all the tests, this approach may make some sense, especially if coupled with health promotion practices.

Also, for those diseases affecting only a small fraction of the population, an individual approach seems more appropriate. (After all, should the entire nation be discouraged from eating bread, because a small fraction of people is allergic to wheat?)

However, in dealing with diseases of epidemic proportion, the individualized approach is expensive, inefficient, and impractical. As national policy it would be a disastrous mistake. We should not be so smitten with our technological capabilities that we buy the mirage of health and not the real thing.

145

> *And while the scientists debate, as Clancy and Jacobson point out, the ordinary person must figure out what to do. During the hearings of the Senate Select Committee that put out the original Dietary Goals, Senator Hubert Humphrey (who was even then dying of cancer) engaged in a wonderful, garrulous dialogue with a physician about what an ordinary citizen ought to do. It is a perfect confrontation between the medical/clinical model and the needs of the public — represented here by a U. S. Senator.*

DIET RELATED TO KILLER DISEASES*

Dialogue between Dr. Jerome L. Knittle and Senator Hubert H. Humphrey

Senator Humphrey: Isn't it a fact our life style has changed, so that we have a heavy meal in the evening?

Before I came to Washington, I always thought supper was around 6 o'clock. But something happened here, we don't have any suppers. They have dinners, and then you have an hour of drinking before your dinner. So you really don't, on this social circuit here, have a meal around here until around 9 or 9:30.

Of course that curses the life of most of us in public life. It is really a serious health problem. And plus the fact that many times the food is not any good anyhow.

I would like to ask you this question: What kind of a diet would you suggest for those who eat out? I gather that a larger number of Americans are eating out all of the time. There are more and more people eating at McDonald's, Burger Chef and Burger King, and they are eating Big Macs and the Whoppers. And the kids want a milk shake or french fries. Then there is the pizza parlor and fish and chips.

How can you have a proper diet if you are doing that all of the time? I mean it isn't like my Mom, who was home cooking, making bread and biscuits. I thought we had a pretty good diet at home simply because mother didn't know how to make all those fancy dishes.

I never heard about additives. We had our own garden and our own vegetables. Mother made the bread, and we bought our fresh meat. We knew what we were getting until I got to the big city.

What do you do for the person who is obese, who eats out, is a middle-income office worker.

---

*"Diet Related to Killer Diseases," *U. S. Senate Select Committee on Nutrition and Human Needs*, July 27 – 28, 1976, pages 146 – 148.

What kind of a diet would you suggest, and how do you get these companies to have any kind of a diet? I mean look at the menu, and sometimes you would be better off if you asked for poison.

Dr. Knittle: I will take a whirl at it, because I think you are pushing the emphasis too much on the server of the food.

I daresay if you went to the Department of HEW cafeteria, where I have eaten, you will find a display there that if you eat the whole thing, you know, it would as you say poison you.

Senator Humphrey: I was giving a dramatic emphasis.

Dr. Knittle: If you ate everything your mother put on the table you may have become obese — the point I am trying to make is I think there is a certain amount of responsibility in the individual.

Senator Humphrey: Right. But how do we know? For example, I haven't eaten yet today, I had to grab a hurried breakfast, my life does not permit anything normal and regular, I suppose I will have dinner tonight at 11 o'clock.

When I go to eat, what am I supposed to eat?

Dr. Knittle: I would have to know a number of things about you, Senator, I think this is a very important point. Namely, you can't make a menu for 200 million people. It is a very individual kind of thing.

Senator Humphrey: But aren't there some basics you can suggest?

Dr. Knittle: If you want to get a certain amount of protein, a certain amount of vitamins, a certain amount of carbohydrate and fat. There is a argument on what the carbohydrate source should be. But the fact remains it is an educational program, it is an educational program not in just telling people what they should do or not do. I am taking care of people who are 400 pounds, and they know more about calories than you and I, and yet they can't maintain their diet.

The problem is we don't know enough about behavioral problems in terms of why is it that when you go on the circuit and a man comes out with the chicken in cream sauce, why you can't just eat half of the chicken and none of the cream sauce, because you know this is x number of calories and I have already taken in x number of calories today and I know what my energy expenditures are.

It is really individualization.

Senator Humphrey: We are not communicating. I don't disagree with you at all. I am just saying I want to go down to the Senate dining room, I am Hubert Humphrey. I am supposed to know enough about how to select a meal. I haven't the slightest idea of what to eat.

Dr. Knittle: That is what I am saying, what I would have to do in terms of the medical aspect, I would want to know a little more about Senator Hubert Humphrey's intake and what is excessive to him. I daresay Senator McGovern can eat more calories than you and I. Everyone has a different level of consumption.

Senator Humphrey: But aren't there any norms?

147

Dr. Knittle: There are no hard and fast rules, . . . it is not such a simple thing.

There are individual variations. That is what I tried to bring out in my testimony, namely, that it is not as simple as just saying we are going to go to every McDonald's and give a certain number of calories.

If you ate the best of food, but had 200 or more calories per day more than your particular metabolic processes need, you would indeed get fat.

Senator Humphrey: Of course. We are not communicating again.

Dr. Knittle: You would have to live within your own capacity. . . .

Senator Humphrey: I am perfectly aware of the fact that there are no simple answers and all of us respond differently.

Our children are all different. You can have the family, they all have the same diet and you have different weights, they react differently to food. We know that.

But there has to be some norm. There have to be certain things that you can get guidance on. . . .

Afterword

It is hard to avoid the impression that the fight over dietary guidelines is drawing to a close. A revised version of "Nutrition and Your Health: Dietary Guidelines for Americans" was released by the Departments of Agriculture and Health and Human Services late in 1985. Despite months of vigorous attack from opponents of the idea that the government should offer any dietary advice beyond "moderation and variety," the recommendations emerged quite intact.

Why did we think we needed guidelines at all? The General Accounting Office report with which we began this section pointed out that the need for guidelines arose because the nutritional standards we already had did not deal with macronutrients or dietary patterns, subjects on which the public seemed to be asking for guidance. What the professionals are quarreling over is whether we know enough to give the public what it seems to be asking for.

Ought nutritionists to be giving the public advice about their intake of such major food components as fats, fibers and complex carbohydrates? Do we know enough about the relationships between the balance of these substances in our diets and the diseases that afflict us to urge on the U.S. public a changed pattern of intake?

In covering this debate we have, of course, tried to include selections that laid out the major arguments pro and con dietary guidelines. You will have noticed, however, that advocates on both sides are passionately convinced of their causes, and that in this controversy we ourselves have strongly-held views (see the Gussow speech). Nevertheless, we will as usual try our best to be objective in pointing out the issues you need to think about.

We begin with some of the minor areas of disagreement and conclude with an airing of the central issue — whether or not there is a need for, or a knowledge base adequate to, the general adoption of dietary goals.

In their attacks on the Goals and Guidelines, the critics have identified what they believe will be some negative side effects of establishing dietary goals for the country as a whole. Three major ones are: that the goals will have a negative impact on segments of the food industry; that they will have a discouraging effect on funding for nutrition research; and that they will promote faddism.

Opponents of the proposed guidelines argue that it is wrong to recommend compositional changes in the diet without considering the impact such recommendations will have on certain segments of the food industry. The economic health of food producers, they say, is one of the things nutritionists ought to take into account in giving advice. Telling people to eat less meat, whole milk, eggs and sugar, for example, may harm the groups that produce these foods. Those who support the guidelines, on the other hand, argue that nutritionists are not obliged to consider the interests of the food industry when they are trying to decide what is best for the public health.

Rapid change has characterized the food industry in the last 40 years, as new products and processes displaced old ones. When bad weather caused a shortage of a raw material, or public enthusiasm replaced one product on the supermarket shelves with another, the food industry adapted. (See Chapter 5 on Health, Natural and Organic Foods for an excellent example of such adaptation.) Since the food industry is always responding to, and creating, consumption shifts, there is no reason to think that it would be less adaptable to alterations in the national diet that might occur in response to professional advice.

There are two relevant corollaries to this concern over producers, however, both having to do not with the effect of dietary advice on the food industry, but with the effect of the food industry on dietary advice. Critics of the Dietary Goals have expressed alarm at recommendations for what they called "radical long term . . . change in the American diet." Yet as Mark Hegsted among others has pointed out, the diet we are being urged not to change is one of "blind emergence" planned for no nutritional purpose.

Our national diet is a "happenstance of affluence, the productivity of American farmers and the influence of the food industry." In other words, the many people and events who have

149

changed our eating habits over time, notable among them the food industry, have paid essentially no attention to whether these changes would make things better. (Whether things *are* better, as some of the Dietary Goals' critics suggest, will come up later.)

Moreover, the food industry that helped to shape our present diet continues to do so — with no particular nutritional goal in mind. Harper is probably correct that "those from the fruit, vegetable, cereal, fisheries and nutritional supplement industries . . . would benefit substantially if the recommendation to reduce consumption of whole milk, meat and eggs were to be adopted." And he is at least partially correct in his implication that this is *why* those groups supported the Goals.

It is probably equally correct to suggest that self interest accounts for much of the opposition to the Goals on the part of the milk, meat and egg producers. As the Gussow excerpt makes clear, potentially affected producer groups will be heard from, and their pained or delighted cries, alas, may make it harder to hear and interpret the available scientific facts.

It is difficult to identify the voice of truth when contending self-interests are each claiming it as their own. All of which illuminates the reality that food producers must, and will be taken into account whenever food policy decisions are made in the United States. Nutritionists, who are much less numerous and much less powerful, probably don't need to protect them.

A second underlying dispute appears to center around the question of whether issuing dietary guidelines will undermine funding for nutrition research. Opponents of the goals seemed concerned that recommending a preferred dietary pattern on the basis of present knowledge will signal funders that we have completed the research agenda necessary to define the perfect human diet. In the excerpt reprinted here from "Toward Healthful Diets," the Food and Nutrition Board expresses quite explicitly its concern about "diverting resources away from an investigation of the underlying causes of these diseases toward unproven action programs." If we already know what to do, they seem to be saying, who will support more research?

Such a concern is justified, especially in a time of federal fiscal stringency. Research dollars are hard to come by and nutrition has been relatively neglected in the funding competition for biomedical research. Defenders of the goals also recognize the necessity to urge continued support for research.

But trying to get nutrition research supported by refusing to admit that we already know something may be as counterproductive as it is unfair to the public. As Hegsted implies, nutrition research seems more likely to be supported in the long run if we are able to demonstrate that it has produced something useful. Meanwhile, members of the public, who need to eat everyday, would probably appreciate getting our best present advice, even if we later change our minds.

Finally, some opponents of the Dietary Goals have suggested that endorsement of such goals by nutritionists would encourage dietary faddism. "The rationale for the Dietary Goals," Harper writes, "bears a striking resemblance to that of the nutrition healers who recommend large doses of vitamins to prevent colds, influenza, and cancer and large doses of vitamin E to ensure sexual potency and freedom from heart disease and aging." Olson asserts too that "inappropriate dietary intervention" will offer opportunities to "quacks and charlatans to sell inflated values for health foods, nostrums and even dangerous drugs such as laetrile." In short, the critics seem to be saying, promoting the notion that nutrition is linked to health encourages "faddism."

Since the goals and guidelines talk only about foods and macronutrients, it is hard to imagine what sorts of nostrums they might be used to promote. Recommendations to reduce intakes of fat, cholesterol, sugar and sodium, and to increase intakes of fresh fruits and vegetables, whole grains and other sources of complex carbohydrates hardly constitute the stuff of a National Enquirer headline. And while fiber does run the risk of becoming a fad (thanks not to the health food industry but to major breakfast cereal manufacturers), there are certain built-in limitations as to how much of it can be consumed, even by the most ardent "faddist."

To link nutrition to disease avoidance is always to risk the possibility of being misunderstood and, as both sides in the debate warn, it is important not to overpromise benefits from dietary change. We will all die eventually no matter what we eat. But to refuse to become involved in dietary guidance because any specific association between diet and health may be exploited is to risk being professionally useless (as Chapter 6 on Nutritional Supplementation illustrates).

Finally, as Hegsted points out, not to offer guidance to the public is to suggest by implication that the present American diet, "estimated to provide about 40% of calories as fat, about 20% of calories as sugar, 500 to 700 mg. of cholesterol per day and 8 to 10 g of salt, is the best diet that can be recommended for Americans." Frankly, he adds, "I find it inconceivable that anyone familiar with the literature can arrive at [such a] conclusion."

That comment of Hegsted brings us from the edges to the center of the controversy. Is there evidence that the diet Hegsted describes is harmful to our health? Conversely, is there evidence enough that a changed dietary pattern might change our pattern of disease to justify giving guidelines to the general public?

Those who support the guidelines argue that the answers to both those questions are "yes"—yes we already know enough to

151

recommend that presently healthy Americans should modify their diets in an attempt to modify their risks. Those who oppose the guidelines answer "no" — no there is not enough scientific information available to go beyond the generalities of the Basic Four, and it is inappropriate to recommend that presently healthy Americans should change their diets in the hope of avoiding diseases that are at most only partially nutrition related.

It will come as no surprise to those of you who have read this far that the debate here is not about facts, but about policy. As Clancy points out, everyone has essentially the same facts. It is on the question of what attention should be given to the various facts that the contending groups differ.

Clancy's paper is helpfully simple. Opponents of the goals, she points out, are thinking from a medical model which puts a greater emphasis on treatment than on prevention, and depends on clinical studies to test hypotheses in presumably well-controlled experiments.

Notice, in this regard, the emphasis put by the critics on treatment. We cannot "impose a regimen," Olson insists, until we have demonstrated its effectiveness through a clinical trial — like those held for new drugs or operations. If the goals were to be adopted, Harper warns, "programs would be directed toward guidelines for 'nutritional treatment' of diseases that are not primarily nutritional." The American Medical Association finds the guidelines similar to therapeutic diets.

Arguing that diet-disease relationships are incompletely understood, Olson acknowledges that a doctor might treat a patient with an "incompletely understood" condition. But he points out that the physician in that case knows a lot about the individual patient he is treating. In contrast, those who promote dietary change have "no direct contact with any subject and only a statistical view of the disease problem."

There is a great deal of confusion here between prevention and treatment. Those who propose dietary guidelines are not claiming to treat illness but to prevent it, and the diseases in question — heart disease, cancer, diabetes, hypertension — do not appear to be preventable through immunization, like smallpox or polio, or through the provision of a single nutrient, like scurvy and pellagra, the examples Olson uses.

Where the "killer diseases" are concerned, however, we are dealing not with treatment but with prevention, and the time frame is, of necessity, much longer. "Toward Healthful Diets" acknowledges that prevention is preferable to treatment, but only if the prevention intervention is "effective and safe." However, the only example of a tried (and therefore true) prevention measure it gives is immunization; no equivalent intervention is possible where the "killer diseases" of our era are concerned.

What the critics want are clinical trials providing the kinds of inarguable proofs that we have regarding the effectiveness of the polio vaccine. But it is impossible to get equivalent levels of proof-of-effectiveness when you have a long-term intervention (ideally for a lifetime) involving multiple causes, and a complex dietary modification whose desired end point is a reduced *risk* of a range of conditions — coronary artery disease, cancer, hypertension, diabetes . . .

Consider the fact that the tobacco industry still brings forward arguments rejecting the association between tobacco and lung cancer (after all, not everyone who smokes gets lung cancer). Yet in this case we are dealing with a single clear-cut cause, tobacco, and a single clearly defined effect, lung cancer. How will we achieve even an equivalent certainty on questions such as: How much fat of what kind consumed over how long a period of time may predispose which proportion of the population to cardiovascular disease or cancer? — all other things being equal (which they never are).

Even when positive outcomes occur, it is difficult to relate them to specific interventions. As Harper and Leveille both note, cardiovascular disease has been declining. Is this decline the result of popular adherence to recommendations made years ago by the American Heart Association and others to reduce intake of saturated fat and cholesterol, or is it the result of getting hypertensives into treatment, reducing smoking, increasing exercise, or the cumulative effect of all these things (and others) which have occurred over the time period in question?

The Multiple Risk Factor Intervention Trial (MRFIT), which was an attempt to prove the effects of dietary change (among other factors) on heart disease risk, had its results confounded by the fact that men in the "control" group, with which the dietary change group was compared, also changed their diets. This sort of artifact of reality is bound to disturb any attempt to measure the preventive effects of long-term dietary change on the incidence of major chronic diseases.

Interventions which involve long-term compositional changes in the diet are very different in scope from trials of lime juice in the diets of potentially scorbutic sailors. "Of course there are no unequivocal data," as an impatient scientist once commented. "All these conditions are multifactorial. They are caused by interactions among different substances. The body does not use one nutrient at a time. I suppose it only goes to show that if you are a toxin, there is safety in numbers." (Personal communication.)

We noted in the RDA chapter that growing awareness of interactions among the nutrients was now making it much harder than we had previously thought to specify rational numbers for the RDAs. Since the macronutrients as they occur in foods are

153

much more compositionally diverse, and consumed in much greater amounts, trying to control diets and run clinical trials with them is simply more daunting by a factor of thousands.

That being the case, the critics argue, you have not proved the need for dietary modifications. As Clancy says, if you begin from the medical stance that the average American diet is OK unless proven otherwise, i.e., by the development of risk indicators, then action cannot be taken based on population statistics. The stance of the supporters of the guidelines is quite different. They make use of epidemiologic statistics, put an emphasis, as we have noted, on prevention, and recommend modifications in lifestyle (so long as there does not appear to be a realistic possibility for harm). Guidance should be given, they argue, if a prudent person would modify his or her own diet based on the known facts.

But what are the facts? Is it true, as the critics of the goals and guidelines argue, that the increase in life expectancy over the last half century, the marked decrease in infant and child mortality, and the achievement of nearly the genetic maximum in height among Americans supports the argument that the U.S. diet "may be *the* best in the world today"? Is it true that "a far stronger case can be made for concluding that the changes in our food supply during this century have been associated with improved health rather than with deteriorating health"?

As Harper (whose statement that is) would be the first to point out, correlation is not causation, and the increased life expectancy, growth and infant survival of the last half century cannot be confidently attributed to any improvement in the food supply. Nor is there evidence that maximum growth contributes to a long and healthy life.

Much of the improvement in infant survival, which has a major impact on improved life expectancy, must be attributed to improved medical technologies for helping infants survive premature or otherwise troubled births. The availability of antibiotics has reduced mortality from infectious diseases, and much of the reduction in the incidence of heart disease and stroke, which the critics of the goals cite as evidence of our improving food supply, has come about, as we have noted, during a period when many of the measures thought to be beneficial in these conditions have been widely adopted — among them blood pressure control, and reduced cholesterol and saturated fat consumption. Furthermore, all the ways in which we intervene to extend the lives of those who are already unhealthy — coronary bypass operations, kidney dialysis, blood pressure lowering drugs and the like — have also had an unmeasured effect on extending lifespan.

In short, just as the supporters of the goals cannot prove for a certainty that adherence to them will reduce the risk of degenerative disease, the opponents of the goals cannot prove that the indicators of improved health have anything to do with the present quality of our diets.

Is it then inappropriate to recommend any change? As Hegsted points out, absolute increases in life expectancy are not the issue. The issue is how to improve our health from here on out. Seven or eight out of ten people now die of cancer, cardiovascular disease or diabetes, Hegsted notes, so the issue is, "What are the possibilities of modifying that risk?"

The critics, you should note, never specifically praise a high-fat, high-cholesterol, low-fiber diet as healthy. They merely suggest that because we are doing well, we shouldn't take the chance of changing our diets without the kind of nutritional certainty that we have in regard to the RDAs. Yet you will recall from Chapter 1 that there are very real limits to what we know for sure about the setting of RDAs. We change the RDA, Hegsted notes, even though scientific evidence is not available to show that populations consuming 60 or more mg. of vitamin C are better off than populations consuming 45 mg. of vitamin C, or vice versa. In fact, most nutrition recommendations to the public must be made, and, as we have seen, are made on the basis of incomplete and often weak data.

Until people stop asking nutritionists what they ought to eat, (which nutritionists would surely not wish them to do), we must simply give out the best advice we can, let people know it is based on incomplete information, and change our advice as the evidence changes. As for the Dietary Goals and Guidelines, once again, you will have to decide for yourselves.

We believe the risks of dietary change are minimal — that on this ground the critics have not made their case. If you agree that "adequate evidence exists to say the prudent person would modify his or her diet," you will simply have to decide whether to be prudent.

4 Animals and/or Vegetables: Asking the Right Questions about Meat

When we were young nobody we knew was a vegetarian. Vegetarian restaurants were those funny places close to the wrong part of town where they served mock chicken breasts (made of soybeans) and fake liver paté. Then there were Kosher restaurants where meat was not allowed, but only because milk products were on the menu. Nobody could even imagine a restaurant that banned not only meat, but milk, chicken, fish, cheese, eggs . . . what on earth would you eat?

Well, things really have changed. It wasn't too long ago that the great grey New York Times (February 20, 1985) carried a "health" story headlined, "Meat: It's Not Always a Villain." The story went on to say that among a "small but growing group of Americans" it had become fashionable to give up red meat.

"Small, growing, and increasingly visible" is probably the right way to put it, since the notion that vegetarianism can not only be good for you, but fun and fashionable as well seems to be the theme of more and more women's magazine articles, newspaper stories and celebrity bios. The question among many people is no longer, "Are you a vegetarian," but "What kind of vegetarian are you?" — vegan? ("I don't touch anything that comes from animals"), lacto-ovo vegetarian? ("It's OK so long as you don't kill anything that walks, swims or flies") or simply semi-vegetarian? ("I'm using meat as a condiment")

What is happening? Why are people giving up meat, and is there a sensible way to decide whether you ought to? Now that calling yourself a vegetarian doesn't automatically rank you with the "kooks," it has become possible to ask some rational questions about the practice of eating meat not at all or in moderation. Two important questions are: Is it healthier? Is it better for the environment?

Is meat eating consistent with the kind of diet that can best prevent the occurrence of common degenerative diseases? Is it consistent with the kind of diet that best protects the ecological systems upon which our health and the health of our planet depend?

As for the philosophical issue of whether animals have rights not to be killed for food except in emergencies, we will not pursue that debate here. For those who want to look into it, we recommend two books: *The Case for Animal Rights*, by Tom Regan (1983, University of California Press) and *Rights, Killing and Suffering: Moral Vegetarianism and Applied Ethics*, by R. G. Frey (1983, Basil Blackwell Publisher Limited).

We suspect you will find yourself examining your own diet as you read this chapter. The question of whether or not to eat meat appears to provoke a response from everyone, sometimes a very emotional one. We hope that these readings will broaden your

157

understanding of just what the practical arguments are about. Once again, what you do about your own eating practices is a matter for you to decide.

- Thomas Jefferson:

I live so much like other people, that I might refer to ordinary life as the history of my own. [L]ike my friend the Doctor, I have lived temperately, eating little animal food, & that, not as an aliment so much as a condiment for the vegetables, which constitute my principal diet. *

- George M. Briggs (Professor of Nutrition; Dept. of Nutritional Sciences; University of California, Berkeley):

Among the healthiest persons in the United States are those who consume meat. I see a considerable amount of nutrition literature, and I have not seen any research yet that discourages me from recommending one or two servings of meat a day as a routine part of a good diet of normal persons. **

---

*Cortez F. Enloe, Jr. "The end of the beginning. Part two: The visionary fox." *Nutrition Today.* 12:6 – 11, 31 – 40, September/October 1977.

**George M. Briggs. "Muscle foods and human health." *Food Technology.* 39:54, 56 – 57, February 1985.

> *We begin our discussion of whether animal flesh should be part of our diets with a piece by Harlow Hodgson, a retired land management scientist with the Department of Agriculture. Although it has become popular in recent years to condemn meat eating on environmental grounds, Dr. Hodgson argues that cattle, sheep, goats and other ruminant animals not only enhance the quality of our diets, but the quality of our environment as well. Animals, he argues, are not our competitors but our benefactors.*

MAN'S BENEFACTOR*

Harlow J. Hodgson, Ph.D.

A dog may well be man's best friend, but the ruminant must certainly be his greatest benefactor in the animal kingdom. No other animal, including man himself, can produce so much from so little. Man needs machinery of all kinds, lots of fossil fuel, and the choicest soil on the face of the earth in order to produce crops of vegetables that provide him nutrient energy. But not so the ruminant. Give this fellow animal a range that supports only coarse grass, a little water, and without much outside help it will manufacture the richest, most delectable protein, structural fats, vitamins, and minerals known. Thus, cattle and their cousins make land that's not suitable for anything else, and that means about 75 per cent of all the land on earth, useful for mankind.

These are facts seldom realized, seldom appreciated, but hard and true.

Food production is essentially an energy transformation process. Solar energy is transformed by green plants into chemical energy stored in seeds, leaves, stems, roots, and tubers. All green plants — such as crop plants, trees, and range plants — are known as the primary producers. Animals that consume primary production and convert it to a variety of products that man can use are known as secondary producers.

The rate of primary production is increased when the plant's environment is made more favorable. This is why farmers use fertilizers, irrigation, cultivation, pest control, etc. Similarly, the rate of production by secondary producers is increased as the amount of digestible energy consumed per unit of time is increased.

---

*"Man's Benefactor," by Harlow J. Hodgson, Ph.D. *Nutrition Today*, March/April 1979, pages 16–25. Williams & Wilkins, Baltimore, MD. Used with permission.

Solar Energy Converters

Of all primary production on earth, only a small portion can be used directly by man as food. This consists chiefly of seeds, roots, and tubers — products generally low in fiber and high in digestible energy. Even with major food crops such as rice, wheat, and maize, at least half of the energy of primary production is in plant parts that man cannot use directly as food. They are high in cellulose, hemicellulose, and lignan, which man's digestive apparatus cannot handle. Usually these plant parts are left behind at harvest time and, thus, are known as crop residues. In addition, almost one-third of our cropland in the United States is used to grow hay, silage, and pasture. This is essential for erosion control and good soil management. Finally, much of the earth is covered with forest and range land, which produce essentially no primary production useable by man as food. . . . On a world basis, only 11 per cent of the land area is capable of producing the kind of primary production that man could use directly. In the United States, the cropland area is 21 per cent of the total land area. So, most of the world's primary production is in a form man simply isn't built to digest.

Nature developed an efficient means of utilizing the tremendous volume of primary production unuseable as food by man. Ruminant animals evolved into a large number of separate species, some of which occupy nearly every ecological niche from desert to rain forest, from the arctic to the tropics, and from the sea to the highest mountains. They became essential parts of successfully functioning ecosystems.

Man domesticated a few of these ruminant species beginning about ten thousand years ago. Most of the agricultural systems man developed include ruminant animals as food producers or draft power. They produce meat and milk, two of the highest quality foods known and among the most highly prized by man. In fact, about 85 per cent of the world's population desire more meat and milk in their diet. Such foods are important sources of the highest quality protein, energy, minerals, vitamins, and fats. . . .

There are immense populations of domesticated ruminants on earth. They are the major food source in some parts of the world, but of minor importance in other places. In 1976 there were 2.8 billion domesticated ruminants, or nearly three for every four humans. Of these, 1.2 billion were cattle; there was a like number of sheep; and the balance were goats, water buffaloes, camels, yaks, alpaca, and other ruminants. In the United States we have 122 million cattle, plus about 15 million sheep and goats; or about two ruminants for every three people. Interestingly, since 1961 – 65, the world cattle and human population both have increased by 23 per cent — an indication of man's strong reliance on ruminants for food and draft power. . . .

Livestock do not compete with vegetables, fruits, and cereal grains for land. These wholesome primary foods and ruminants in fact complement each other. Nature just made our ecosystem that way. The primary and secondary food producers are essential. This is true because of the nature of the earth's soil.

Vegetables and other primary producers require arable soil, and the amount of this soil is limited. There is not enough to provide food for more than a fraction of the people on earth. This must be why Nature put fish in the sea that convert waterborne nutrients into human food and why She put ruminants on the range because they can eat range grass and turn it into food for man.

A herd of cattle can live on range lands that can't produce anything else but the grass that he eats. On ranches he is a peripatetic forager, eating undergrowth in timber lands and scrub in creek beds. He can wander around the nooks and crannies of hill country and other areas that can't be farmed, pulling out the sweet grasses and making them into milk and protein. Without him, the waste land would truly go to waste.

Consider the situation here in America where farmers have the most sophisticated means in the world for getting food from the soil. Right now, only 21 per cent of our land can be coaxed into producing the primary foods. On the other hand, there is nearly 28 per cent more permanent pasture and range land, all suitable for producing food from ruminants, than there is cropland. And, here we're fortunate because the situation world-wide is even less hospitable for growing vegetables and other primary crops. Taken as a whole on the entire earth, only 11 per cent of the land mass is cropland. More than twice that amount of land is suitable for raising ruminants, and that's not counting the waste land and forest where cattle can graze. . . .

Biologic Disposals

Ruminants do more than just use our waste land. Consider the amount of our refuse they convert to food for us. They are marvelous converters of nature's and man's waste products into nutritious foods. As such, they are essential disposal agents for the straw left after the wheat has been harvested, for cuttings, rejects, culls, and other refuse of fruit and vegetable farming. The refuse from citrus packing and processing provides cattle and other ruminants with essential vitamins and other nutrients. In some areas, ruminants thrive on the leftovers from sugar cane harvest. In others, the "schlempe" or slops that remain after sugar has been extracted from sugar beets are fabulously rich in betraine, glycocyamine, and other protein building blocks that cattle convert to protein. In some areas, ruminants thrive on seeds.

In the cotton growing districts, the bulk left over from cotton ginning has been found to be a useful feed for cattle. Ruminants can also convert sawdust and even shredded newspaper into human food. This **161** ability to use the land we cannot use and to relieve man of the problem of getting rid of an enormous amount of waste products not only solves a huge practical problem, but also materially reduces the cost of all human foods everywhere.

The greater the cropland area, the greater the volume of crop residues and processing by-products that are only convertible to food by ruminant animals. If they are not so consumed, they present disposal problems of enormous proportions.

So it is clear that every farm animal contributes in one way or another to the balance of the plant-to-animal-to-food-for-man chain. The ruminants play the major role because they have a unique digestive system that enables them to consume that which man must reject. Chickens and pigs are mono-gastric with digestive systems quite similar to man. Accordingly, they must have feeds that are low in fiber. Much of their food could be digested by man, but cattle, sheep, and other ruminants are quite another thing. . . .

Benefactors, Not Competitors

In the final stage of growth, before the animal is said to be finished and ready for slaughter, beef cattle are sent to feed lots where additional protein and fat are laid on by using high-energy feeds, principally corn. This keeps meat prices down, increases the nutritive value of the end product, and makes the beef tastier and tender. As mentioned earlier, this is a nutritionally sound and economic investment of the 15 to 20 per cent of cropland that the system requires. Farmers will strive to use feeds with high energy content as long as it is economic to do so. The exception to this is feed for breeding herds of beef cattle and sheep where, for much of the year, only maintenance levels of feeding are required.

Ruminants can use, but do not require, concentrate feeds such as grain and by-products that contain large amounts of digestible energy in starch, sugars, fats, and proteins and minimal proportions of fiber — cellulose, hemicellulose, and lignin. The high energy content of concentrates makes them desirable feeds when they are available in quantity and at low cost.

Animal production has been criticized in recent years as consumers of grains that could otherwise be used for human consumption. Most of the grain consumed is corn and sorghum for which there is not much human demand as food in the United States or in many other countries. However, grain is becoming increasingly important in export markets, in industrial uses, and is being mentioned as a raw material for alcohol production for use in fuels. Thus, there are competitive markets for grains. The amount fed to cattle depends upon price — consumption is greatest when prices are low, and moderate price increases rapidly decrease consumption. The livestock feed mar-

162

ket then is a great stabilizer that ensures a market for grain and tends to cause production to be maintained at fairly constant levels to meet whatever markets are most competitive.

Forages provide most of the feed for ruminants in the United States. . . .

What Ruminants Provide

World population growth accentuates the pressures on agricultural landscapes for more food. Marginal areas are brought into production of food crops and usually unsound management results in substantial increases in soil erosion from wind and water. The productive capacity of the resource is diminished. This trend is currently advancing at a rapid pace in the United States and world-wide.

The production of forages and ruminant livestock is very often the most economical and practical method of protecting the productive capacity of our soil resources. Not only are soil losses minimized but the export of nutrients (energy) from properly managed forage-livestock systems is less than in the case of grain systems for direct human consumption. Properly managed forage-livestock systems are probably the most ecologically sound food production systems we have.

Ruminants provide a variety of products used by humans. Best known, at least in the United States, are meat, milk, and wool. Also produced are hair, skins, fertilizer, fuel, and many inedible by-products including pharmaceuticals, glue, buttons, soaps, plastics, and many more. While our chief concern here is about the relation of the ruminant to food, in some areas of the world ruminants are enormously important for other contributions, and they too should be mentioned. For example, the contribution of ruminants to draft power offers some interesting figures. In India, for example, cattle and water buffalo provide milk for the farmer and his family and the people living in cities. And, not only are they, in most cases, the source of the security of a sound capital investment, they've produced more than 54 per cent of the energy used in that nation's agriculture. In fact, it has been said that without cows and water buffaloes to do the hauling, India—the great subcontinent—would have to import more than a billion dollars worth of gasoline and diesel oil a year.

To increase food production in much of the developing world, additional cultural energy in some form must be infused into the production system. Ruminant power may well supply much of that energy while consuming renewable primary plant products non-consumable by man. . . .

The already large contribution of forages and ruminant animals in food production can be greatly expanded in the future by using nonarable land resources together with forage production on arable land as **163** needed for sound soil management. This expansion would not only multiply the world's food supply but also increase its nutritional quality. Ruminants should not be viewed as competitors with humans but, conversely, as benefactors. . . .

> *Well-known author Frances Moore Lappé disagrees with many of the arguments put forward by the author of the previous selection. Arguing that our meat-centered diet puts an enormous demand on our finite natural resources, she concludes that we can't go on like this. The excerpt is from the latest revision of her 10-year-old bestseller,* Diet for a Small Planet.

LIKE DRIVING A CADILLAC*

Frances Moore Lappé

. . . A grain-fed-meat centered diet *is* like driving a Cadillac. Yet many Americans who have reluctantly given up their gas-guzzling cars would never think of questioning the resource costs of their grain-fed-meat diet. So let me try to give you some sense of the enormity of the resources flowing into livestock production in the United States. The consequences of a grain-fed-meat diet may be as severe as those of a nation of Cadillac drivers.

A detailed 1978 study sponsored by the Departments of Interior and Commerce produced startling figures showing that *the value of raw materials consumed to produce food from livestock is greater than the value of all oil, gas, and coal consumed in this country.* Expressed another way, one-third of the value of *all* raw materials consumed for all purposes in the United States is consumed in livestock foods.

How can this be?

The Protein Factory in Reverse
Excluding exports, about one-half of our harvested acreage goes to feed livestock. Over the last forty years the amount of grain, soybeans, and special feeds going to American livestock has doubled. Now approaching 200 million tons, it is equal in volume to all the grain that

---

*Diet for a Small Planet, 10th Anniversary Edition. Reprinted by permission of Frances Moore Lappé, and her agents Raines & Raines, New York. Copyright 1971, 1975, 1982 by Frances Moore Lappé. Pgs 66–68.

is now imported throughout the world. Today our livestock consume ten times the grain that we Americans eat directly and they outweigh the human population of our country four to one.

These staggering estimates reflect the revolution that has taken place in meat and poultry production and consumption since about 1950. . . .

. . . Our cattle still graze. In fact, from one-third to one-half of the continental land mass is used for grazing. But since the 1940s we have developed a system of feeding grain to cattle that is unique in human history. Instead of going from pasture to slaughter, most cattle in the United States now first pass through feedlots where they are each fed over 2,500 pounds of grain and soybean products (about 22 pounds a day) plus hormones and antibiotics. . . .

In addition to cattle, poultry have also become a big consumer of our harvested crops. Poultry can't eat grass. Unlike cows, they need a source of protein. But it doesn't have to be grain. Although prepared feed played an important role in the past, chickens also scratched the barnyard for seeds, worms, and bits of organic matter. They also got scraps from the kitchen. But after 1950, when poultry moved from the barnyard into huge factorylike compounds, production leaped more than threefold, and the volume of grains fed to poultry climbed almost as much.

Hogs, too, are big grain consumers in the United States, taking almost a third of the total fed to livestock. Many countries, however, raise hogs exclusively on waste products and on plants which humans don't eat. . . . In the United States hogs are now fed about as much grain as is fed to cattle.

All told, each grain-consuming animal "unit" (as the Department of Agriculture calls our livestock) eats almost two and a half tons of grain, soy, and other feeds each year.

What Do We Get Back?

For every 16 pounds of grain and soy fed to beef cattle in the United States we only get 1 pound back in meat on our plates. The other 15 pounds are inaccessible to us, either used by the animal to produce energy or to make some part of its own body that we do not eat (like hair or bones) or excreted.

To give you some basis for comparison, 16 pounds of grain has twenty-one times more calories and eight times more protein — but only three times more fat — than a pound of hamburger.

Livestock other than cattle are markedly more efficient in converting grain to meat; . . . hogs consume 6, turkeys 4, and chickens 3 pounds of grain and soy to produce 1 pound of meat. Milk production is even more efficient, with less than 1 pound of grain fed for every pint of milk produced. (This is partly because we don't have to grow a

165

new cow every time we milk one.)

Now let us put these two factors together: the large quantities of humanly edible plants fed to animals and their inefficient conversion into meat for us to eat. Some very startling statistics result. If we exclude dairy cows, the average ratio of all U.S. livestock is 7 pounds of grain and soy fed to produce 1 pound of edible food. Thus, of the 145 million tons of grain and soy fed to our beef cattle, poultry, and hogs in 1979, only 21 million tons were returned to us in meat, poultry, and eggs. *The rest, about 124 million tons of grain and soybeans, became inaccessible to human consumption.* (We also feed considerable quantities of wheat germ, milk products, and fishmeal to livestock, but here I am including only grain and soybeans.) To put this enormous quantity in some perspective, consider that 120 million tons is worth over $20 billion. If cooked, it is the equivalent of 1 cup of grain for every single human being on earth every day for a year. . . .

The Feedlot Logic: More Grain, Lower Cost

On the surface it would seem that beef produced by feeding grain to livestock would be more expensive than beef produced solely on the range. For, after all, isn't grain more expensive than grass? To us it might be, but not to the cattle producer. As long as the cost of grain is cheap in relation to the price of meat, the lowest production costs per pound are achieved by putting the animal in the feedlot as soon as possible after weaning and feeding it as long as it continues to gain significant weight. This is true in large part because an animal gains weight three times faster in the feedlot on a grain and high-protein feed diet than on the range. . . .

The Livestock Explosion and the Illusion of Cheap Grain

If we are feeding millions of tons of grain to livestock, it must be because it makes economic sense. Indeed, it does "make sense" under the rules of our economy. But that fact might better be seen as the problem, rather than the explanation that should put our concerns to rest. We got hooked on grain-fed meat just as we got hooked on gas-guzzling automobiles. Big cars "made sense" only when oil was cheap; grain-fed meat "makes sense" only because the true costs of producing it are not counted.

But why is grain in America so cheap? If grain is cheap simply because there is so much of it and it will go to waste unless we feed it to livestock, doesn't grain-fed meat represent a sound use of our resources? Here we need to back up to another, more basic question: why is there so much grain in the first place?

In our production system each farmer must compete against every other farmer; the only way a farmer can compete is to produce more. Therefore, every farmer is motivated to use any new technology — higher yielding seeds, fertilizers, or machines — which will grow more and require less labor. In the last 30 years crop production has virtually doubled as farmers have adopted hybrid seeds and applied ever more fertilizer and pesticides. Since the 1940s fertilizer use has increased fivefold, and corn yields have tripled.

But this production imperative is ultimately self-defeating. As soon as one farmer adopts the more productive technology, all other farmers must do the same or go out of business. This is because those using the more productive technology can afford to sell their grain at a lower price, making up in volume what they lose in profit per bushel. That means constant downward pressure on the price of grain.

Since World War II real grain prices have sometimes fluctuated wildly, but the indisputable trend has been downward. . . .

But neglected in this explanation of the low price of grain are the hidden production costs which we and future generations are subsidizing: the fossil fuels and water consumed, the groundwater mined, the topsoil lost, the fertilizer resources depleted, and the water polluted.

Fossil Fuel Costs
Agricultural production uses the equivalent of about 10 percent of all of the fossil fuel imported into the United States.

Besides the cost of the grain used to produce meat, we can also measure the cost of the fossil fuel energy used compared with the food value we receive. Each calorie of protein we get from feedlot-produced beef costs us 78 calories of fossil fuel . . . Grains and beans are from 22 to almost 40 times less fossil-fuel costly.

Enough Water to Float a Destroyer
. . . According to food geographer Georg Borgstrom, to produce a 1-pound steak requires 2,500 gallons of water! The average U.S. diet requires 4,200 gallons of water a day for each person, and of this he estimates animal products account for over 80 percent.

"The water that goes into a 1,000-pound steer would float a destroyer," *Newsweek* recently reported. When I sat down with my calculator, I realized that the water used to produce just 10 pounds of steak equals the household consumption of my family for the entire year.

. . . To produce 1 pound of beef protein can require as much as fifteen times the amount of water needed to produce the protein in plant food.

Minding Our Water

Irrigation to grow food for livestock, including hay, corn, sorghum, and pasture, uses 50 out of every 100 gallons of water "consumed" in the United States. Other farm uses — mainly irrigation for food crops — add another 35 gallons, so agriculture's total use of water equals 85 out of every 100 gallons consumed. (Water is "consumed" when it doesn't return to our rivers and streams.)

Over the past fifteen years grain-fed-beef production has been shifting from the rain-fed Corn Belt to newly irrigated acres in the Great Plains. Just four Great Plains states, Nebraska, Kansas, Oklahoma, and Texas, have accounted for over three-fourths of the new irrigation since 1964, and most of that irrigation has been used to grow more feed. Today half of the grain-fed beef in the United States is produced in states that depend for irrigation on an enormous underground lake called the Ogallala Aquifer.

But much of this irrigation just can't last.

Rainwater seeps into this underground lake so slowly in some areas that scientists consider parts of the aquifer a virtually nonrenewable resource, much like oil deposits. . . .

When most of us think of California's irrigated acres, we visualize lush fields growing tomatoes, artichokes, strawberries, and grapes. But in California, the biggest user of underground water, more irrigation water is used for feed crops and pasture than for all these specialty crops combined. In fact, 42 percent of California's irrigation goes to produce livestock. Not only are water tables dropping, but in some parts of California the earth itself is sinking as groundwater is drawn out. . . .

The Soil in Our Steaks

Most of us think of soil as a renewable resource. After all, in parts of Europe and Asia, haven't crops been grown on the same land for thousands of years? It's true, soil should be a renewable resource; but in the United States, we have not allowed it to be. . . .

. . . Few would dispute that our topsoil loss is a national catastrophe, or that in the last two decades we have backpedaled on protecting our topsoil, or that in some places erosion is as bad as or worse than during the Dust Bowl era. Few dispute that excessive erosion is reducing the soil's productive capacity, making chemical fertilizers ever more necessary while their cost soars. The only dispute is how many billions of dollars topsoil erosion is costing Americans and how soon the impact will be felt in higher food prices and the end of farming on land that could have been abundant for years to come. . . .

Robin Hur is a mathematician and Harvard Business School graduate who has spent the last year documenting the resource cost of livestock production for his forthcoming book. "How much of our topsoil erosion is associated with crops destined for livestock and over-grazing of rangeland?" I asked him. "Most of it — about 5.9 billion tons," he calculates, including erosion associated with exported feed grains. This is true not only because feed crops cover half of our harvested acres, but because these crops, especially corn and soybeans, are among the worst offenders when it comes to soil erosion. . . .

168

Fertilizers: Becoming Import-Dependent

To determine a price for grain which reflects all its costs would also mean looking at the fertilizers required to mask our lost fertility and continually increase production. Higher yields and continuous cropping deplete soil nutrients, so that ever greater quantities of fertilizer must be used. This vicious circle caused our nation's use of chemical fertilizer to increase fivefold between the 1940s and the 1970s. . . . Corn, the major national feed grain, which occupies about 23 percent of all our cropland, uses more fertilizer than any other crop — about 40 percent of the total.

Because fertilizer has been relatively cheap, farmers have been encouraged to apply ever greater quantities in their desperate struggle to produce. As with topsoil and groundwater, we squander fertilizer resources today without considering the consequences tomorrow. One of the consequences of our heavy consumption of fertilizer is increasing dependence on imports. . . .

Livestock Pollution

Some people believe that although we feed enormous quantities of high-grade plant food to livestock with relatively little return to us as food, there is really no loss. After all, we live in a closed system, don't we? Animal waste returns to the soil, providing nutrients for the crops that the animals themselves will eventually eat, thus completing a natural ecological cycle.

Unfortunately, it doesn't work that way anymore. Most manure is not returned to the land. Animal waste in the United States amounts to 2 billion tons annually, equivalent to the waste of almost half of the world's human population. Much of the nitrogen-containing waste from livestock is converted into ammonia and into nitrates, which leach into the groundwater beneath the soil or run directly into surface water, thus contributing to high nitrate levels in the rural wells which tap the groundwater. In streams and lakes, high levels of waste runoff contribute to oxygen depletion and algae overgrowth. American livestock contribute five times more harmful organic waste to water pollution than do people, and twice that of industry, estimates food geographer Georg Borgstrom.

Cheap Water for Cheap Grain

In a true accounting, the two bushels of topsoil washed away with every bushel of corn grown on Iowa's sloping land would be seen as a subsidy to our cheap grain. In other words, if we were to use all of the conservation measures we know of to prevent this erosion, the cost of producing our grain would go up, as it would if we were to add in all of the costs of dredging the soil from our waterways or charge for feedlot pollution. Failing to account for these costs amounts to hidden subsidies. But in addition, you and I as taxpayers are paying *direct* subsidies right now.

169

Our tax dollars have paid for more than one-half of the net value of all irrigation facilities in the United States as of 1975. Since the turn of the century the federal government has sponsored 32 irrigation projects in 17 western states where 20 percent of the acreage is now irrigated with the help of government subsidies. A recent General Accounting Office study concluded that even though farmers are legally required to repay irrigation construction costs, in the cases studied the repayments amounted to less than 8 percent of the cost to the federal government. . . .

Cheap water encourages farmers to grow livestock feed. "Because water is so cheap, its use is based on its price and not its supposed scarcity," observes *Fortune*. "Many farmers . . . use inferior land to grow low value crops that require large amounts of water, like alfalfa and sorghum" for feed. . . .

Tax Benefits at the Feedlot, Too

Besides directly and indirectly subsidizing the feedlot system by keeping the price of grain low, we taxpayers also subsidize the feedlot operations themselves. Tax laws, favoring feedlot owners and investors in feedlot cattle shift the tax burden onto the rest of us. . . .

Agricultural economists V. James Rhodes and the late Joseph C. Meisner of the University of Missouri offer this observation of tax favors to feedlot operations:

"Subsidies to large-size feedlot firms, indirect though they be, would tend to lead to survival and growth of those firms on a basis of other than economic efficiency. . . . If the nation seeks to subsidize beef production, direct grants to feedlot firms is an alternative. Then, true economic costs of the subsidies would be more apparent. However, in a world of growing concern for energy supplies, the beef industry would seem to be a most unlikely recipient of national subsidy."

A Fatal Blindness

After reading this account of the resource costs of our current production system, you probably are amazed that more people are not aware and alarmed. I am continually amazed. Again and again I have to learn this lesson: often those with the most information concerning our society's basic problems are those so schooled in defending the status quo that they are blind to the implications of what they know.

As I was preparing this chapter I came across a book that read as if designed to be the definitive rebuttal to *Diet for a Small Planet*. Three noted livestock economists conclude that "total resource use in this [livestock] production has decreased dramatically." To arrive here, they had, of course, to ignore such hidden costs as I've just outlined — the fossil fuel used, the water consumed (including groundwater that is irreplaceable), the topsoil eroded, and the domestic fertilizer depleted as we attempt to make up for our soil's declining fertility. They

170

also ignore feedlot pollution and hidden tax subsidies. All this I would have expected. What really shocked me was their attempt to prove that we are producing more meat using *less* resources. Their evidence? A decline in labor used and a dramatic drop in acres devoted to feed grains between 1944 and about 1960, while meat production rose. What they fail to tell us is that about one-third of our total cropland was released from feed-grain production between 1930 and 1955 by the rapid replacement of grain-consuming draft animals by fuel-consuming tractors. *Thus, much of the decline in feed-grain acres had nothing to do with increased efficiency of meat production.* Just as appalling, these economists ignore the fact that livestock eat more than feed grains. Since 1960 there has been a spectacular rise in soybean use as animal feed. Tripling since 1960, acres in soybeans now exceed two-thirds of total acres in feed grains. (Almost half of those acres are used to feed domestic livestock, the rest for export.) Soybeans are not even mentioned by these economists as a resource in livestock production.

While it is useful to keep these gross oversights in mind for the next time we feel cowed by an "authority" questioning *our* facts, they sidetrack us a bit from the basic argument used by such defenders of the status quo. Most economists defend our current meat production system by arguing that feeding grain to livestock is the cheapest way to produce meat. The fatal blindness in this argument is attention only to price. As we have seen, the price of our grain is an illusion. It results from the powerlessness of farmers to pass on their costs of production and the fact that so many of the costs of production — topsoil and groundwater, for example — carry no price at all.

In writing this chapter I came to realize more clearly than ever that our production system is ultimately self-destructive because it is self-deceptive; it can't incorporate the many costs I've outlined here. It can't look to the future. And it blinds those closest to it from even seeing what is happening. Thus, the task of opening our eyes lies more heavily with the rest of us — those less committed to protecting the status quo. As awakening stewards of this small planet, we have a lot to learn — and fast. . . .

> *The next reading lays out several of the environmental problems indirectly caused by our collective hunger for meat. In it James Nations and Daniel Komer tell us how our love for fast food hamburgers contributes to the destruction of tropical rainforests in Central America — and why that should be of concern to us as well as to Central Americans.*

RAINFORESTS AND THE HAMBURGER SOCIETY*

James D. Nations and Daniel I. Komer

Few Americans associate fast food hamburgers or TV dinners with the eradication of Central America's tropical rainforests. But for more than 30 years, the United States' appetite for cheap, imported beef has been a critical factor in the future of those forests. Tropical rainforests throughout Central America (including southeastern Mexico and Panama) are being replaced by pasturelands to produce beef, much of which is consumed by U.S. citizens.

This cycle of destruction of rainforests and use of the land to produce beef for export involves international bank loans to support cattle industry development, U.S. Department of Agriculture inspections to control undesirable ingredients, and the continuation of a socioeconomic system that concentrates landholdings — and thus power — in the hands of the few.

The destruction of rainforests in other areas of the world is sometimes even more dramatic than in Central America — as in the Amazon Basin where bulldozing, burning, and chemical defoliation destroy immense tracts of forest each year. But nowhere is the loss of biological diversity more severe, and nowhere is the United States' unwitting role in deforestation more apparent, than in the case of Central America.

Almost two-thirds of Central America's lowland and lower mountain rainforest have been cleared or severely degraded since 1950. At current rates of destruction, most of the remaining forest will be eradicated during the next 20 years, leaving only impoverished remnants in national parks and reserves. Despite the grim ecological consequences of such a prospect, some hope remains to break this cycle. Because the causes of deforestation in Central America are so apparent, the measures required to halt it are also obvious.

---

*"Rainforests and the Hamburger Society," by James D. Nations and Daniel I. Komer. *Environment* 25:12–20, April 1983. Reprinted with permission of the Helen Dwight Reid Educational Foundation. Published by Heldref Publications, 4000 Albemarle St., N. W., Washington, DC 20016. © 1983.

Logging, then Colonization

While some scientists and many Latin American politicians blame the slash-and-burn agriculture of Indian and peasant farmers for the destruction of Central America's tropical forests, in reality the problem results from a combination of local, regional, and international activities. In fact, forest conversion in Central America usually occurs in stages.

During the first stage, logging companies enter the forest to extract valuable hardwoods such as mahogany and tropical cedar. . . .

But the damage wrought by commercial logging is not so much the result of what foresters remove from the forests as what they leave behind — namely, the roads they construct to enter and exploit the area. Road construction introduces the second stage of deforestation: colonization. For down these roads, like leafcutter ants on a forest trail, come landless peasants from other areas of the country. . . .

. . . To understand the colonists' role in deforestation, one must ask why these families enter the rainforest in the first place. The answer is simple: because there is no land for them elsewhere.

Behind that answer are several underlying factors, among them inequitable land distribution and population growth. Central American government officials promote jungle colonization projects or tolerate "spontaneous" colonization partly because doing so temporarily relieves pressures for land reform in other areas of the country, thus reducing demands to break up and redistribute large estates and company holdings. . . .

Population growth is an equally important force behind rainforest colonization in Central America. . . . In Central America, as in the rest of the world, 90 percent of the expected population growth during the next 20 years will take place in areas that are now covered, or formerly were covered, by tropical forests. . . .

Export Beef Production

With colonization comes the third stage of tropical deforestation in Central America. During this final stage, land cleared by Indian and immigrant farm families is absorbed by individuals or companies who use it to produce export crops — sugar cane, bananas, pineapples, coffee, oil palm, or beef cattle. In Central America, the most dominant and most destructive of these export crops is beef. . . .

. . . Rather than recognizing tropical rainforests as valuable natural resources, many Central American politicians view them as obstacles to national development. Not only do they fail to conserve nationally owned forest lands, but they also provide legal and financial incentives to peasant farmers and cattlemen to colonize and clear these forests. In many of the Central American countries, in order to gain title to a

173

plot of federal forest land, the colonizing individual must simply "improve" it by clearing it of vegetation. Because individuals can obtain generous loans from government and commercial banks to raise beef cattle, they simply transform the rainforest into pastureland.

By any of these methods of converting forest to pasture, the end result is the same. After 7 to 10 years of beef cattle yields, the effects of overgrazing and torrential rains turn the rainforest's nutrient-poor soils into eroded wastelands. When this happens, the rancher must find new cropland or rainforest to transform into pasture. In these various ways, beef cattle producers are expanding their operations throughout the rainforests of Central America, destroying forests, wildlife, and agricultural production with equal disregard.

The tragic senselessness of converting Central America's rainforest into pastureland is evident on several levels. The stocking rate (the number of animals per unit of land) on newly cleared rainforest land is a mere one head per hectare during the first year. Within five to ten years, this rate drops to five to seven *hectares per head* as nutrient-leaching and erosion impoverish the soil. Studies of pasturelands cleared from rainforest in eastern Chiapas, Mexico — where the soils are better than most in the region — demonstrate that the average beef yield is 22 pounds of meat per hectare per year. By contrast, the traditional agricultural system of the Lacandon Maya, the area's indigenous inhabitants, produces up to 13,000 pounds of shelled corn and 10,000 pounds of root and vegetable crops per hectare per year. Moreover, the Lacandones produce these yields for five to seven consecutive years on a single forest plot before they allow the areas to regrow for another cycle of food and forest five to ten years later. Even then, rather than abandon their harvested plots, Lacandon farmers plant these areas with three crops — citrus, rubber, cacao, avocado, papaya — in a system of traditional agroforestry that both conserves the rainforest biome and enhances its regeneration as a renewable resource.

Clearly, if Central America's rainforests were being eradicated to produce food for a hungry world, as some researchers contend, then systems more productive than extensive cattle production could be utilized. Indeed, food production systems practiced by traditional rainforest Indians are, without exception, more productive than the pasturelands that are replacing these systems.

Even the sad yield that pastures do produce in the Central American tropics carries no benefits for local populations, either Indians or immigrant colonists. The U.S. Department of Agriculture (USDA) has pointed out that as beef production increases in Central American countries, per capita beef consumption actually declines in the individual countries. . . .

Behind this illogical situation lies a simple fact: the expansion of Central America's beef cattle production is largely a response to the lucrative beef import market in the United States. As beef cattle pro-

174

duction expands in Central America, beef exports expand accordingly. Because foreign companies can pay higher prices for beef than can domestic consumers, local beef prices increase, leaving many Central American families unable to afford the luxury of beef. This problem is compounded by population growth, which means that, each year, more and more people are competing for the meat that does remain within the country. . . .

But U.S. imports of Central American beef introduce more than cheap beef into American diets. They also bring some undesirable ingredients, such as toxic residues of chlorinated hydrocarbons, found in DDT and other agricultural pesticides. . . .

The Search for Solutions

Despite its complexity, the multifaceted problem of rainforest destruction, undermined Central American food production, and toxic residues in beef imports is a problem with simple solutions. At some point, the Central American governments will realize that transforming their rainforests and agricultural land into beef for export is a poor use of their nations' natural resources. . . . Changes will take time, and that time will take its toll on Central America's remaining rainforests. Each year that current patterns persist means another 4,000 km^2 of tropical rainforest eradicated. Until the parties involved take definite action toward solving the problem of deforestation at its roots, one of the most important steps toward preserving the region's tropical rainforests is to educate the American public about the social and ecological consequences of their eating habits. Americans must be made aware that when they bite into a fast-food hamburger or feed their dogs, they may also be consuming toucans, tapirs, and tropical rainforests.

*Our guarantee that the meat and poultry we consume is safe
and wholesome is a federal inspection system that has operated since shortly after the turn of the century. Does the system
work as promised? That's what the Department of Agriculture
asked the prestigious National Academy of Sciences to find
out. The conclusions of their Meat and Poultry Inspection Program panel are summarized in this selection.*

The excerpt that follows, from the Environmental Nutrition
*newsletter, conveys a sense of the problems facing any inspec-
tion system that attempts to cope with modern animal production methods.*

MEAT AND POULTRY INSPECTION: THE SCIENTIFIC BASIS OF THE NATION'S PROGRAM*

*Committee on the Scientific Basis of the Nation's Meat and Poultry
Inspection Program*

. . . The responsibility for ensuring the safety of meat and poultry products was conferred upon the USDA through a mandate in the Federal
Meat Inspection Act of 1906 and subsequent acts and amendments.
These documents directed the USDA to inspect meat and poultry products that enter commerce and are destined for human consumption.
. . . Toward this goal, FSIS [Food Safety and Inspection Service] personnel inspect meat and poultry products animal-by-animal and pro-
cess-by-process in slaughterhouses and processing plants.

Slaughter inspectors rely almost completely on sight, smell, and
touch to discern abnormalities in animals and carcasses. This procedure was designed primarily to protect consumers from grossly visible
lesions or diseases. Although this labor-intensive system tends to ensure safe and wholesome products with respect to such lesions, its
efficiency came under scrutiny by FSIS as science and technology advanced and the understanding of risks to human health became more
defined.

In 1906, acute infections were the leading causes of human mortality and morbidity. Today, more than 60% of all human deaths in this
country each year are due to cardiovascular disease and cancer. . . .
Also, through improved controls and deliverance of health care to
farm animals, certain animal diseases have been virtually eradicated.
The importation of diseased animals into the United States has essen-

Meat and Poultry Inspection: The Scientific Basis of the Nation's Program; Chapter
1: "Executive Summary." National Academy Press, 1985. Used with permission.

tially been prevented, and diseases that can be transmitted from animals to humans have been curtailed or in some cases practically eliminated.

Simultaneously, the production of meat and poultry products has become increasingly complex. In contrast to the few basic cuts of fresh meat and poultry available early in this century, there is now a great variety of raw, canned, cured, dried, fermented, and frozen products. The technological growth that made these products possible has contributed to the greater need for sophistication in determining the origin and path of food-borne microbial infections. Finally, environmental contaminants and the increasing use of chemicals in animal feeds and to some extent in processed foods have led to the presence of chemical residues in meat and poultry, some of which may be sources of potentially deleterious effects. . . .

Major Conclusions and Recommendations

The meat and poultry inspection program of the FSIS has in general been effective in ensuring that apparently healthy animals are slaughtered in clean and sanitary environments. FSIS has made progress in reducing risks to public health from conditions that can be observed during antemortem and postmortem inspection and that can be evaluated during processing. However, substantial challenges continue to confront the agency. Some aspects of the inspection system are poorly defined in terms of objectives relevant to public health. . . .

Public Health Risks Related to Biological Agents

It is well established that species of *Salmonella* and *Campylobacter* are major causes of diseases transmissible to humans through the consumption of meat and poultry products, and the committee concluded that current postmortem inspection methods are not adequate to detect these organisms. For example, meat and poultry were implicated in 1,420 of the 2,666 food-borne disease outbreaks from known sources reported to the Centers for Disease Control (CDC) between 1968 and 1977. . . .

Of particular concern to the committee is the risk presented by food-borne microbial infections to susceptible subgroups such as young children and the elderly. Pathogenic microorganisms reside in the gastrointestinal tracts and on external surfaces of food-animals and cannot be detected by the usual organoleptic procedures (i.e., sight, smell, and touch) used during inspection. . . .

Public Health Risks Related to Chemical Agents

The committee concluded that although significant strides have been made in protecting the public against exposure to hazardous chemicals in meat and poultry, the fundamental design of FSIS's residue

177

monitoring program needs to be improved to ensure maximum protection. In particular, the committee questions the adequacy of sampling size and procedures, the basis for and the utility of tolerance levels for chemicals, and the basis for setting priorities for testing chemicals.

. . . Because millions of animals are slaughtered annually (e.g., between 36 million and 40 million cattle alone), the chance of any animal being sampled in the United States is minuscule. Furthermore, because of the increasing number and variety of contaminating residues that may constitute possible health hazards, especially to susceptible subgroups in the population, and because the overall contamination rate of less than 1% may be considerably higher for certain food sources or consumer groups, the committee questions whether the size of the sampling plan is adequate. . . .

Production of Food-Animals

The committee concluded that the most effective way to prevent or minimize hazards presented by certain infectious agents and chemical residues in meat and poultry is to control these agents at their point of entry into the food chain, i.e., during the production phase on the farm and in feedlots. However, FSIS cannot exercise such control because it has no jurisdiction in those areas. Environmental contamination and improper use of feed additives fall within the purview of other government agencies such as the Food and Drug Administration and the Environmental Protection Agency. The problem is compounded by the absence of an effective national surveillance system for monitoring the disease status of food-animals and by an inadequate mechanism for tracing infected or contaminated animals back to their source.

Currently, the probability of successfully tracing a diseased or contaminated animal to the producer is very low (approximately 10% for cattle and 30% for swine). . . .

. . . Contamination at the farm creates a significant problem that is difficult for the inspection system to control by traditional inspection methods. Once animals reach the slaughterhouse, the line speeds and economic concerns necessitate sampling for residues on a very limited basis, and mostly with technology that is still quite imperfect and is not yet adequate to alleviate the problem. . . .

ANTIBIOTICS IN OUR FOOD SUPPLY*

. . . In September of 1984 the Centers for Disease Control (CDC) published a study in *The New England Journal of Medicine* that made front-page headlines. For the first time, scientists had evidence linking human illness to drug-resistant bacteria in meat. Although the possibility of this occurring had been theorized, based on a chain of known events, the link to human disease had never been proven. To do so is very difficult, because of the complex sequence of events involved.

The CDC study linked antibiotic-resistant bacteria present in hamburger meat to the Salmonella poisoning of 18 individuals in Minnesota, Iowa and the Dakotas. One man died after presumably contracting the disease from another individual, as a result of inadequately sterilized hospital equipment. An important factor was revealed during the CDC investigation — 12 of the 18 patients had been taking antibiotics for other unrelated symptoms just prior to becoming ill. Although the antibiotics were initially suspected as the cause of the disease, it was later determined that they were in fact catalysts for the illness. The antibiotics taken by the patients killed off other bacteria that might have competed with the Salmonella bacteria, thus allowing the Salmonella to flourish. The antibiotics were not effective on the Salmonella bacteria — as were none of the antibiotics subsequently administered to the patients — because the Salmonella was an antibiotic-resistant strain. This was a dramatic example of just what can happen when such bacteria infect humans.

Just how do bacteria become resistant to these drugs? Scientists have known for years that routine use of an antibiotic will kill some bacteria, but also will cause a "survival of the fittest" situation, allowing hardier strains to live on. Since killing the majority of bacteria is an obvious benefit of the antibiotic, the risk of breeding "super" bacteria must be weighed against this. And the antibiotic useage that must be examined is not just in animals. Many critics of a ban on medicated feed argue that the real problem is the over-prescribing of antibiotics by physicians. Most experts in the field acknowledge that human use needs to be severely curtailed if these drugs are to have any effect on future illnesses.

But the fact remains that 40% of the antibiotics produced in this country are fed to animals. Most of this is — and has been for 30 years — routinely added to animal feed in subtherapeutic doses. This is standard practice in most livestock and poultry operations. Besides preventing bacterial diseases from developing, the antibiotics increase the rate of weight gain in the animals, for reasons that are not understood. Obviously this provides an economic benefit to farmers and ultimately to consumers.

---

*"Antibiotics in Our Food Supply." *Environmental Nutrition,* 8:1 – 2, January 1985. Used with permission.

Occasionally, farmers feed animals therapeutic doses of antibiotics to treat specific illnesses. It has been assumed by many that these non-routine large-dose feedings are the real danger because significant levels of residues can remain in the animal. As a result, the U.S. Department of Agriculture requires that animals fed antibiotics (in feed or administered therapeutically) must wait a specified period of time before slaughter. This regulation addresses the residue problem, but not the problem of drug-resistant bacteria that may have flourished in the animal in response to the medicated feed.

That animals (and humans) receiving antibiotics have increased numbers of antibiotic-resistant bacteria in their digestive tracts is well-known. It is also known that resistance to antibiotics is a threat to any bacteria-caused illness. What had not been demonstrated before was the link between these two facts; that the drug-resistant bacteria in animals causes resistance to antibiotics in humans. The recent CDC study has shown that this cause/effect relationship can and does exist.

Does all this mean antibiotics in animal feed will be banned? Not necessarily, however it does give the FDA some ammunition. In 1977, the FDA sought to ban penicillin and tetracycline in animal feed (these are two of the most widely-used animal antibiotics and, not un-coincidentally, the two most important antibiotics for humans as well). The proposed ban has been held up at the congressional level ever since, due to pressure by legislators from farm states. . . .

Proponents of the ban argue that it would leave farmers free to substitute other antibiotics and perhaps force them to rely less on drugs as a crutch for the overcrowded, unsanitary conditions of many operations. Critics of the ban note that England enacted such legislation on medicated feed in 1970, but resistant bacteria are still a problem there because of therapeutic use of antibiotics in animals and humans.

The American Council on Science and Health (ACSH), an independent scientific organization, contends that a major problem is not imminent, because we have seen no evidence of epidemics breaking out among those with closest exposure to the animals — or for that matter, in the animals themselves. The ACSH opposes a ban because consumers would absorb the resulting increase in economic cost. In addition, critics argue, the indiscriminate use of antibiotics in humans is a far more serious problem. Both sides agree the medical profession needs to address this issue more openly and take steps to limit abuse of these drugs. Likewise, it seems prudent to do what we can to limit animal useage, at least to those antibiotics not quite so crucial to human survival as tetracycline and penicillin.

> *To conclude this discussion of the health and safety issues in-volved in how animals are raised for human food, we turn to writer Orville Schell. Coming as it does from a man who is both a rancher and a writer who has done his homework, this view on the matter seems to us to be particularly thought pro-voking.*

MODERN MEAT*

Orville Schell

Over the past several decades, the ways in which livestock are pro-duced in the industrialized world have undergone a dramatic trans-formation. Antibiotics, new feed technologies and hormones have all played a major role in this transformation. While the short-term bene-fits in the form of greater efficiency in mass production and thus low-er meat costs to consumers are undeniable, assessing the long-term risks has been a much more elusive undertaking. In many instances drugs and chemicals have been approved before the long-range conse-quences of their use are completely understood. Frequently the stu-dies that might have helped establish the degree of such risk have not been done, or have only been done incompletely because of the im-mense costs they entail. But just as often it has been impossible to do conclusive testing because the state of our scientific knowledge has not been sufficiently advanced. Instead, we have often allayed our fears with short-term studies that, though important, are too incom-plete to tell us all we need to know. It is true that each time a hog consumes a subtherapeutic dose of tetracycline, a cow ingests a small quantity of printer's ink or insecticide, or a steer is implanted with a hormonal pellet the consequences to humans is probably negligible. But when the use of these compounds is extended over millions of such episodes and continued for decades, the cumulative effects may present a whole different magnitude of effect. . . .

Almost anyone familiar with farmlife or the livestock industry has witnessed instances of carelessness and misuse of animal drugs and chemicals. Livestock may be treated right up to slaughter time with no observance of federally required withdrawal times. Drugs approved for only one species of animal may be used on an "extra label basis" for another. Large overdoses may be given on the assumption that if a little is good, a lot is better.

---

*Modern Meat, by Orville Schell. Chapter 5: Conclusion, pp. 323–327. Random House, Inc. 1984. Used with permission.

Many of those who handle animal drugs, veterinarians included, are carelessly exposing themselves and their fellow workers to contamination. Their cavalier attitude is frequently startling. On one occasion, for instance, I witnessed a Texas cowboy pick up a syringe as if it were a water pistol and shoot a co-worker in the face with estradiol cypionate, an injectable estrogen . . . used to abort animals or induce them to expel mummified fetuses. On another occasion, I witnessed an experienced cattlewoman repeatedly douse her hands and arms with the highly toxic grubicide Coumaphos (an organophosphate) while pouring it on the backs of cattle, where it kills the grubs of heel flies and lice by being dermally absorbed into the animal's system.

Many cattlemen seem almost to cultivate a disregard for caution around potentially dangerous drugs and chemicals, as if prudence might be misinterpreted as timidity or unmanliness. A corollary of this kind of machismo is the cattleman's often-haughty disregard for government inspectors, who are viewed not as protectors of the public health but as bothersome fuddy-duddies, sent forth from the disdained, and possibly socialistic, world of "big government" to spy and intrude on private enterprise.

Cattlemen are people of a practical rather than scientific bent. They are more concerned to know *if* a drug is effective rather than *how* it is effective. And, working outside as they do where the wind blows free across vast open spaces and where there are relatively few signs of man's encroachment on the environment, minuscule amounts of anything can easily seem trivial, and the consequences of carelessness insignificant.

Habitual carelessness easily turns into lawlessness. And . . . not only is the potential for the lawless use of animal drugs real, but government regulatory agencies are often ill equipped to handle it when it does occur. . . .

Although there are many areas in which it would behoove us all to be wary of blindly accepting the ever-increasing use of drugs and chemicals in the husbandry of meat animals, it also behooves us to remember that a fearful concern that leads to the rejection of all of these new livestock technologies will be as blind as one that leads to embracing them indiscriminately. Certain feed-additive antibiotics — such as those that are not used for human therapy, or those few that curiously do not generate R plasmids — can be a great asset to livestockmen if used judiciously. Certain hormones, such as those prostaglandins that are very short-lived, and even certain growth-promoting hormonal implants ultimately may prove not to pose unreasonable risks to humans when used properly in meat animals. And when the shock of thinking about cows eating ethylene and propylene pellets wears off, we may actually wish to applaud such new technologies as Dr. Erle Bartley's amazing plastic hay.

But in those cases where the consequences of continued widespread use are still not yet clearly known, or where reputable scien-

182

tists have provided evidence that continued use may prove injurious to us or to our environment, we will be ill advised to blunder wrecklessly on, business-as-usual.

The use of penicillin and tetracycline feed additives, which we once believed we could feed to animals with no ill consequences to humans, now appears to be compounding a serious problem by decreasing the efficacy of these very drugs for human use. Like the air we breathe, the water we drink and the food we eat, we find that bacteria are not the exclusive province of any one country, any one part of the body, any one person or even any one species of animal. They are more like an unseen matrix connecting all forms of life. The discovery of the specific mechanisms by which resistance to antibiotics is transferred between living things reminds us that in spite of our biological diversity we are all, in the last analysis, inextricably joined.

"The vulnerability of microorganisms to antibiotics is a kind of commons — a resource, which, as we consume it by the use of antibiotics for nonmedical purposes in animals, is now diminished in man," noted Donald Kennedy, a biologist who is president of Stanford University and was commissioner of the FDA under President Carter when that agency last attempted to regulate the use of penicillin and tetracycline for feed-additive use. "The benefit of using these drugs routinely as over-the-counter products to help animals grow faster, or in prophylactic programs, does not outweigh the potential risks posed to people."

The sex hormones with which almost all beef cattle are now raised in this country may not pose such a well-documented and clear-cut danger as penicillin and tetracycline feed additives. In their case, it is not so much what we already know about them but what we do not yet know about their widespread and often indiscreet use that gives cause for concern.

"One can easily appear Luddite about the use of hormones in meat animals," says Samuel S. Epstein, M.D., professor of occupational and environmental health at the School of Public Health, University of Illinois Medical Center in Chicago. "Even though the consequences of their use are unclear, one can still look at them by way of analogy to our experiences with other hazardous drugs and chemicals. Over the last forty years we have paid such a terrible price for refusing intelligently to assess the risks of new technologies before leaping into them. We have too often perturbed natural systems for short-term gains, but with disastrous long-term consequences. And quite apart from science, I feel instinctively that it is a terrible mistake to interfere with anything as delicately poised as the endocrine system, with so little information about where it is leading us."

"When it comes to using drugs and chemicals in meat animals, we find ourselves in a situation in which our problems are well ahead of our answers," says Dr. Jere Goyan, dean of the Pharmacy School at the University of California in San Francisco, reflecting on his tenure

183

as commissioner of the FDA after Donald Kennedy. "We just have not yet developed the science to back up reasonable regulations and safeguards in advance of their use. And until that time, if we are going to err, it would seem wise to me to err on the side of safety."

> Will we be driven by these stories of unregulated drugs to give up meat? Probably not says anthropologist Marvin Harris. We're programmed to like animal foods, he concludes, probably for nutritional reasons.

MEAT HUNGER*

Marvin Harris, Ph.D.

. . . Less than 1 percent of the world's population voluntarily spurns every type of flesh food, and less than one-tenth of 1 percent are bona fide vegans. Involuntary rather than voluntary abstinence characterizes the animal food patterns of people in less developed countries. This can be seen from the changing proportions of plant and animal foods in relation to improvements in per capita income. The Japanese experience should be taken as a harbinger of Asian things to come: between 1961 and 1971 Japanese consumption of animal protein rose 37 percent while plant protein consumption fell by 3 percent. On a worldwide basis the consumption of grain by livestock is rising twice as fast as the consumption of grain by people. Within most societies, developed as well as underdeveloped, the higher the income bracket, the greater the proportion of animal products in the diet. . . .

Many different kinds of cultures, from hunter-gatherer bands to industrial states, exhibit similar preferences for animal food. . . .

Virtually every band or village society studied by anthropologists expresses a special esteem for animal flesh by using meat to reinforce the social ties that bind campmates and kinfolk together. Far more often than plant foods, animal products must be shared reciprocally between producers and consumers. . . .

The preoccupation with meat has another side to it. Meat hunger can be a powerfully disruptive as well as harmonious force. In band and village societies, especially those which do not possess significant

*Good to Eat: Riddles of Food & Culture, Chapter 2: "Meat Hunger," by Marvin Harris. Simon & Schuster, Inc., New York, NY. 1985. Used with permission. Pp. 24–31.

domesticated sources of animal flesh, eggs, or milk, lack of success in the hunt may lead to quarrels, a split in the community, and the outbreak of warfare between neighboring camps and settlements. . . .

A preoccupation with animal flesh also dominates the foodways of more complex societies. It is no accident that chiefs and heroes the world over celebrate their victories by hosting feasts and bestowing large portions of meat on followers and guests. Nor is it an accident that priestly castes such as those described in the Hebrews' Book of Leviticus or the Hindus' Rig Veda made ritual slaughter and consumption of domestic animals a principal focus of their sacraments. The very idea of sacrifice, fundamental to the formative doctrines of Christianity, Hinduism, Judaism and Islam, arose from the sharing of meat in the camps and villages of prehistoric times. With the domestication of herds and flocks, meat, blood, and milk had to be shared with the ancestors and gods, just as hunters had to share the day's catch with each other, to create a web of mutual obligations, to prevent jealousies and strife, and to preserve communities that embraced both the invisible rulers of the world and their earthly creations. . . .

All these cultural convergences and recurrences support my theory that animal foods play a special role in the nutritional physiology of our species. In addition we seem to have descended from a long line of meat-hungry animals. Not so long ago anthropologists believed that monkeys and apes were strict vegetarians. Now, after closer and more meticulous observation in the wild, most primates turn out to be omnivorous just like us. And many species of monkeys and apes are not only omnivorous, but they further resemble humans by making a big fuss when they dine on meat.

Being rather small creatures, monkeys prey mostly on insects rather than game. But they expend much more time on capturing and eating insects than anyone previously believed. This has cleared up a long-standing puzzle about the way monkeys feed in the wild. As they make their way through the forest canopy, many species of monkeys send down a constant rain of half-chewed pieces of leaves and fruit. Further study of the morsels they consume versus the morsels they discard indicates that they are not being sloppy but finicky. Monkeys do a lot of sniffing, feeling, exploratory nibbling, and spitting out before they pick the fruit they want. But they are not looking for the perfect, ripe, unblemished Garden of Eden apple; they are trying to find the ones with the worms inside. In fact, some Amazonian species are more interested in the insect larva than in the fruit. They open a weevil-infested fig, eat the weevil, and discard the fig. Some eat both fruit and larva, spitting out the portion that hasn't been spoiled. Some simply ignore fruits that show no signs of insect-induced decomposition. . . .

We now also know that several species of monkeys not only consume insects but actively pursue small game. Baboons are especially keen hunters. During a single year of observation in Kenya, Robert

185

Harding saw baboons kill and eat forty-seven small vertebrates including infant gazelles and antelopes. Baboons normally spend most of their time in the wild eating plant foods. But as among many involuntary "vegetarian" human populations, the reason baboons consume only small quantities of meat may be more a matter of necessity than choice: they have difficulty finding and capturing suitable prey. Whenever there is a choice, claims William Hamilton, the baboons he has observed in Namibia and Botswana prefer to feed on animal matter first; roots, grass seeds, fruits, and flowers second; and leafy materials and grass third. During seasons when insects were abundant, Hamilton found that baboons spent as much as 72 percent of the time eating them.

The most startling discovery about nonhuman primate meat eating is that chimpanzees, our closest relatives in the animal kingdom, are devoted and fairly effective hunters. (So much for the ever-popular theory that humans are unique "killer apes.") On the basis of a decade of observation on Gombe National Park in Tanzania, Geza Teleki estimates that chimpanzees use about 10 percent of their time to hunt small mammals — mostly young baboons, other kinds of monkeys, and "bushpigs." Also at Gombe, R. W. Wrangham observed chimpanzees capturing and eating colobus monkeys, bushpig, bushbuck, redtail monkeys, blue monkeys, and baboons in descending order of frequency. Teleki estimates that the adult males eat noninsect meat about once every two weeks. Chimpanzee hunters frequently cooperate with each other. As many as nine chimpanzees, mostly males, position and reposition and coordinate their movements, sometimes for an hour or more, to surround their quarry and effectively prevent its escape. After capturing their prey, chimpanzees typically spend several hours tearing the carcass apart and eating it. Many individuals get a share. Some "beg" for morsels by holding the palms of their hands upward under the chin of a dominant male; some snatch pieces from one another, and dart in and out to recover dropped fragments — behavior that seldom occurs when they dine on plant foods. Through one means or another, as many as fifteen different individuals — mostly males — share in eating a single prey animal.

I do not see how it can be either arbitrary or coincidental that animal foods evoke special behavior among so many human groups as well as among our primate cousins. But this does not mean that I believe humans are compelled by genetic programming to seek out and consume such foods, the way lions or eagles and other true carnivores are driven to eat meat. There is too much variation in the ratios of plants to animals in the foodways of different cultures to support the idea that we instinctively recognize animal foods as something we *must* eat. A more plausible explanation is that our species-given physiology and digestive processes predispose us to learn to prefer animal foods. We and our primate cousins pay special attention to foods of animal origin because such foods have special characteristics which make them exceptionally nutritious. . . .

186

> *We turn now from the question of whether modern livestock flesh is wholesome to the equally knotty and much more discussed question of whether, as Harris suggested, it is nutritionally advantageous for humans to eat meat. We lead off this section with a defense of red meat from a writer for* ACSH News & Views.

THE RED MEAT IN OUR DIET — GOOD OR BAD?*

Delia A. Hammock, M.S., R.D.

Red meat. The food that once symbolized strength, vigor, virility, and success is now getting top billing as a life-shortening villain.

While there have always been those few who shunned meat for moralistic or religious reasons, today everyone from starlets to athletes has jumped on the anti-meat bandwagon, making it very fashionable to say "I don't eat meat" in a tone that would suggest that eating a thick, juicy, charbroiled steak is an act of immorality, lunacy, or suicide.

Meat-eating has become an emotional issue fueled by myths, half-truths, and distortions which have left many Americans confused or misinformed about the value or ramifications of red meat in their diets. . . .

. . . According to the NLSMB [National Live Stock and Meat Board] calculations, Americans actually ate 91.12 pounds of cooked red meat in 1982, or about four ounces per person per day.

Nutrients in Red Meat

This average four ounce portion of meat represents a total of 327 calories or about 16 percent of the 2,000 calories a typical adult female consumes each day. . . .

For good nutrition, a food that contributes a proportion of a person's caloric allotment should contribute at least a similar proportion of the person's daily nutrient needs. . . . Red meat carries its weight nutritionally. While some of these nutrients, such as protein, can readily be obtained from non-meat sources, others are not so easy to come by.

Vitamin B_{12}, for instance, is only found in animal foods, so true vegetarians must rely on supplements or fortified cereals. Of course

---

*"The Red Meat in Our Diet — Good or Bad?," by Delia A. Hammock, M.S., R.D. *ACSH News & Views*, 6:6–7, September/October 1985. American Council of Science and Health, New York, NY.

red meat isn't the only source, but it is near the top of the list. You would have to eat about 23 ounces of roasted chicken, 9 ounces of cheddar cheese, 20 ounces of plain yogurt, or 7 ounces of flounder to obtain the amount of B_{12} found in 4 ounces of meat.

Iron deficiency is probably the most common nutrient deficiency in this country. Red meat is one of the best sources of food iron. Not only does it have a higher percentage of iron than most other foods do, but about 50 percent of the iron in red meat is "heme" iron which is much more readily absorbed by the body than the "nonheme" iron present in fruits, vegetables, grains, soy products, and fortified foods. . . .

Zinc is closely linked to protein, but adequacy of protein does not assure adequate zinc. Not only does zinc content in different types of protein vary greatly, but the availability (i.e., solubility and absorbability) of the zinc also varies widely. Red meat has a high zinc content and availability. . . .

Red Meat and Fat

Of course most of the attention given to meat in the last few years has had little to do with its contribution of essential vitamins and minerals. Instead, red meats have been singled out by the public as a major fatty culprit in several "modern" diseases, including obesity, atherosclerosis, and some types of cancer. . . .

Red meats are . . . a major contributor of fat to the diet. But the latest USDA nutrient profiles for red meat show that it is significantly lower in fat and calories than it was 30 years ago when the last composition studies were done. Changes in breeding and feeding techniques have resulted in 10 percent fewer fat calories in beef, while pork has less than half the fat it once had.

The 4 ounce portion of meat that the typical American eats each day contains 213.3 calories as fat or 10.7 percent of the calories in a 2,000 calorie diet. Less than 5 percent of these total fat calories come from saturated fats. And this estimate is based on the assumption that 50 percent of the fat on the meat will also be eaten. Trimming away more fat would reduce fat intake even further.

For those following a low-fat diet, this moderate amount of meat can easily fit into recommendations by the American Heart Association to reduce dietary fat to 30 percent of total calories with saturated fat accounting for less than 10 percent of total calories.

And what about cholesterol? Actually, one average 4 ounce meat serving contains 87 mg of cholesterol — almost the same as in 4 ounces of roasted turkey (84 mg) and less than in the same amount of roasted chicken without skin (100 mg).

Cutting out red meats will reduce dietary fat and cholesterol, but the cost in vitamins and minerals could be high for individuals who

188

are presently eating only moderate amounts of these nutrient-packed foods. A better way to cut back on fat and/or cholesterol intake without decreasing the nutrient density of the diet is by choosing lean cuts of meat and removing all trimmable fat, selecting lowfat milk and dairy products, and reducing consumption of oils, shortenings, and fat-containing salad dressings and table spreads.

Red Meat and Dieters

The high nutrient density (ratio of nutrients to calories) of red meats also makes them an excellent choice for those counting calories. For instance, a 3 ounce serving of cooked lean beef contains only 192 calories, but it provides even a higher concentration of vitamins and minerals than the fattier cuts.

But, again, moderation is the key. A 3 ounce serving of lean meat will easily pay for itself nutritionally on a calorie-restricted diet, but a 16 ounce prime sirloin will not. The nutritional importance of a food depends not only on its nutrient content, but also on the quantities in which it is eaten and the composition of the rest of the diet. No food is perfect. Excessive consumption of any food or beverage is unwise.

Red meat, or any other single food, is not essential in the diet for anyone — man, woman, or child. It is, however, an easily obtained, easily prepared, nutritious food which a majority of Americans enjoy. It doesn't deserve to be made a scapegoat for all the health problems that trouble modern Americans.

189

*If red meat eaters are healthy, are those who avoid it less so?
Is abstaining from meat an invitation to nutrient deficiency?
The answer of the American Meat Institute, a trade industry
association, is, not surprisingly, "yes." This excerpt from*
Answers to Predictable Questions Consumers Ask About Meat
*deals with vegetarianism as a potential nutritional hazard.
In the selection that follows, nutritionist Bonnie Liebman
offers a more balanced view of the pros and cons of meat
avoidance.*

MEAT AND NUTRITION*

Consumer Affairs Committee, American Meat Institute

Q: Is vegetarianism healthful?

A: It is difficult to obtain sufficient calcium, zinc and vitamin B_{12}
from an all-plant diet, so a plant diet is not recommended for growing
children. It is also difficult to obtain the right balance of essential amino acids (building blocks of protein) needed by the body, but the
proper balance can be achieved if foods are carefully chosen to complement each other for their amino acid contents.

Q: What nutrients are missing from the diet of the strict vegetarian?

A: The nutrients calcium, vitamin D, riboflavin, vitamin B_{12}, available zinc and iron, and high quality protein have been identified as
being low in the strict vegetarian's diet.

---

*"Meat and Nutrition," *Yellow Pages: Answers to Predictable Questions Consumers
Ask About Meat.* Pg. 41. Consumer Affairs Committee. American Meat Institute, © 1982.
Used with permission.

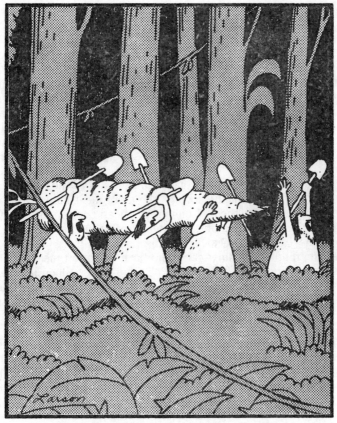

Early vegetarians returning from the kill

"The Far Side" cartoon by Gary Larson is reprinted with permission of Chronicle Features, San Francisco.

191

ARE VEGETARIANS HEALTHIER THAN THE REST OF US?*

Bonnie Liebman, M.S.

To many Americans, the word "vegetarian" conjures up an image of a 60s era flower child eating brown rice, vegetables, and soybeans grown organically in the back yard. In fact, vegetarianism is far older and more common than most people think. Much of the world's population currently eats vegetarian or largely vegetarian diets. The vegetarian movement was founded in the sixth century BC by Pythagoras. Its purposes were not only to foster hygiene and kinship between humans and animals, but also to protest the self-indulgence of ancient Roman society.

Today, the Western world follows in the path of the Romans. Generally, the more affluent the society, the more meat its people consume. In this country, the $37 billion American fast food industry thrives on the sale of hamburgers, steaks, roast beef and franks. "Real" men eat meat and potatoes, not quiche.

Yet the number of Americans who have sworn off meat is considerable. According to a 1978 Roper Poll, nine to 10 million people consider themselves vegetarians. Though reasons for being vegetarian include economic constraints as well as religious, ethical, and political beliefs, more and more people are eschewing meat to protect their health.

Though all who claim to be vegetarians should avoid meat, fish, and poultry, not all 10 million vegetarians have the same eating habits. Those who eat milk products (lacto) and eggs (ovo) are called the *lacto-ovo-vegetarians.* The Vegetarian Information Service in Bethesda, Maryland, estimates that over 90 percent of American vegetarians are lacto-ovo.

Vegans or *strict vegetarians* avoid all animal foods, including eggs and dairy products.

People who follow a Zen macrobiotic diet eat mainly whole grains, legumes, vegetables, and other staples of the Eastern world. Technically, macrobiotic followers may not be vegetarians — many eat small amounts of fish, meat, eggs, and milk products. But from a nutritional standpoint, macrobiotic and vegan diets are quite similar.

Is vegetarianism truly "the way to superior health," as some claim? Or is the National Live Stock and Meat Board correct when it says "an increase in malnutrition has been noted among youths who have switched to diets with little or no foods of animal origin?"

Unfortunately, as with so many other nutrition issues, the debate

*"Are Vegetarians Healthier Than the Rest of Us?", by Bonnie Liebman. *Nutrition Action, 10:8–11,* June 1983. Used with permission.

is often clouded by conflicting emotions, scientific opinions, and economic interests.

"We tend to scoff at vegetarians, call them the nuts among the berries, but the fact is, they're doing much better than we are," says Dr. William Castelli, director of the federal government's Framingham Heart Study in Massachusetts.

Even the ordinarily conservative American Dietetic Association recently recognized that "a growing body of scientific evidence supports a positive relationship between the consumption of a plant-based diet and the prevention of certain diseases."

In contrast, the National Live Stock and Meat Board believes that "from a health standpoint, people are better off including meat and other animal products in their diet," according to Board nutritionist, Dr. Burdette Breidenstein.

The meat industry may insist on denying the health benefits of vegetarian diets, but research on heart disease, cancer, high blood pressure, diabetes, and obesity argues otherwise. The research shows that vegetarians are lowering their risks of developing a host of the most serious diseases confronting our society. That they eat less fat, particularly less saturated fat, and more grains, legumes, and vegetables, appears to make them healthier than the average American.

Heart Disease

"The vegans have cholesterol levels so low, they'd never get a heart attack," says Dr. William Castelli, referring to a group of macrobiotic vegetarians in Boston. "Their average blood cholesterol level is about 125, and we've never seen anyone at Framingham with a cholesterol level below 150 have a heart attack."

For more than a decade, researchers have known that lacto-ovo vegetarians have lower blood cholesterol levels than non-vegetarians, and vegans have even lower levels. These findings come as no surprise. After all, vegans eat less saturated fat, less cholesterol, and more fiber than lacto-ovos, who in turn eat less than meat-eaters.

More recent studies indicate that vegetarians enjoy a further protection against heart disease: the percentage of their blood cholesterol carried in high-density lipoproteins (HDL) is higher than in meat-eaters.

But skeptics want evidence that vegetarians have lower heart attack rates, not just lower cholesterol levels. That means following a sizable number of people for several decades. Now the data are finally at hand. In Loma Linda, California, Drs. Roland Phillips and David Snowdon have monitored the health of 25,000 Seventh Day Adventists (SDAs) for over 20 years. About half of the SDAs are lacto-ovo vegetarians. The rest eat meat, though somewhat less often than most Americans. Cigarette smoking is rare in both groups.

193

According to Phillips:

- older male SDAs (aged 55 and above) who eat meat six or more times a week are twice as likely to die of heart disease as vegetarian SDAs;
- younger male SDAs (aged 40 to 54) who eat meat six or more times a week run four times the risk of a fatal heart attack than their vegetarian brethren;
- meat-eating SDA women over 55 run 1.5 times the risk of a fatal heart attack encountered by female vegetarian SDAs.

The lower heart attack rate in younger male vegetarians means that heart disease strikes later in life in these men than in meat-eaters. A vegetarian diet seems to have no effect in younger women, says Snowdon, because premenopausal women — vegetarian or not — seem to be protected from heart disease by hormonal factors.

In November, 1982, English researchers reported similar results after comparing over 10,000 vegetarians and omnivores. The more meat people ate, the greater their risk of heart attack.

While this evidence is impressive, meat-lovers needn't cringe at the thought of going "cold turkey" forever. Abundant evidence suggests that eating less saturated fat and cholesterol is the *real* key to preventing heart attacks. Though meat is the largest source of fat in the American diet, it is far from the only one.

Eliminating meat will have little impact on fat consumption if high-fat dairy foods take its place. Though most vegetarians eat less fat than omnivores, lacto-ovo delicacies can be just as fatty as the typical meat-laden menu. . . .

Cancer

"I simply don't have an explanation yet," says Phillips when asked why SDA vegetarians are only about *one half* as likely as other Americans to develop colon or rectal cancer. His most recent data, as yet unpublished, indicates that something other than the lack of meat in their diets is responsible. If meat consumption were directly associated with cancer, the more meat one consumed, the more likely one would be to develop cancer. Phillips' data says that is not the case.

Compared to the average American, SDAs also have less breast, prostrate, pancreatic, and ovarian cancer. As with colon and rectal cancer, the reasons are unclear.

However, Phillips and Snowdon note that SDA vegetarians don't just eat less meat — they also eat more beans, whole grains, vegetables, and fruits than non-vegetarians. The fiber, vitamins A and C, or other substances in these foods — such as indoles in cruciferous vegetables or protease inhibitors in legumes — might prevent vegetarians from developing cancer.

194

In other words, say Phillips and Snowdon, simply dropping meat from your daily menu is no guarantee that you have skirted our most dreaded disease. However, eating a typical SDA vegetarian diet, complete whole grains, vegetables, fruit, and legumes appears to offer some protection.

Moving closer to a vegan diet may be even more prudent. While the cancer rates of SDA vegetarians are noteworthy, they pale in comparison to Japanese rates. The Japanese suffer only one-fifth as much breast and colon cancer as we do. Until recently, only 10 percent of the calories in their largely vegan diets came from fat. (Now that McDonald's and other Western foods have invaded, the level of fat has jumped to about 20 percent.). . .

Obesity

Will you lose pounds by curbing your appetite for meat? If you continue to eat eggs and dairy products, the answer is "maybe." If you cut out all animal foods, the answer is "probably."

Most studies show that on the average lacto-ovo vegetarians are slightly leaner than meat-eaters. According to Phillips, only 15 percent of SDA vegetarians are overweight, compared to roughly 30 to 40 percent of SDA meat-eaters. But all researchers agree that vegans weigh less than omnivores by between eight and 20 pounds, depending on the study.

High Blood Pressure

In 1974, Frank Sacks, then a graduate student at Harvard Medical School, reported on the results of his study looking at 210 macrobiotic vegetarians living in Boston area communes. The macrobiotics, who were predominantly vegans, had surprisingly low blood pressures — only 106/60 millimeters of mercury for those aged 16 to 29. The U.S. average for 18- to 24-year-olds is 117/73.

Sacks doesn't believe meatless meals are directly responsible for the low blood pressure findings. "My opinion is that the most important thing about a vegetarian diet for blood pressure is that it causes people to lose weight," he explains.

As for lacto-ovo vegetarians, some researchers have found that these people have slightly lower blood pressures than meat eaters; others have found no significant difference.

Diabetes

The typical vegan's diet is surprisingly similar to the high-complex carbohydrate, high-fiber (HCF) diet now being used to treat adult onset diabetics. . . .

If the HCF diet can completely control this common form of diabetes, might it also prevent the condition from developing in the first

195

place? No studies have compared the number of American vegetarian diabetics to the number of omnivore diabetics. To date, one can only say that lacto-ovo diets *may* and vegan diets *are likely* to prevent diabetes, if for no other reason, than because they help keep people lean.

Mutagens in Fried and Broiled Meat

"Our working hypothesis," says Dr. John Weisburger, of the American Health Foundation in Valhalla, New York, "is that mutagens in fried and broiled meat *initiate* and that high-fat diets *promote* cancers of the breast, prostate, and colon." Weisburger and co-workers are trying to isolate the mutagens formed when meats are browned. Microwave cooking produces no mutagens. Nor are foods other than meats much of a problem. "Toasted bread, fried potatoes, and similar foods contain some mutagens, but meats contain one thousand times more," he explains.

Dr. Weisburger's colleague, Dr. B. S. Reddy, found mutagens in the stools of about 20 percent of people eating standard American diets. Of the 11 SDA vegetarians he tested, none had mutagens in their stools. Weisburger emphasizes the preliminary nature of his work. Meanwhile, meat eaters might consider cooking their meat in a microwave to avoid creating mutagens.

Pesticide Residues

Meat-eaters are more likely to consume certain agricultural and industrial chemicals linked to cancer than vegetarians. One class of insecticides — the chlorinated hydrocarbons — accumulates in the body fat of animals and humans. Therefore, eating fatty foods, such as meats, cream, whole milk and cheeses, increases exposure to these chemicals. Two of the most well-known are dieldrin and DDT. According to a 1979 study by the Environmental Defense Fund, the breast milk of vegetarian women contains lower levels of chlorinated hydrocarbons than the breast milk of meat-eating women.

Moreover, FDA analyses show that two industrial chemicals, PCBs (polychlorinated biphenyls) and PCP (pentachlorophenol) accumulate primarily in these food groups: the Meat, Fish, and Poultry group, the Dairy group, and the Oils and Fats group.

But before vegetarians breathe a sigh of relief, they ought to know that dozens of other chemicals remain in the fruits, vegetables, grains and potatoes they eat. Most of these, the organophosphate insecticides, are less dangerous because they break down sooner than the chlorinated hydrocarbons. Nevertheless, vegetarians get their share of chemicals they haven't asked for. . . .

Osteoporosis

Roughly 15 million Americans, mostly post-menopausal women, have bones so brittle that they are likely to crack spontaneously, causing the person to fall and break a hip. Now at least one study suggests that lacto-ovo vegetarians aged 55 and above have a reduced risk of osteoporosis, because their bones have more mineral mass than those of meat-eating non-SDAs.

There may be several reasons why SDA vegetarians suffer less osteoporosis, even though their lacto-ovo diets contain no more calcium than meatier fare. Conceivably, the high protein content of meaty diets might cause the body to excrete excess calcium. . . . Also, more frequent exercise or other aspects of Adventist lifestyle might strengthen their bones. . . .

When it comes to heart disease, cancer, obesity, high blood pressure, diabetes, and osteoporosis, vegetarians seem to be better off than meat-eaters. But what about reports such as these?

* In 1966, the Grand Jury of Passaic, New Jersey, warned the public that the Zen macrobiotic diet had caused severe nutritional deficiencies in six young adults, four of whom died;
* In 1978, vitamin B-12 deficiency was found in a six-month-old infant breast fed by her 26-year-old vegan mother;
* In 1979, rickets — a bone disease caused by lack of vitamin D — was found in four pre-school children of vegan parents.

These sad tales might suggest that we all should eat three meat-packed meals a day. But a closer look at vegetarian diets reveals quite a different picture. In fact, nutritional deficiencies are no more common in lacto-ovo vegetarians than in omnivores. When deficiencies occur, they most commonly appear in vegans, and particularly vegan children. Yet even these problems can be averted with careful planning. As for Zen macrobiotics, most followers consume far more nutritious and varied diets than the very restricted regimens that injured or killed the six New Jersey residents in the mid-60s.

Dr. Johanna Dwyer, director of the Frances Stern Nutrition Center at Tufts University Medical School, has carefully examined the health of children from macrobiotic and lacto-ovo vegetarian families in Boston. "There is nothing inherently wrong about vegetarian or vegan diets," she asserts. "Both can be safe with proper planning."

The American Dietetic Association agrees: "A total vegetarian diet can be planned to be nutritionally adequate, if attention is given to specific nutrients which may be in less available form or in lower concentration or absent in plant foods."

197

Vegans, especially vegan children, might have trouble getting enough vitamins D and B-12, calcium, zinc, iron, riboflavin, or calories. . . . Vegetarian diets have an equal amount if not more of other nutrients than most meat-filled cuisines.

While vegan diets do require some attention, lacto-ovo diets are probably no more difficult to plan than meals with meat. Moreover, this "planning" should be kept in perspective.

As Dr. John Scharffenberg, associate professor of applied nutrition at Loma Linda, has pointed out: "A vegetarian diet is easily formulated — in fact, more easily than a meat diet. With a meat diet, one has to consider how to restrict the cholesterol and saturated fat, how to get adequate fiber, and how to increase the carbohydrates according to present national recommendations. . . . Our sense of proportion should not get distorted. The number of children acquiring atherosclerosis and the potential for what is killing more than half of us is so much greater in families on the usual American meat diet than is the number of potential rickets cases from vegetarian families.

In other words, the benefits of vegetarian diets probably outweigh the risks. But one needn't shun meat completely to get those benefits. Simply cutting back on meats and fatty dairy products and eating more plant foods should lead to healthier and longer lives.

Nutritionist George Briggs sees no harm in 2 servings of meat a day. Nutritionist Bonnie Liebman probably wouldn't go that far, but agrees that some meat in the diet is certainly OK. We close this section with a piece from American Health, *a popular magazine whose editor, Joel Gurin, notes that Americans are cutting down voluntarily on their meat consumption primarily for health reasons — an eating trend that a majority of health professionals would probably applaud.*

ARE YOU A SEMI-VEGETARIAN?*

Joel Gurin

. . . Most people don't have the willpower to live an entirely meatless life, even if they wanted to. But a growing number of *semi-vegetarians* — people who eat less meat, more vegetables — are becoming a decisive force in shaping the nation's taste in food. And it's possible that their way of eating may be the healthiest of all.

*"Are You A Semi-Vegetarian?," by Joel Gurin. Reprinted with permission from *American Health: Fitness of Body and Mind.* 4:37–39, 41–43, July/August, 1985. Copyright 1985 American Health Partners.

Recent Gallup surveys done for *American Health* show that semi-vegetarianism is a major trend. Late last year, in a survey on the impact of the health movement, Gallup found that 24% of us now eat less meat than we used to. That's 40 *million* adults. And fully 44% eat more fruits and vegetables. . . .

Now a second-stage poll on food habits shows the reasons for the shift. *American Health* had Gallup phone 1,033 Americans in January to ask about their dietary beliefs. Right away, they made it clear they are not hard-line vegetarian purists. Only 3.7% of Americans now say they consider themselves to be vegetarians.

But tens of millions of us, the new survey shows, agree in principle with the movement away from meat. A clear majority, 52%, believe that "no one really needs to eat meat more than once or twice a week." More than a third (37%) believe that "vegetarians are probably healthier than most Americans." And a whopping majority of 72% *disagree* with what used to be the standard notion: "The vegetarian diet — one without any meat, poultry or fish — is just a fad that will pass." (Possible error: 4%.)

An Epicurean Revolution

The greening of the American diet is well under way. But if we're witnessing a nutritional revolution, it's one that's been led by a small cadre: the true vegetarians. Simply by living without meat, and thriving, they've made it possible for millions of others to consider greener meals.

Nutritionists and doctors have studied vegetarians, and found that they're generally well-nourished — and have less chronic disease than the rest of the population. Doctors have recently tested vegetarian diets as a treatment for heart disease, hypertension, early-stage kidney disease and other ills. And they've told the whole population to eat more complex carbohydrates, less protein and less fat — in other words, a semi-vegetarian diet.

The health evidence is so persuasive that it's become the main motivation for new converts to vegetarianism. That's a change. Most people used to become vegetarians "to solve the world hunger problem, or for spiritual reasons or animal rights," says Paul Obis, founder and editor of *Vegetarian Times* magazine. . . . But now, he says, health has become the number-one reason his readers have given up meat.

If it were just good for you, like cod liver oil, meatless fare wouldn't be catching on. But today's vegetarians have also shown that meatless meals don't have to be ascetic.

Vegetarians are now producing a chic, fresh, tasty cuisine that even semi-vegetarians can enjoy. . . . Even some airlines are now creating good-tasting vegetarian meals, and United reports that requests 199 for meatless dishes have quadrupled in the last few years. Perhaps most important, vegetarian cookbooks have undergone a renaissance. There are now books on Chinese, Indian and Italian meatless cookery, and home-grown best-sellers with rich illustrations and gourmet recipes. . . .

Finally, just as vegetarian recipes are getting more popular, so are "vegetarian" foods — soy products developed as meat or dairy substitutes. Some food marketers believe that tofu (derived from soybeans) may soon become as popular a "health food" as yogurt. . . .

Protein: No Longer a Bugaboo

Vegetarians have become our nutritional pacesetters by bringing together health and taste in a new way. It's a recent match, and one that became possible only with changes in nutritional knowledge. These changes have liberated vegetarian chefs.

In the '60s and '70s, vegetarians were careful to make sure they ate "complementary" proteins. A decade ago, in *Diet for a Small Planet*, Frances Moore Lappé described the basis for this concern. . . .

Today, however, many vegetarians have become much less concerned about balancing their proteins. In her tenth-anniversary reissue of *Diet for a Small Planet* (Ballantine, $3.50), Lappé even includes a *mea culpa* for her earlier crusade. "In combating the myth that meat is the only way to get high-quality protein," she now writes, "I reinforced another myth. I gave the impression that in order to get enough protein without meat, considerable care was needed in choosing foods. Actually, it is much easier than I thought."

Here's why. First, nutritionists have generally de-emphasized protein over the last several years. Protein is so plentiful in America that most of us — meat-eaters, anyway — could eat half as much protein as we do and still meet our bodies' needs. Eating too much protein may even be detrimental, putting a strain on your kidneys or draining calcium from your bones.

It's also become clear that eating meat isn't the only good way to get your protein. The protein in eggs and milk is actually more balanced and digestible than that in meat. MIT research has shown that soy protein is perfectly adequate as a sole protein source. And hardly any vegetables or grains are *completely* lacking in essential amino acids; they just have more of some than they do of others.

Finally, even if you are concerned about balancing your amino acid intake, Lappé says now, you don't need to eat complementary foods at the same meal. You can eat the foods three or four hours apart, and their amino acids will still complement each other in useful ways.

200

The Case for Semi-Veg

Although the protein controversy may be resolved, other dilemmas of vegetarianism are not. Most of all, nutritionists are concerned about the low levels of "trace elements," such as iron and zinc, in meatless meals. . . .

Even meat-eaters are turning out to have deficiencies in some of these elements, particularly iron. And certain groups of vegetarians may be at special risk. Vegetarian runners, for example, may be particularly susceptible to iron deficiency (as well as amenorrhea in women.)

Despite this concern, most vegetarians *are* well fed, particularly if their diets include eggs and dairy products. . . .

From a nutritionist's point of view, though, the *ideal* diet for most of us might be one that's largely vegetarian, but with just enough meat, poultry or fish to supply those hard-to-get vitamins and minerals. Meat isn't only a ready source of minerals, it may also enhance the nutritional value of other foods you eat it with.

Iron, for example, is found in both meat and plant food. But meat contains an unidentified "meat factor" that makes iron from *other* sources easier to absorb. . . .

For most Americans, then, a semi-vegetarian diet may be the choice for both taste and health. And we may be headed for a style of eating that's quite different from either traditional vegetarian cooking or traditional American fare.

"It's a matter of being selective," says Bonnie Liebman, Director of Nutrition with the Center for Science in the Public Interest. "Instead of sitting down to a New York steak, people might settle for a little bit of beef in a salad. They could start thinking of meat as a condiment rather than a main course."

Afterword

Most meat eaters would probably prefer not to dwell on the fact that what they have on their plates is a piece of a once-living animal. Where flesh eating is concerned, we're all vulnerable to unexpected emotions. As you prepare to enjoy a succulent chunk of steak, you really aren't interested in details about the steer's character and home life. Once the emotional issue of taking life is set aside, the remaining questions are more subtle, but no less divisive.

Hodgson's excerpt that begins our chapter praises animals as users of waste land and waste materials. They are not competitors with humans, he says, but benefactors.

201

Actually, they are neither. The sense of "intention" that infuses both of those descriptors is unnecessarily divisive. Most of us do not believe — although Hodgson seems to — that everything on earth has quite literally been put here for our benefit. Arguing that there is not enough arable soil on earth to provide food "for more than a fraction of the people on earth" (which is not true), Hodgson asserts that "this must be why Nature put fish in the sea that convert waterborne nutrients into human food and why She put ruminants on the range because they can eat range grass and turn it into food for man." In fact, it is highly doubtful that She had any such thing in mind.

Whatever one's religious beliefs, it is clear that most animals were here first. They are living creatures sharing the planet, who occupy ecological niches different than ours. And they are most assuredly not "competitors" with us in the "them or us" sense. Our "unnatural" expansion in numbers, it must be understood, has made us competitors with *them;* the available resources were theirs first — if that is the issue. But it is not.

Both humans and domestic animals have expanded in numbers well beyond the capacity of any "natural" system to support them. There are more domestic animals on earth than could possibly survive in a natural setting — many more than there are humans — and there are more humans than could possibly survive without organized agriculture. Therefore, all human food systems, whether or not they contain animals, are inherently *unnatural* — and in them humans and animals depend upon each other.

The first real issue, then, is whether or not our livestock-containing food system is sustainable, and whether animals contribute to or detract from that sustainability. Animal-containing food systems *can* be sustainable, as is shown by the existence of such systems in Africa and Asia, which are hundreds or even thousands of years old. The question here is whether American meat, especially the beef that predominates in our diets, is produced in a manner compatible with the long-term health of the environment. On that issue there is marked disagreement.

It is true, as Hodgson points out, that ruminant animals can utilize plants, and therefore land, that humans could not otherwise make use of. And it is also true that in our livestock systems, ruminants (animals that chew the cud and make their own amino acids from poor quality nitrogen sources) serve as what Hodgson calls biologic disposals — making use not only of traditional hays and straws, but of organic wastes left over from the processing of fruits, vegetables and other animals (as well as some less savory materials such as newspaper, discarded Fritos, and cardboard dust from milk cartons). There is no competition here — these are not substances humans would otherwise use as foods.

And with both food and feed grains presently in surplus in the

U.S., it is difficult to argue that the grain and soybeans cattle do consume are being snatched from the mouths of the starving. (Why there is surplus food in some parts of the world and starvation in other parts is a different issue, beyond the scope of this chapter.)

So let us back off from that other emotional issue of whether animals are eating what rightfully belongs to humans elsewhere. That is the sort of moral dilemma that you will have to decide in terms of your own value system, not on the basis of facts alone. Let us simply ask whether humans, by raising animals, are putting an unacceptably large demand on the environment of the U.S. and the world.

Lappé, Nations and Komer all say "yes." Producing the enormous amount of feed grains animals consume yearly in the U.S., Lappé argues, is putting an unsustainable drain on agricultural resources — mining and polluting our irreplaceable ground water, wasting our precious topsoils, and polluting air, soil and water with pesticides and other agricultural chemicals.

A study published in 1986 which looked at the question of how many people and animals the natural resources of the U.S. could sustain over time, concluded that resource limitations would make it increasingly difficult for Americans to continue to produce and eat their meat-heavy diet very long into the 21st century — because, as Lappé indicated, such a large percentage of the soil erosion in this country is caused by the production of corn and other animal feeds. (John Gever, Robert Kaufmann, David Skole and Charles Vörösmarty. *Beyond Oil: The Threat to Food and Fuel in the Coming Decades.* 1986. Cambridge: Ballinger Publishing Company.)

Cattle stress the environment even before they are brought into feedlots to be given grain and soybeans to eat. They cause harm even when they are "grazing." "No other activity covers so much land area in this country," one observer has pointed out, "as cows eating grass." (Philip L. Fradkin. The eating of the West. *Audubon*, January 1979.) He notes that 63% of the total land area in the continental U.S. has been or is being grazed — and the animals are eating not merely grass, but whatever greenmatter is edible.

Nations and Komer add the observation that beef cattle are "the most dominant and destructive of the export crops" presently being raised in Central America. Grazing animals have historically been destroyers of the earth's fertility — goats eating their way through the last edible shrub are a classic symbol of desertification around the world.

But cattle on the present scale are a new threat, at least partly because the relative wealth of the United States allows us to eat not only our own beef, but that raised by poor people and

203

pulled into our rich markets by their enormous debts and our great wealth. They need to sell us something just to keep up the interest payments on their debts. Too often that "something" is food. The result, as Nations and Komer point out, is that our imported beef comes to represent the destruction of toucans, tapirs, and Central American rainforests, as the latter are turned into short-lived pasture for exportable beef.

Rainforest beef carries not only the burden of wildlife extinction, but a burden of pesticide residues as well, often pesticides barred as hazardous in the U.S. and exported by us to countries with less strict regulations than our own. Domestic beef, however, may carry as heavy a burden of residues.

Antibiotics and hormones are used not only to keep down levels of disease, but to keep the animals growing rapidly on as little feed as possible. Almost half of all antibiotics used in the U.S. are fed to animals; their ability to keep down disease in spite of the stress of crowded conditions is what actually permitted the development of confinement feeding. The excerpt from *Environmental Nutrition* confirms the potential hazard of this — chronically-fed antibiotics may generate resistant strains of bacteria, and this resistance may spread to other bacteria (salmonella in the case cited), thus rendering major antibiotics useless against human illnesses.

As we were putting together this chapter, a Congressional committee came out with a report documenting the Food and Drug Administration's (FDA) loss of control over these and other drugs. (U.S. House of Representatives Committee on Government Operations. *Human Food Safety and the Regulation of Animal Drugs.* 1985. Washington: U.S. Government Printing Office.) The news is fairly shocking even to those who would otherwise dismiss as hysterical all questions about the safety of American meat. As the hearing record shows, only a small percentage of the 20,000 to 30,000 drugs used in livestock are even listed with the FDA. The illegal use of animal drugs is so widespread, as one FDA staff person testified, that companies are reporting one another's violations.

This means that ensuring the safety of the meat supply is a much more difficult task than our present inspection system is designed to deal with. As the excerpt from the National Academy of Sciences (NAS) shows, "slaughter inspectors rely almost completely on sight, smell, and touch to discern abnormalities in animals and carcasses." But much of what may be questionable about the meat supply is unlikely to be visible, smellable, or tangible.

The eyeballing of carcasses that has been the center of the inspection process may be almost irrelevant. Although it usually comes as stunning news to the ordinary observer that an inspec-

204

tor might be asked to examine 105 chickens per minute, the number may not really matter. Technological changes, as the NAS report comments, have complicated the paths of potential foodborne microbial infections and increased the likelihood of contamination of meat and poultry with residues of environmental contaminants and animal feed chemicals. None of these potential hazards can be dealt with by inspectors making use of eyes, noses and fingers.

Present sampling methods designed to pick up contamination have a "minuscule" chance of picking up a contaminated animal, and even if such a diseased or contaminated animal were picked up by the monitoring system, the probability of "successfully tracing" that animal back to its producer (to encourage changes in the practices that led to contamination) is as low as 10% for cattle and 30% for swine. Finally, as the Congressional report made clear, for many of the chemicals whose residues are of interest, tests do not exist to detect them if they are present.

In many cases illegal use of drugs may have nothing to do with intentional lawlessness. Rancher and writer Orville Schell notes that what is involved is often simply "habitual carelessness" on the part of "machismo" cattlemen, working in wide open spaces where the problem of pollution seems both remote and trivial.

Although his own book vividly describes some of the more unpalatable waste products fed to cattle for the gratifying weight gains they inexpensively produce, Schell urges us to avoid "fearful concern" that would lead us to reject "all these new livestock technologies." But we would be equally ill-advised, he warns, "to blunder recklessly on, business-as-usual." The appropriate attitude is, at a minimum, one of caution. "Our problems," he quotes one knowledgeable observer as saying, "are well ahead of our answers."

Given the dramatic changes in the ways animals are raised, given monitoring that probably does not protect us from potentially hazardous residues, and given our lack of knowledge about the risks to human health produced by such residues — or by the compositional changes in meat produced through changes in animal husbandry — some people choose simply to give up animal flesh altogether. Others opt to reduce their exposure to whatever may turn up in meat by eating less of it.

Will most people give it up entirely? This may be difficult, says anthropologist Marvin Harris. We hunger for meat, as have all people in all times, even those who don't have a chance to eat much of it. A very small percentage of humankind is vegan — usually for powerful religious reasons.

Are there nutritional reasons for this meat hunger? Nutritionist Delia Hammock argues that there are. Meat is a healthful food, she points out, carrying a heavy and needed load of vitamins and minerals, and the "typical" American portion need not be so high in fat as to be dangerous.

Those who eat meat are "among the healthiest persons in the United States," agrees nutritionist Briggs in one of our opening quotes. But nutritionist Liebman's article suggests that the people they are "among" are vegetarians, who appear to be even healthier. Vegetarians "are lowering their risks of developing a host of the most serious diseases confronting our society." The serum cholesterols of vegetarians are lower than those of meat eaters, she shows, and those of vegans lower even than that; and their HDL levels (the good cholesterol) are higher.

A long-term study of Seventh Day Adventists shows that those who do not eat meat have fewer heart attacks and lower rates of rectal, colon, breast, prostate, pancreatic and ovarian cancer. Fewer vegetarians are overweight or have high blood pressure.

So it is clear that you don't have to eat meat to be healthy. And though the article on cattle raising with which we opened this chapter seemed to suggest that the majority of the world subsists on animal products, the reality is that most of the world's protein comes from plants, not animals, and many of the world's peoples live on diets with few, or no, animal products.

Many of these people, it is true, are malnourished, but this is not because they are vegetarians. Many of them are vegetarians for the same reason they are malnourished — because they are poor and cannot afford meat or eggs or milk. They are malnourished not for lack of meat but because they cannot get enough of the diet they do eat, because they are hungry. More immediately relevant to us is the fact that many of the world's great cultures, and great cuisines, have grown up around food patterns that were very meat restricted.

That vegetarianism or even a move toward semi-vegetarianism long seemed so "radical" in the United States reflects the fact that we have been rich enough in land and resources to have a meat-centered diet. And in meat eating, as in many other aspects of our lives, we have simply gone too far. In the period following World War II, beef consumption, which had dipped to its lowest point in the century in the middle of the Great Depression, began a steady climb that took it from an average of 2.2 oz per day in 1950 to a high of 4.2 oz per day in 1976.

It is now declining. But since our per capita consumption per day still exceeds three ounces of cattle flesh, we have clearly not "demoted" meat as Tudge urged, in Chapter 2, to the status of a condiment. We have, on the average, begun to cut down on our portions. The vegetables edged off our plates after World War II by those ever larger steaks are making a comeback. Though we will probably never become a vegetarian society, it may well be that our romance with heavy flesh-eating is over.

206

5 Health, Natural and Organic: Foods or Frauds?

There are many things nutritionists do not agree about, but some areas of disagreement generate much more heat than others. This chapter is about one of those. "Health foods," "organic foods" and "natural foods" are among the most heat-producing terms in our profession; some nutritionists get angry just hearing the words. In fact, when the Federal Trade Commission several years ago proposed banning the use of the words *health, natural* and *organic* in food advertising, many nutritionists testified that they *should* be banned — including professionals who in other circumstances would be appalled by any proposal that the government might actually outlaw a *word!*

What on earth could produce such emotion? On the most obvious level, the argument is about the literal meanings of words. Many nutritionists question whether we can even agree on what the words *health, natural* and *organic should* mean when they are applied to food. They claim that these terms are intrinsically meaningless or misleading and should not be used at all. Other nutritionists think that the terms can (and should) be officially defined, that they are only meaningless because they have been so misused.

We have tried in this chapter to give you some sense of the debate, beginning with a few items intended to show you the problem everyone is trying (in different ways) to deal with. Clearly there is a problem; the question is how can it best be solved?

We follow with some abbreviated excerpts from a report by the staff of the Federal Trade Commission, which originally proposed the ban on the terms *natural, organic* and *health.* Their opinion was written after extended hearings when all sides of the argument had been presented. After laying out their conclusions, we present two points of view that differ from the staff recommendation — in opposite directions.

The argument is not confined to definitions, however. Even if terms like *organic* and *natural* could be defined, are such products worth buying? Here again passions run high. Is organic agriculture, as many nutritionists claim, something worth supporting; or is it, as others argue, a cruel delusion in a world that cannot be fed by organic methods? Are "organic" and "natural" foods overpriced frauds? Do they always cost more? And what are we paying *for:* are "organic" or "natural" foods freer of chemicals, tastier, more nutritious, or in some other mysterious way "better" than ordinary supermarket foods?

We hope the selections in this chapter will help you to answer these questions, to come to your own conclusions about the attitude you ought to convey when people ask you for your advice or opinion on these matters. We also hope that the selections will stimulate you to keep reading and thinking about these issues; all the answers are not yet in.

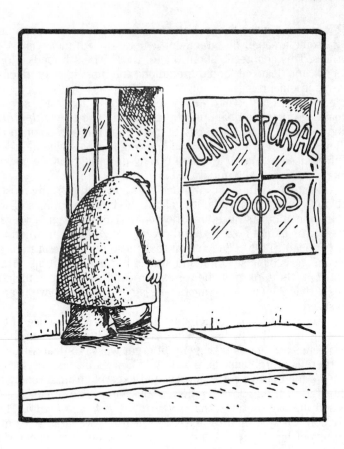

> *When the organic food craze of the 1970s reached its zenith among Manhattan swingers, writer Julie Baumgold wrote a wonderfully irreverent essay for* New York Magazine *on the progression of one health foodist from peanut butter and jelly to : . . Well, see for yourself. We have excerpted it here to suggest that some questionable ideas and activities, however mistaken, are sometimes best treated with humor rather than outrage.*

CAN CRUNCHY GRANOLA BRING NEW MEANING TO CITY LIFE?*

Julie Baumgold

. . . Consider our man: Mr. California.

Adelle Davis comes upon him like a temple bell. . . . Someone leaves *Let's Eat Right to Keep Fit* or *Let's Get Well,* . . . in his guest room, and there are the answers, naked as protein. Is he tired? Is he a grouch? After the first chapter he is at the health food store.

It is one of the old, pre-Frenzy places without the clever California name. A faint film of what is hopefully chaff rises in the air. Fat cats rumble in the windows. . . .

Around Mr. California is all this ugly food. Grown in manure, with a dabble of fungus and mold, organic food is very romantic. It is low and raw and quick to rot. By definition nothing is "refined." Dispirited little green apples with nature's own brown flaws, tatterings of lettuce, which, like some ugly people, apologize for their looks with their taste. A lot of fat people are vigorously shopping around him.

So it starts — the Peanut Butter and Jelly Cycle. Mr. California, whose sustenance was peanut butter and jelly, discards his Skippy jar after carefully running his finger around the rim for the last buttery dregs. Now in the Early Adelle Davis Phase, he eats big breakfasts, high protein and liver and greens and Tiger's Milk and a daily spoonful of unrefined cold-pressed vegetable oil. During this stage no one should sit next to him at dinner because he has that wild convert's gleam in his eye. . . . He eats all the parsley and has a funny way of looking at gravy blood.

Mr. California now sniggers at Chocks and One-a-Day and swallows a whole alphabet of vitamins; he bristles when he sees the asterisk on his vitamin bottle and reads, "No Minimum Daily Requirement in Hu-

*"Can Crunchy Granola Bring New Meaning to City Life?", by Julie Baumgold. *New York Magazine,* 4:39–45, June 28, 1971. Used with permission.

man Nutrition Has Been Established," knowing that it is part of the Conspiracy, that top-level plot between the FDA and the AMA and the drug companies to keep him and nature apart — to block the use of chiropractic medicine, mega-vitamins, and nutrition in favor of drug therapy.

Mr. California is reading Herbert Bailey's *The Vitamin Pioneers* and *Vitamin E — Your Key to a Healthy Heart*, talking about the Shute doctors in Canada and enjoying a wonderful sex life. . . . He takes wheat germ oil, bioflavinoids, kelp tablets, bone meal tablets, Brewer's yeast, which makes him gag enthusiastically, desiccated liver tablets. . . .

Mr. California owns a Juicer and a Brownie's Discount Card. People smile at him at The Good Earth. During a ten-day rice purge recommended by Georges Ohsawa in *Zen Macrobiotics*, he also reads *You Are All Sanpaku* and other cultist books. A rational being until now, he becomes a brown ricer and abandons vitamins. . . . He knows artificial foods make him artificial; fruits, though cleansing and sustaining, make him sweet and gushy, and animal flesh (even organic range-fed flown-in beef) makes him truculent and nasty, albeit kind of snappy and fast. He soon hears, however, that with macrobiotics his vegetables are overcooked and heat kills the vitamins and he is not getting enough salads and fruits and liquids.

Mr. California now starts Eliminating. First flesh, which is easy when you think of all those scared animals with their endocrine glands gushing out adrenalin before the ax. Then chicken, because he's heard that a friend of Bob Dylan's wife was walking home with a chicken and some of its juice fell on his foot and burned a hole right through his boot. Then fish, which has changed his body odor. He becomes a Vegetarian who doesn't eat "products" like eggs, even fertile ones from chickens who scratched for their own food and never tasted a hormone. He goes on Grains, crunches up rice cakes with wheat grass juice, and feels like a sponge stuffed with lead pellets. He is now a Fruitarian under the tutelage of what is left of a man who has lived for ten years in the Andes on nothing but fruit; he learns that papaya is the purest thing you can eat and it slides through the body in only seven minutes. Finally Mr. California fasts.

Then he's into the Highly Peculiar Stage. He "does" ginseng, which he gets . . . in the form of a tiny $21 red root which looks like a man on a cross and tastes like bad earth. . . . Ginseng is so violently exotic that the plant seeks a radioactive soil to grow in and only after seven years produces a tiny blue flower that glows in the dark. It can thus be gathered only at night, and since it is so trembly that it closes at the hunter's footsteps, it must be shot with a bow and arrow. There is also miso, a black Japanese paste which is buried for at least three years in wooden barrels and which smells and tastes like naked protein or an old sneaker abandoned for at least three years. . . . Finally, he is in the Ultimate Vitamin Stage where he considers vitamins "addictive." Phosphoaminolipide no longer affects him like the litany of

212

a Far Eastern religion. Instead his D comes from going naked in the sun; A from pressed carrots; C from rose hips. Like everyone in Hollywood, Mr. California has abandoned his Dairy Diet because he knows that milk protein causes phlegm and mucus. And now that meats, poultry, fish, eggs, dairy have been eliminated he finds himself come full cycle to . . . breads and jam and nut butter.

So here is his friend Bonnie, flat out on her sinner's bed, popping jelly beans and speed for breakfast, whose lunch at high teatime is a dollop of hydrogenated Skippy and Smucker's, or perhaps Shedd's Peanuto (stripes of grape jelly alternating with stripes of peanut butter) in a jar with a purple circus elephant on the label . . . and Mr. California spreading his Tibetan Barley Bread with Natural Organic Blenheim Apricot and a dab of Unsalted Raw Sesame Butter or Elam's Natural Peanut Butter or Nuts 'n' Seed. . . .

Mr. California had a discount card at Brownies, a Manhattan health food store. In Youngstown, Ohio, he might have gone to a health food store owned by Max Huberman. This is an excerpt from Mr. Huberman's testimony before the Federal Trade Commission, given when Mr. Huberman was President of the National Nutritional Foods Association, an organization of health food store owners. His mini-survey of his own customers tells us something about the people (other than Mr. California) who go to health food stores, what sorts of beliefs they hold and what sorts of products they spend their money on.

TESTIMONY BEFORE THE FEDERAL TRADE COMMISSION*

Max Huberman

. . . Since the central tenet of our philosophy is complete freedom of choice for our consumers in the selection of dietary preferences and life styles, we must examine these in order to place the issues before us in proper perspective. Rather than giving you my own articulation of this consumer mood, let me present it here to you as it was presented recently to me by some of my own customers.

---

*Max Huberman, testimony before the Federal Trade Commission. FTC, 1976–77. *Rulemaking Record of the Proposed Trade Regulation Rule on Food Advertising, Phase I Public Record Number 215–40.*

On the afternoon of Friday, October 22, 1976, at my Health Food Store in Youngstown, Ohio, I informally interviewed approximately twenty patrons who entered the premises. Orally, I posed a series of . . . questions to those who had the time to respond.

The questions I posed were as follows:

1. What does the term "natural food" mean to you?
2. What does the term "natural ingredient" mean to you?
3. Why do you prefer natural foods?
4. What does the term "health food store" mean to you? . . .
5. What items do you seek to obtain in a health food store? . . .

After eliminating almost identical responses and selecting a balanced cross-section of daily consumers, I present here the recorded verbatim responses from the following five persons:

1. An 18-year-old girl college student.
2. A retired railroad worker.
3. A male school teacher.
4. A tire salesman.
5. A middle-aged housewife.

This is not presented as a formal poll or scientific survey by any means. However, my firm is typical of the thousands of other "momma-poppa" health food stores, and I assure you that these on-the-spot, off-the-cuff and unrehearsed responses which I have recorded fairly reflect what we health food dealers encounter in the course of any day's business transactions.

To the first question — "What does the term 'natural food' mean to you?" — the following were the responses:
College Student: "Foods grown or processed without harmful chemicals."
Retired Railroad Worker: "To me, 'natural foods' mean honest foods. If you wax an apple or color an orange that isn't even ripe, they may look prettier but they are phony and unhealthy."
Schoolteacher: "It means just what it says. As far as I'm concerned, if the food isn't natural, it just isn't food."
Tire Salesman: "I guess it means just what you people sell. I just started on this stuff a few months ago. My wife's been after me to cut down this gut of mine — I'm on the road a lot and I never eat right when I'm on the job. I can't afford to be sick. Natural foods may not be so fancy but they taste better and they sure are life savers for me."
Housewife: "Real instead of fake; closest to nature."

The following were the responses to the question — "What does
the term 'natural ingredient' mean to you?":
College Student: "The contents are safer and more nutritious."

Railroad Worker: "It means that a loaf of bread or mixed cereal is made from items as close to nature as possible, instead of cooked up in a laboratory with chemical substitutes."

Schoolteacher: "Well, like this package of cereal here, like the label says: 'Whole oat flakes, dried apple flakes, whole wheat and rye flakes, dried raisins, turbinado sugar, crushed hazlenuts and almonds, wheat germ, honey and nothing else. That's what I call 'natural ingredients.'"

Tire Salesman: "I've been reading quite a bit about the food additives. I have learned to read labels. If I can't pronounce it, I won't eat it. To me, 'natural ingredients' are safer ingredients."

Housewife: "The kind of ingredients I don't have to worry about if my kids eat the food. If the label says 'vanilla flavor' in the package, I want real vanilla, not some chemicals. I also want natural colors in the food."

To the question: "Why do you prefer natural foods?", note the following responses:

College Student: "I'm concerned about my health and diet. I'm getting married and a healthier mother will have healthier children. That's reason enough to stay away from junk foods."

Railroad Worker: "I was raised on a farm. I know what free scratching chicks, fertile eggs, real bread and home-made ice cream should be, and all our fruits and vegetables were organically grown. I'm almost 80, and I feel damn fine. I want to stick around a lot longer. That's why I favor the natural foods."

Schoolteacher: "I see so many of my students with their messed-up complexions, their sniffles, bad teeth, bad tempers. Their bad diet has plenty to do with their bad behavior and bad health. It's no different with adults either. Natural foods make the big difference. I won't gamble with my health."

Tire Salesman: "Like I told you, I can't afford to be overweight and sick. I've only made some gradual changes away from my old eat-everything style, but I can already feel the difference. I sleep better and I have much more pep. Starting to slim down, too."

Housewife: "I've learned that natural foods help keep us all well. I've got a big family. Natural foods mean better health for all of us."

Responses to question four — "What does the term 'health food store' mean to you?" — were as follows:

College Student: "It's a place to get food, vitamins, supplements as natural as I prefer them to be and plenty of variety too."

Retired Railroad Worker: "A place to get honest food and honest answers to my questions."

Schoolteacher: "Where else am I going to find such an assortment of really natural foods — I mean, honest-to-goodness natural foods?"

Tire Salesman: "To me, health foods and natural foods are the same. The more natural, the better."

215

Housewife: "It's my headquarters for good values. I don't get to many health food stores besides this one, but I like the kind of people that run them. There's just no place like a health food store."

To question five — "What items do you seek to obtain in a health food store?" — I obtained the following responses:

College Student: "Vitamins and fresh unsprayed fruits and vegetables and knowledgeable people about the products. I prefer natural vitamins and I feel better about those in a health food store."

Retired Railroad Worker: "I grow what I can, but in winter I depend on you to supply some of the produce. I don't eat much, but I like to try different things you stock. Also, I take certain vitamins you carry."

Schoolteacher: "I'm mostly interested in dried fruits and organic nuts, the latest health magazines, natural bakery items. For years, I've been taking a one-a-day vitamin just for insurance. It's only available in health food stores. I would never want to be without it."

Tire Salesman: "I'm still new to a lot of this, so I'm sort of groping around. My wife and I have been reading and learning and switching over to different things. No more coffee, for instance. We've been trying different coffee substitutes and nice fruit teas like mint and sassafras, delicious! Say, what the hell happened to sassafras? My wife tried baking bread but finds it easier to just buy the good bread from the health food store. Incidentally, I've been to about five or six health food stores and I'm pleased at the patience and help I get from you health food people wherever I go. And nobody tries to sell me anything I don't want."

Housewife: "Just about everything except toilet paper. That, I still get at the supermarket." . . .

> *When the Federal Trade Commission first proposed to regulate food advertising a decade or so ago, they suggested that the terms* organic, natural, *and* health *should be entirely banned from food advertising as indefinable. A number of people came forward to object. It was relatively easy, they said, to construct a definition of an organic food. The term* natural *had fewer defenders — even though it made many people uneasy to think that in an increasingly artificial world nothing could be called* natural. *The most articulate defender of the term was Annette Dickinson, whose testimony on the matter is presented here.*

STATEMENT BEFORE THE FEDERAL TRADE COMMISSION*

Annette Dickinson

I am Annette Dickinson, Director of Government Affairs for a trade association of nutrient supplement manufacturers, the Council for Responsible Nutrition. . . . I consider it particularly important that the term "natural" be retained and if possible defined. . . .

I believe that those of us who care about basic, traditional foods are in danger of losing our freedom of choice in the marketplace, as traditional foods are gradually replaced by new products. I believe that the term "natural" has sufficient selling power not only to encourage consumers to buy "natural" products, but also to encourage manufacturers to produce more truly "natural" products. I would like to see the term used in this way as an incentive for the production of more basic, minimally processed foods, free of artificial ingredients. . . .

In attempting to define "natural foods," I believe it is helpful to consider that there is a hierarchy of processes used on food, ranging from trivial to severe. These processes can be grouped to some extent, and a series of decisions to accept or reject each group of processes as appropriate or inappropriate for "natural foods" will result in the outlines of a definition.

First, assuming that the source of all natural foods will be plants and animals, one must decide whether the term "natural" will apply to the treatment the food receives after harvesting, or whether the term will include the methods of agriculture used to produce the raw plant or animal. In the references I have cited, it seems clear that a dis-

---

*Annette Dickinson, testimony before the Federal Trade Commission. FTC, 1976–77. *Rulemaking Record of the Proposed Trade Regulation Rule on Food Advertising, Phase I Public Record Number 215–40.*

tinction is drawn between "natural" and "organic," with the former applying only to post-harvest processing and the latter applying to the methods of culture.

Second, one must decide whether any processing at all will be accepted for products labeled as "natural." While I believe that the term "natural" implies minimum processing, as well as the absence of synthetic ingredients, *some* basic processing should be allowed, including at least treatments which primarily accomplish the removal of inedible portions of the product. These would include washing, skinning, shelling, plucking, seeding, and coring.

Third, one must decide whether to accept certain physical treatments which may result in some waste of edible portions, but which fundamentally do not alter the makeup of the raw product. These would include peeling, cutting, slicing, dicing, grinding, and mashing.

Fourth, one must decide whether it is acceptable for a "natural" food to be heated (including cooking) or cooled (including freezing). Since presumably "natural foods" will not be permitted to contain preservatives, I believe heating and cooling should be permitted to accomplish minimal preservation.

Fifth, one must decide whether the traditional process of fermentation may be permitted. Even though fermentation results in considerable changes in the raw materials, I believe fermentation should be accepted as a "natural" process, since it is so well established that it is recognized as one of the oldest forms of food preservation known to man.

Sixth, one must decide whether "natural" foods may be partitioned into their component parts. Partitioned foods have been described . . . as those purified components which are separated from the whole, intact, basic food. The partitioning of foods would include the pressing of seeds and nuts to produce purified oils, or the pressing of fruits to produce juices, or the separation of whole milk into cream and skim, or the separation of ground whole wheat into the bran, germ and endosperm. The decision about partitioning is perhaps the most troublesome aspect of defining the term "natural," for partitioning may result in either a loss or a concentration of nutrients, fiber and flavor. It may be possible to permit partitioning of "natural" foods only in those instances where the partitioned end product contains all or most of the indigenous nutrients in the whole food, but even this solution is not complete. Some consumer surveys may be necessary to determine the strength of various consumer expectations regarding "natural" partitioned foods.

Seventh, one must decide whether to accept relatively severe physical and chemical treatments such as dehydration, distillation, extraction, hydrolysis and enzymolysis. I believe that a consumer survey would show that most of these processes are not perceived as appropriate for "natural" foods, yet some of these are specifically permitted by FDA for natural flavorings. This is one instance in which it may be necessary to resolve conflicts between existing regulations and any new definitions that may emerge.

Eighth, one must decide whether two or more individual "natural" foods may be combined to create formulated natural food products. Such formulated products may be simple, as in the case of mixed nuts, or rather complex as in the case of whole wheat bread or clam chowder. One alternative may be to allow only single-component foods to be marketed outright as "natural," but to allow formulated products made from two or more natural ingredients to be labeled "made from all natural ingredients."

If it is decided to permit products made up of two or more ingredients to be called "natural," then a number of complications are introduced which may need to be handled individually. The status of added salt, for example, would need to be decided. The addition of flavorings, colorings and nutrients would need to be handled in some uniform way.

These judgments are complex, but no more complex than judgments made by FTC, FDA and other regulatory agencies in other proceedings. It is well within the competence of either the FTC or the FDA to promulgate a reasonable uniform definition of "natural" foods as an aid to those consumers who want to seek out such products and as an incentive to manufacturers to direct more of their efforts toward producing foods which are minimally processed, which are free of synthetic ingredients, and which retain all or most of their indigenous nutrients, fiber, color and flavor.

> *Most of the issues over which we battle in nutrition never come to formal trial. But the merits of defining or banning "natural," "organic," and "health" as descriptions of food were chewed over by lawyers, witnesses and a law judge — and ultimately by the Federal Trade Commission staff. Here, drastically cut in length but with its principal arguments intact, is part of the staff's 1978 report presenting its conclusions about the definability of these terms — and the desirability of defining them.*

NATURAL AND ORGANIC FOOD CLAIMS AND HEALTH AND RELATED CLAIMS*

Federal Trade Commission Staff

1. §§437.6(a) and (b) — Natural Food Claims

a. Evidence
The record demonstrates that the designation of specific foods as "natural" is highly controversial. As will be shown, the term is ill-defined and frequently abused. Nonetheless, so-called "natural" foods have been — and continue to be — heavily promoted, with considerable success. . . .

Existing scientific and regulatory standards. . . .The record makes it abundantly clear that there is no generally accepted definition, either regulatory or scientific, which delimits the appropriate use of the term "natural" as applied to food. In the absence of such a definition, the term can be — and in fact has been — used by advertisers to suit their own purposes in promoting and selling various food products. . . .

Many nutritionists, food technologists, and other scientists who testified at the hearings were of the opinion that it is scientifically inappropriate to designate any particular food as "natural" because the term is not only undefined, but also undefinable. In this connection, several experts testified that, in the scientific sense, virtually all foods are "natural," as opposed to artificial or synthetic. While totally synthetic or artificial foods may be possible in the future, today's foods, according to this viewpoint, are either "natural" or manufactured from "natural foods."

---

*"Natural and Organic Food Claims and Health and Related Claims," by the U.S. Federal Trade Commission. Proposed trade regulation rule on food advertising. *16 CFR Part 437*, Phase I. Staff report and recommendations. September 25, 1978, pages 206–251.

Despite rather considerable resistance among many scientists to the use of the term "natural food," it was generally recognized that two major elements — minimal processing and the absence of artificial or synthetic ingredients or additives — were integral to the concept. Indeed, even experts who considered the term undefinable were aware of this usage.

Moreover, although many scientists opposed the use of the term "natural," it should be emphasized that many other experts testified that the term has scientific validity. Those who took this position were concerned that our diets were becoming increasingly dependent upon fabricated, highly processed foods. In their view, it is important that consumers eat a variety of foods, and that some foods in the diet be "natural" (i.e., relatively unprocessed) foods. . . .

To reiterate briefly . . . First, it is clear that the term "natural" refers to the processing of a food after it has been harvested, as distinguished from the term "organic," which refers to the method of growth. Second, there is widespread agreement that a "natural" food should be subjected to only minimal processing after harvest. Finally, a "natural" food is generally recognized as not containing artificial additives or other artificial ingredients.

Of these criteria, serious problems are presented only by the second one. Most of the witnesses who believed that the term "natural" was undefinable premised this conclusion upon their inability to clarify the term "minimal processing." . . .

Illustrative advertising claims. The record amply demonstrates the diverse and inconsistent usages and meanings of the term "natural" in food advertising. Indeed, in the absence of regulatory standards, it appears that advertisers have used the term whenever, and wherever, it suited their purposes to do so.

Among other things, the term "natural" has been applied to foods which run the gamut insofar as extent of processing is concerned. For example, some advertisements use the term to describe unprocessed fruits and vegetables, such as bananas . . . and grapefruits. . . . Dairy products such as milk . . . and cottage cheese . . . are described as "natural," despite the fact that at least some processing (e.g., pasteurization, homogenization, etc.) is obviously involved. At the other extreme, highly processed products such as instant bouillon, frozen onion rings . . . yogurt chips, . . . and vitamin and mineral supplements . . . are also characterized as "natural."

Advertising claims are equally confusing and inconsistent with regard to the presence of additives in a "natural" food. For example, the claim that a food is "natural" has been made for orange juice that contains "no additives," . . . cereal that has "no preservatives," . . . and another cereal that has "no artificial preservatives." Presumably, both of these cereals could contain artificial flavors or colors and still fall within this self-serving definition of "natural." Finally, still another

221

"natural" cereal is vitamin fortified, meaning that vitamins have been added. . . .

Furthermore, there are advertisements which characterize foods as "natural" even though they are processed and contain synthetic additives. Both Kellogg's All-Bran . . . and Post Grape Nuts. . . are described as "natural," but they have been processed to a considerable degree and fortified. The All-Bran package indicates that the product also contains BHA and BHT, chemical preservatives. Similarly, Mrs. Paul's onion rings are fried in batter and frozen, and thus are highly processed. They also contain additives. Nonetheless, they are characterized as "natural" simply because the onion ring inside is sliced, rather than diced and re-formed. . . .

Consumer understanding. . . . The record clearly reflects that consumers are confused in at least two respects: they lack understanding of the term "natural food," and they misunderstand it by confusing it with the term "organic." . . .

A significant number of consumers believe that a "natural food" is one which is grown by "organic" methods. Yet this understanding is clearly incorrect since it does not comport either with scientific understanding or with the way "natural" foods are manufactured. Thus, the expectations of many consumers are violated under any of the current usages. . . .

Notwithstanding the widespread consumer confusion regarding the term "natural food," it is noteworthy that the record also indicates that some consumers appear to have at least a general grasp of the term. Both the testimony and the consumer research reflect some agreement among consumers that a "natural food" should not contain additives and, to a lesser degree, agreement that it should be only minimally processed. . . .

Quite apart from the issue of consumer confusion, the record also demonstrates that substantial numbers of consumers perceive "natural" foods to be nutritionally superior to, and/or safer than, their non-natural (or "unnatural") counterparts. Experts in consumer psychology testified that such inferences were readily drawn by consumers, a conclusion also reached by numerous other witnesses, including scientists and consumer representatives. Thus, the weight of the testimonial evidence clearly establishes that the term leads consumers to infer that there is something special about a "natural" food which makes it superior to a food which is not so characterized. . . .

Scientific evidence regarding perceived superiority. As has been demonstrated, advertising has represented — and a significant number of consumers believe — that "natural" foods are superior on nutritional and/or safety grounds to their non-natural counterparts. Yet the nutritionists, food technologists, and other scientific experts who testified at the hearings consistently stated that such was simply not the case.

Hence, it must be regarded as scientifically established that "natural" foods are not inherently superior, either in terms of nutrient content or safety, to foods which are not so characterized. . . .

2. §§437.6(c) and (d) — Organic Food Claims

a. Evidence

As with the term "natural," the advertising of specific foods as "organic" (or "organically grown") is the subject of considerable dispute. . . .

Existing scientific and regulatory standards. The record demonstrates that there is a well-established scientific definition of the term "organic," namely, a material containing the element carbon. Thus, as was repeatedly emphasized, virtually all foods are "organic" in the only sense in which that term is scientifically meaningful. Similarly, since all soil contains some organic matter, all crops could be considered "organically grown."

In the face of this accepted scientific meaning, most scientists were reluctant to conclude that the term "organic" could legitimately be used in any other manner. Nonetheless, most of the scientific witnesses who addressed this issue were aware that the designation of a food as "organic" (or "organically grown") had come to be used, generally outside the scientific community, to refer to the method by which the food had been grown. Specifically, it was recognized that the term "organic food" (or "organically grown food") generally encompassed concepts such as the use of organic material and the non-use of artificial fertilizers or pesticides during the growth process. Thus, while scientists are largely unwilling to accept this use of the term as scientifically meaningful, they are nonetheless generally aware of the concepts involved.

Despite questions raised by many scientists as to the sufficiency of existing definitional standards, several witnesses from the organic foods industry maintained that a viable and accepted definition of the terms "organic" and "organically grown" already exists. That definition, which was developed by the editors of *Organic Gardening and Farming,* an organic foods magazine, states as follows:

"Organically grown food is produced on humus-rich soil whose fertility has been maintained with organic materials and natural mineral fertilizers. No pesticides, artificial fertilizers or synthetic additives are used in the production of organic foods."

However, witnesses representing other segments of the food industry were less certain of the existence of, and adherence to, any uniform definitional standards, and concluded that there was considerable conflict in these respects.

223

Finally, it should be noted that . . . at least one state, Oregon, has already adopted a definition of the term, and several others are apparently moving in this direction. . . .

In conclusion, with the exception of Oregon and perhaps a few other states, there are no regulatory standards governing the use of the term "organic food." However, the standards set forth in the Oregon definition (and in the *Organic Gardening* definition) appear to be those which representatives of the organic foods industry agree should be applied. Moreover, the general concepts contained in these definitions are recognized, albeit often reluctantly, by the scientific community. . . .

Consumer understanding. The record convincingly establishes that there is significant consumer confusion regarding the use of the terms "organic food" and, to a somewhat lesser degree, "organically grown food." . . .

(1) when asked to define the term "organic" (or "organically grown"), consumers give widely dispersed responses, which is indicative of confusion; and (2) a substantial number of consumers incorrectly infer that these terms are concerned with processing and food additives. . . .

This does not mean, however, that there is a complete lack of understanding among all consumers. To the contrary, the record reflects that a significant number of consumers recognize that the term "organic" is concerned with some aspect of the method of growth. Although most of those consumers who exhibited some understanding of the term were unable fully to define it, they were nonetheless able to set forth at least one element related to the concept (e.g., use of organic fertilizers, non-use of artificial fertilizers or pesticides). It can therefore be said that at least some consumers have expectations regarding "organic" food which are generally consistent with definitions such as the Oregon definition or the definition suggested by *Organic Gardening.* . . .

Regardless of how well they understand the term "organic" as applied to food, many consumers infer that a food described in this fashion is inherently superior, in terms of nutrient content and/or safety, to ordinary "non-organic" food. This fact was attested to by a number of witnesses with a wide variety of backgrounds, and is also reflected in the consumer research. . . .

Scientific evidence regarding perceived superiority. Given the existence of consumer beliefs that "organic" foods are higher in nutrient content and/or safer than other foods, the next question to be resolved is whether those beliefs are accurate. . . .

The vast preponderance of the evidence indicates that "organic" foods are not nutritionally superior to ordinary foods. Thus, the inference of nutritional superiority, which a significant number of consum-

224

ers draw from the use of the term, is false.

Turning to the issue of relative safety, the first matter to be considered is whether either form of fertilizer poses toxicity problems. Although questions were raised about the safety of synthetic or inorganic fertilizers, soil scientists and nutritionists concurred that, with proper use, both types of fertilizer are perfectly safe to use on crops which are intended for human consumption. . . .

The major question addressed with regard to safety was whether "organic" food is safer by virtue of the non-use of pesticides. Scientists who testified in this area agreed that there was no inherent danger of accumulation of harmful substances in foodstuffs due to the regular use of pesticides. . . .

Of equal importance is the fact that the non-use of pesticides does not mean that the food produced is necessarily free of residues. Even when a food is not intentionally subjected to pesticides, it may nevertheless contain pesticide residues by virtue of wind-drift, storage conditions, or previous soil conditions. . . .

To summarize briefly, the levels of pesticide residues found in "organically grown" foods are not necessarily lower, let alone *significantly* lower, than those in commercially grown foods. Moreover, even if "organically grown" foods did contain significantly lower levels, the difference could not provide a basis for a superiority claim because all foods containing pesticide residues that are within the established tolerances are safe. . . .

Conclusion. As with the term "natural," the absence of a uniform standard governing the use of the terms "organic" and "organically grown" has led to confusion and deception. By virtue of the lack of uniformity, advertisers have been able to designate their foods as "organic" based upon their own understanding of the term. Not only has this contributed to the confusion, but it has also created the potential for deception in those instances where the consumer's understanding of the term differs from that of the advertiser. . . .

In assessing possible regulatory action to remedy the aforementioned problems, the same three options which were considered in connection with the term "natural" are also available here. Briefly stated, those options include inaction, standardization, and prohibition. . . .

The first option, inaction, would not remedy the actual or potential deception arising out of the unrestricted use of the term. In fact, it is submitted that it is unfair for claims to continue to be made against this background of confusion and misunderstanding.

The original staff proposal would have prohibited the use of the terms "organic" and "organically grown" in food advertising. . . .

Staff has been convinced by the rulemaking record that these terms can be used accurately in accordance with certain standards. . . . Staff has changed its position and now recommends the

225

adoption of standards, consistent with consumer expectations, to regulate the use of the terms "organic" and "organically grown." Staff believes that this less restrictive alternative would be as effective as a prohibition in eliminating deception and unfairness. The adoption of uniform standards, particularly if they are communicated to consumers, will help dispel existing confusion and prevent future deception. Furthermore, this approach recognizes the consumer's desire to use the term "organic" to reflect a life-style choice in the foods he or she eats, despite the fact that, from a scientific standpoint, those foods do not differ from their commercial counterparts. . . .

3. §§437.10(b) — Health Food Claims

a. Evidence

The term "health food" was widely regarded by those participating in this proceeding as the most confusing and misleading of the terms under consideration. The record demonstrates that the term, as applied to any particular food, is inherently deceptive and incapable of qualification. Moreover, the term is both undefined and undefinable. Under the circumstances, the term "health food" stands in stark contrast to the term "natural," where the underlying concept is legitimate and accepted, or the term "organic," where an objectively definable secondary usage has been accepted as meaningful by consumers. As will be shown, there is no alternative but to prohibit the use of this term in advertising.

Existing scientific and regulatory standards. The record amply demonstrates the complete absence of standards governing the use of the term "health food." . . .

All of the scientific experts who testified in this area agreed the term should be prohibited on the grounds that it is undefined, undefinable, and inherently deceptive. Indeed, even those who opposed a ban on the use of the terms "natural" and "organic" concluded that a prohibition was appropriate in this case.

The inherently meaningless and deceptive nature of the term is further illustrated by the fact that no one even sought to suggest standards which might govern its use. . . .

Consumer understanding. The record provides abundant support for two major findings regarding consumer perception of the term "health food." First, it is clear that there is overwhelming confusion surrounding the use of the term. Second, a significant number of consumers interpret the term as implying that the foods described in this manner are more healthful than foods which are not so described. . . .

. . . In contrast to the terms "natural" and "organic," the record

226 demonstrates that there are absolutely no criteria regarding the use of the term "health food" which are generally accepted among consumers. In fact, it is evident that the term is as meaningless to consumers as it is to scientists. . . .

Scientific evidence regarding perceived superiority. The record establishes through expert testimony that no single food is capable of maintaining or ensuring good health, and that all foods are capable of contributing to good health if not consumed in excess. Experts in nutrition repeatedly emphasized that health is a property of an individual, not a food. Moreover, health is dependent upon a number of dietary and non-dietary factors. Insofar as food is concerned, good health rests upon eating a balanced diet involving the right choices and combinations of foods. It is the balanced diet, not the particular foods which constitute it, which is conducive to good health.

In sum, the representation that one food is more healthful than another, or that a food is of some special significance, in and of itself, in ensuring good health, is false and deceptive.

Conclusion. Staff concurs with the Presiding Officer in recommending a prohibition against describing any particular food(s) as "health food(s)." The term "health food" is inherently deceptive in that it falsely attributes special or superior health-giving properties to certain foods. Moreover, the term is not capable of being qualified or defined in any meaningful fashion.

> *In light of nutritionists' general agreement that the term "health foods" should be banned, Denise Foley's article raises some interesting and thought-provoking questions. Even if "health foods" is an indefinable term, would nutritionists not agree that some foods are healthier than others? Are the "superfoods" listed here healthy for everyone? Is it simply stubbornness that makes us resist calling foods we agree are healthy "health foods"?*

THE TOP 25 'SUPERFOODS'*

Denise Foley

There was a time when the phrase "health food" conjured up the image of a monastic meal with all the lip-smacking lusciousness of grass and moon dust.

Today, healthy foods have taken on a whole new mainstream meaning. No longer esoteric edibles available only in health-food stores, they're foods fresh from the supermarket and produce stand, superfoods that medical researchers believe really may make us healthy.

Their evidence? Healthy people like the Eskimos, whose snacks of whale blubber should make them prime candidates for heart disease before 40 but whose fish diet actually seems to protect their hearts from harm; Italy's Neapolitans, whose high-fiber, low-fat natural foods keep them fit; the Seventh-day Adventists, largely vegetarians who serve up a menu for long life.

There's evidence from the laboratory too. Did you know that there is a substance in cabbage and its clan that actually may "trap" cancer-causing agents in your body before they do any harm? Or that carrots, rich in beta-carotene, can decrease your risk of lung cancer? Or that something called a protease inhibitor found in seeds, beans and rice may actually be an antidote to the cancer-causing effects of a high-fat diet?

Like medical research, we turned to the laboratory and to healthy people when we put together our own well-balanced menu of superfoods. We also filled in with some of the foods Mother Nature blessed with a cornucopia of nutrients, such as liver, oysters and green and red peppers. To make shopping easier, we included foods that, with perhaps one exception, you can find in any supermarket. And we offer them now to you with a toast: To your health!

Amaranth

You might not find this little-known grain on your market shelves — yet. Amaranth is a food of the future. It is literally manna to the millions of malnourished people of the Third World because it is remarkably high in protein and lysine, an essential amino acid — far higher than any other cereal grain. It also contains significant amounts of iron and magnesium. And it's versatile. You can use its leaves in salad and its seed for breakfast cereal, snacks or flour for baking.

Bananas

The banana disputes the old theory that if something tastes good it can't be good for you. Bananas are a great-tasting source of potassium, vitamin B_6 and biotin, another B vitamin. A medium banana contains about 100 calories, making it a delicious snack or dessert for dieters.

Beans

If you don't know beans about beans, consider this: In several tests on patients with high blood lipids (a risk factor for heart disease), a bean diet brought down cholesterol and triglyceride levels significantly, with no serious side effects. Beans are also high in magnesium, a good heart mineral, and the B vitamins thiamine, B_6 and riboflavin. They're also an excellent nonmeat source of iron.

Bran

One researcher calls wheat bran "the gold standard" against which the other brans, like oat and corn, are measured. Well, these days the other two are measuring up just fine. In a study of the effects of bran on constipation, corn bran was found to be therapeutically superior to wheat bran, probably because corn bran is 92 percent fiber compared to wheat bran's 52 percent fiber. Another group of researchers, at the University of Texas Health Science Center, also found in a feeding study with rats that corn bran cereal, even though it contained sucrose, helped prevent cavities.

And oat bran has been found to lower cholesterol as much as 13 percent in studies done by James Anderson, M.D., and associates, at the Veterans Administration Medical Center in Lexington, Kentucky.

Cabbage and its Clan

Include broccoli, brussels sprouts and cauliflower in this happy family. They all figure prominently in the anticancer diet prescribed by the National Academy of Sciences a few years ago. They all appear to have some cancer-fighting properties, including vitamin A. And a cooked stalk of broccoli alone has all the Recommended Dietary Allowance of A and twice the RDA of vitamin C, another cancer fighter, as well as calcium and potassium. Cabbage, brussels sprouts and cauliflower contain a substance that has been shown to "trap" certain carcinogens before they do any damage to the body. University of

229

Minnesota researcher Lee Wattenberg, M.D., found that these vegetables enhance a natural detoxification system in the small intestine
that keeps the carcinogen away from susceptible tissues.

Carrots
Carrots are very high in beta-carotene, a precursor of vitamin A that is
associated with a decreased risk of cancer. High in fiber, low in calories, even the crunch in carrots is good, toning and strengthening the
gums.

Citrus Fruits
A group of Florida researchers noticed an interesting statistic. Residents of southeastern Florida, many of whom have backyard citrus
trees, have a lower incidence of colon and rectal cancers than people
in the northern parts of the nation. The scientists at Florida Atlantic
University in Boca Raton believe the secret is in the fruit. They say
the vitamins A, C and E and pectin fiber have a synergistic effect that
may prevent cancer.

Fish
Holy mackerel! Would you believe you could lower your blood pressure and cholesterol and triglyceride levels by eating mackerel and
salmon? Researchers worldwide have discovered that certain types of
fish — those containing eicosapentanoic acid, a fatty acid — protect
against heart disease. They were tipped off by the healthy hearts of
Greenland Eskimos, whose diets were otherwise high in fat. Apparently, it's a special kind of fat, which researchers at the Oregon Health
Sciences University say may be "metabolically unique" and useful in
controlling other fats that can clog the bloodstream.

Garlic and Onions
Bad for your breath but wonderful for the rest of you. A spate of studies found these two odoriferous roots can lower your cholesterol and
their oils inhibit tumor growth in the laboratory. Onions have been
used to slow down platelet aggregation or clumping, which can lead to
deadly blood clots.

Herbs and Spices
Before you throw away your salt-shaker and sugar bowl, consider re-
filling them — with herbs and spices. They're actually more flavorful
substitutes. A couple of dashes of curry powder on fresh roasted nuts
or popcorn and you'll never miss the salt. And as for sweets, the
American Spice Trade Association found that desserts and beverages
with sugar and other sweeteners replaced by spices drew rave reviews
from a panel of tasters. They even loved blueberry shortcake sweet-
ened with fruit juice and cinnamon and creamy custard with reduced
230   sugar and a surprising bay leaf added for sweetness.

Kale, Spinach and the Leafy Greens
Your mother — and the National Academy of Sciences — insisted that you eat your leafy green vegetables. Here's why you should: Greens like spinach contain chlorophyll, a substance that helps plants turn sunlight into food. Chlorophyll also has been found to lower the tendency of cancer-causing agents to cause genetic damage to your body's cells. Spinach and the other greens also contain significant amounts of vitamin A and calcium, although their oxalic-acid content can change calcium into an indigestible compound in the body. Kale, on the other hand, has far more calcium than oxalic acid, so it's a good source of this bone-strengthening mineral.

Liver
Usually found smothered in another superfood, onions, beef liver contains almost every nutrient going. It's rich in iron, zinc, copper, vitamins A, E, K, thiamine, riboflavin, biotin, folate, B_{12}, choline and inositol. Who can ask for anything more?

Melons
Cantaloupes and honeydews are low-calorie treats or high-energy breakfast sources of vitamin C. One two-inch wedge of honeydew, for example, has only 49 calories but supplies more than half the RDA of vitamin C.

Nuts
You can consume a considerable portion of your minimum daily requirement of zinc during an afternoon snack if you're snacking on nuts. Nuts, especially cashews and almonds, are very high in this trace mineral so necessary for cell growth. But don't go nutty with nuts. Zinc notwithstanding, you're also munching a handful of calories, so enjoy them in moderation.

Oysters
Legend has it that oysters are an aphrodisiac. We don't make any claims for that, but oysters are high in zinc, shown to be necessary for proper prostate and sexual functioning and sperm motility. Oysters are also rich in calcium, iron, copper and iodine. But a word of caution. You'll rarely hear us say this about anything else: Don't eat them raw. Oysters tend to pick up bacteria that can make you ill if they're not cooked.

Peppers
Which has more vitamin C, an orange or a pepper? Better bet on the pepper. One of these gorgeous green beauties contains twice the vitamin C of an orange. And an amazing thing happens when peppers age. They turn red — and fill up with a good supply of vitamin A.

231

Poultry

Let's talk turkey. And chicken while we're at it. They're low in calories, low in fat, high in essential nutrients and taste. An average half a chicken breast contains 25.7 grams of protein, just 5.1 grams of fat and only 160 calories. With that you get a side order of vitamin A, riboflavin and niacin, not to mention iron. A chicken leg contains only 88 calories and 3.8 grams of fat. Turkey is equally good news. Three ounces of light meat without skin totals 150 calories, 28 grams of protein and 3.3 grams of fat, with respectable amounts of B vitamins.

Seeds

High in zinc and protein, seeds (such as pumpkin, sunflower and sesame seeds) also contain something called a protease inhibitor, which seems to help protect us against cancer. Protease inhibitors have been shown to prevent liver, mammary and colon cancer in cancer-prone laboratory animals.

Soup

It's not only good food, it's the food that makes you eat less. A study that analyzed the food diaries of 90 patients determined that those who ate soup more than four times a week ate fewer calories a day and lost more weight than those who didn't eat as much soup. In fact, the researchers found, a soup meal contained an average of 54.5 percent fewer calories than a nonsoup meal.

Soybeans

They're good protein — as good as animal sources, say nutritionists at the Massachusetts Institute of Technology. They lower cholesterol, say researchers at Washington University School of Medicine. And there's some indication that soybeans are cancer fighters. Like seeds, soybeans contain protease inhibitors. And soybean products like tofu (bean curd) and miso (soybean paste) tested by researchers in Tokyo seemed to inhibit potential carcinogens called n-nitrosamines in the stomach.

Sprouts

They're more than just a grassy accoutrement to salad and sandwich. Studies show that the ascorbic acid (vitamin C) in some sprouted seeds and beans increases 29- to 86-fold after germination! Mung bean sprouts are especially high in magnesium and calcium. But the best news concerns the wheat sprout. It's been shown to inhibit the genetic damage to cells caused by some cancer-causing agents.

Sweet Potatoes

This superfood is a sleeper that deserves to appear on the dinner table at times other than Thanksgiving and Christmas. Besides being tastier than white potatoes — no relation — they're high in vitamin A,

232

the substance that makes carrots such a potent cancer-fighter. Sweet potatoes are also low in calories. One five-inch potato contains only 148 calories.

Wheat Germ
The B vitamin thiamine is abundant in only a few foods. But one of them is wheat germ, which is also rich in vitamin B_6. This versatile food was once relegated to the breakfast table but is now being used in everything from breads to salads.

Whole Grains
Writer Henry Miller once said, "You can travel 50,000 miles in America without once tasting a piece of good bread." But that was a generation ago, when the only place you could get a piece of good whole-grain bread was at the health-food store or in the kitchen of a wise, healthy cook. Whether it's bread, cereal or brown rice, the whole grains are the way to go. They're an excellent source of dietary fiber, suspected of protecting us from everything from cholesterol to cancer. A recent Welsh study found that people who ate whole-meal bread were less likely to die from cerebrovascular disease.

Yogurt
African Masai warriors eat large portions of fermented cow's milk daily, which makes their already low cholesterol levels drop even lower. In the United States, fermented cow's milk is marketed as yogurt and appears to have a similar effect on American cholesterol levels. When 26 people in a study at Vanderbilt University went on a diet of whole- and skim-milk yogurt, their cholesterol levels dropped significantly. Rich in calcium and all the nutrients in a glass of milk, yogurt is also easier to digest for people who are intolerant to plain milk.

For food scientist Vernal Packard, "health food" is one among many words that has a fuzzy meaning. What on earth is an "organic food"? And what would a "natural food" be?

NATURAL? ORGANIC? WHAT DO THEY REALLY MEAN?*

Vernal S. Packard, Jr., Ph.D.

If you can't define it, then it doesn't really exist. Whether by word or mathematical formula, this truism is a fact of the physical world. That also makes it fact for so-called natural, organic, or health foods. You must first be able to define them, to know precisely what they are. And then, and only then, can you make judgment of their relative worth. This is as true for foods found in "health" or "natural" food stores.

Today, as never before, natural/organic foods defy definition. The name on the label, except in rare instances where a state (such as Oregon) has established a formal legal definition, truly tells you little or nothing. A consumer can only guess at the meaning. And more often than not, it is a guarded secret, closeted in the minds or files of growers or processors, which can imply as many different definitions as there are people in the business. . . .

In the supermarket "natural" may mean absence of artificial colors or flavors — in one food product, that is. In another it may imply an absence of preservatives, or perhaps only "artificial" preservatives.

Ascorbic acid (either naturally occurring or synthetic, who knows?) in food products is okay; BHA and BHT are out. Pure vanilla extract, a natural, is defined into a product. Vanillin, an artificial cousin, is shunned. Or is it? Or a cereal product may be called "natural" and contain no additives, not even health rendering vitamins and minerals. But the product's sugar content may soar above comparable products, the food itself may be "processed" in some manner, and the fat consist chiefly of the hard (saturated) kind.

These are only a sprinkling of potential inconsistencies to be found in any supermarket.

"Health" food stores offer even greater variety and certainly more ingenuity of definition, an ingenuity borne of a compulsion to be set apart from the conventional. When tradition makes inroads on sacred territory, the strict advocate moves out. He or she seeks new identity,

---

*"Natural? Organic? What Do They Really Mean?" by Vernal S. Packard, Jr. *The Professional Nutritionist*, Summer 1978, pge. 1–3. Foremost-McKesson, Inc. Used with permission.

here related to the food eaten. Not that "natural" food stores are fre-
quented only by rebels to the establishment; not any longer.

You will find there consumers interested in something new and
different. Others are seeking special health benefits known only to
themselves. And not a few pay the higher price (two times that of
similar fare purchased in supermarkets, according to more than one
survey) out of unawareness. For those falling in the latter category,
especially the elderly living on fixed incomes, one must feel pity and
not a small sense of outrage.

Historically, natural foods were limited pretty much to products
grown without use of pesticides. They were neither treated nor mixed
with additives of any kind. They were, for the most part, unrefined —
not further processed from the state in which they grew on the land.

But as the "movement" progressed, these standards were sub-
verted. In came a host of qualifications, dependent solely upon features inherent in the food and the imagination of the supplier.

So how bad can it get? Let's take a simple example: milk. Certainly
milk is a product that could be produced under a concept of "natural."
To begin with, the cows would have to be fed natural feed, i.e., feed
untreated with pesticides of any kind. No matter how thick the weeds,
no matter how bad the infestation of corn borer, no pesticides. Well, it
can be done, profitability notwithstanding.

Then, too, "chemicals" get into milk through treatment of animals
with drugs. While regulations specify withholding periods for milk from
cows treated with drugs — antibiotics, for example — a purist would
simply not allow any of it, period.

And how about the containers in which milk is handled on the
farm. Should they be clean? You bet! Diseases like diphtheria, septic
sore throat, tuberculosis, polio, and undulant fever, among others, are
all transmissable through milk as a carrier.

But what kind of cleaning compound should we use? Deter-
gents — aren't they man-made chemicals, synthetics? Seems to me
they are. Well, soap then. But commercial soap? Isn't it processed with
chemicals too? Ah, I've got it! How about home-made soap — lye and
animal fat? We'll clean the milk-handling equipment in soap made
from pure lye and pork fat, just like great-grandmother used to do.
One could also allow beef fat, I suppose. Or any animal fat.

Though come to think of it, isn't the fat of the animal the place
where pesticides like DDT lodge? Perhaps the animal from which the
fat comes also ought to be housed and fed "naturally." That would
take care of that. Don't allow pesticides anywhere on the farm; use
only the fat of those animals pastured on that farm. Good! I like that.

Sanitizers? You use sanitizers to kill any residual bacteria missed
during cleaning. You can't be sure those few aren't disease germs,
either. One really should sanitize equipment. No reason why not, except that some sanitizers currently permitted by FDA for dairy farm
use are synthetics.

Perhaps we should stick with something like hypochlorites —
bleach. They're not synthetics. Or, if worse comes to worse, we could
simply petition FDA to allow use of some "natural" sanitizer. Of
course, then we'd have to prove efficacy and safety. But that costs
money, lots of it. Forget it! We'll stick with hypochlorites.

Pasteurization? That would kill all disease germs. There's certainly
value in that. But I seem to remember reading somewhere that un-
heated milk has some special health-promoting qualities. Some medical
doctor wrote the article. He ought to know. And pasteurization is, after
all, a form of processing. Natural should really be limited to unprocessed — raw — milk. We'll take our chances with disease. I know people
who have drunk raw milk all their lives and never had a day of sick-
ness. Or, if we have to pasteurize it, I guess we could. Some people
might not buy it otherwise. I wonder what temperature we should
use?

And the container: Isn't glass more natural than paper or plastic?
Don't they use "chemicals" in the manufacture of paperboard? Plastics
are *made* of them. . . .

And so it goes, all in the name of definition and personal or ideo-
logical idiosyncracy.

What's more, incongruities and misconceptions abound. For the
"natural" food consumer, bone meal overflows as a rich source of calcium, phosphorus, and fluorine. But mechanically deboned meat, with
a fraction of a percent of bone dust mixed in, meets with cries of outrage and indignation, even though the method could salvage one to
five billion pounds of meaty food a year in the U.S. alone!

Honey can do no wrong. It is *the* natural sweetener. Yet its sweetness stems chiefly from the same sugar found in sugarcane and beet.
And bees that milk sugar from mountain laurel, rhododendron, azalea,
or oleander produce a honey with a deadly potent heart stimulant —
all quite natural. Or where artificial sweeteners are not added, you
now find "natural" sweetener added: sucrose, refined sugar.

Soybean lecithin has health properties unequalled. That same
lecithin, extracted and purified (because the soybean contains at least
five known anti-nutritional compounds) and placed in a product as an
additive, becomes to some a cause of fear and loathing.

In a fruit preserve, where none is needed, comes the label, "no
artificial preservatives added." Sugar itself, like salt, at high enough
concentrations is all a product may need.

And bread without preservatives could well cost you more than
bread with them. Without preservatives the bread gets stale faster; it
may go moldy with the production of poisonous aflatoxins. And
already we in the U.S. return to the grocer 100 million pounds of
bread each year — this in a world nagged by hunger and malnutrition
and threatened always with mass starvation.

Organic foods suffer the same potential for perversion. In the
beginning, and these foods hark back to the turn of the century, organ-

236

ic implied growth of plant crops on soil fertilized only with organic fertilizers. You could now add to that any one or more of the natural food traits already discussed.

In essence, though, this wing of the ideology shunned inorganic chemicals, those balanced soil nutrients made up of nitrogen, phosphorus, and potassium. The emphasis is on the chemical form in which these elements exist.

Yet it matters not to the plant one whit whether the nitrogen, phosphorus, and potassium originate in organic (containing carbon) or inorganic form. It's the nutrients they're after. And so long as they get them in ample amounts at the right time, one source serves equally as well as the other — except that it takes time for organic fertilizer to break down and release the nutrients to the plant. Fine, so long as the nutrients are available when the plant needs them. Add organic fertilizer at the wrong time and it actually *ties up* nutrients.

On the positive side, organic fertilizers do provide materials which tend to improve soil consistency, resulting in better moisture retention. It is for this reason that farmers who use inorganic fertilizers often plow back to the soil a crop of green manure. And certainly there is nothing wrong with the concept of re-cycling waste, be it manure, garbage, compost, or peanut hulls (among many others).

It is when the organic gardener attributes to his produce some special health or nutritional qualities that the movement goes awry. No less than three major scientific studies covering 10, 25 and 34 years, respectively, dispute that claim. No nutrient differences exist in food crops grown under the two different methods — none. Those who suggest otherwise are clearly and grossly in error, whether purposely so or out of innocent ignorance. And to suggest that a deep-rooted plant like alfalfa promises a special nutritional value because it draws its trace elements from a deeper strata of the soil, well . . .

We can only hope that those same enthusiasts of alfalfa come forward as advocates of alfalfa leaf protein. Here is a vast source of high-quality protein, one which the world may some day recognize as part of the answer to a malnutrition problem of immense proportions.

"Health" foods? To that term one must simply say no. It is clearly a misnomer giving to one set of foods more health promotion qualities than another set. Health is derived from eating a balanced diet of foods containing nutrients necessary for life. Balance implies kind and amount. All foods so taken provide health. And nobody has a corner on that market. (Or if the "health" food store does have an edge, it lies in the high cost of its fare, which might just force a few of us, who should, to eat less.)

All this will be meaningless to the more staunch advocates of the movement. Nor is it intended to deter home gardeners from using the best of natural/organic methods in recycling a variety of wastes back through the soil. And any gardener with a hoe and a little sweat can do battle with weeds fully as well as any herbicide known.

Nor are my comments intended to dissuade the movement to simpler ways of living, the back-to-the-land lifestyle. That, too, has its place and its own unique set of values. I am not even suggesting that some natural/organically grown foods do not fit reasonably well the more traditional definitions attached to them. Some do. But many more do not; more so today than at any time in the past.

For this reason the time has come to take some positive steps to clarify the situation. The options, though, are few.

There is education, perhaps, on a massive scale. That would help. And certainly nutrition education is sorely needed. From this standpoint, the natural/organic food controversy could serve as a focal point of interest. In the end, though, education can only go so far.

There comes a point where legal action becomes necessary. In this case a definition would be needed, and on a national basis.

The term "health" food can and should be outlawed. Just as surely there is no basis for assigning to organically grown foods *per se* any special nutritional significance. It does not exist. And there is indeed precedence for ruling out unsubstantiated nutritional claims. FDA does just this for a number of compounds governed by the agency's nutritional labeling regulations.

As for use and meaning of the term "natural," a different problem is posed. With suitable qualifications, greatly restrictive of present usage, the word and the foods could be defined. And there could well be a basis of comparison between these and other foods which in some way might represent a meaningful difference. Indeed, some pesticides, some drugs, some "chemicals" can be to some extent harmful. That these same compounds also provide enormous benefits in yield and quality of foods, for this one case in point, can perhaps be considered beside the point.

We may also choose to disregard the fact that naturally occurring foods, untouched by man-made chemicals, also contain numerous "unsafe" compounds, some as dangerous as to cause paralysis or cancer. We can even overlook the fact that certain additives are beneficial to life, that some are thought now to promote human longevity.

All these matters could well be discounted in favor of precise, meaningful use of the term "natural." One might even define into the word a requirement that such foods be "organically" grown. It could be done. And the word "natural" could well come to mean a food product produced and processed without use of pesticides, drugs, non-naturally-occurring (artificial) additives, etc. Such definition might also disallow use of the word "natural" where it has no true significance.

And then, finally, a costly (to consumers) though effective program could be set up to monitor producer and processor of these foods, just as is done in California in the certification of raw milk supplies for human consumption. All this could be done to assure the public interest. Given leave to a personal opinion, I doubt such effort worth the trouble. But until and unless it is undertaken, confusion and deception will reign unchecked where the terms natural and organic are applied to food.

> *This bit of doggerel, published originally in* Food & Nutrition News *(a publication of the National Live Stock and Meat Board), expresses a common complaint about organic foods. The accusation it makes was put much more directly by a former Secretary of Agriculture who once commented that before we returned the U.S. to organic farming, someone would have to decide "which 50 million of our people will starve." (Fergus M. Clydesdale and Frederick J. Francis. (1977).* Food, Nutrition, & You. *Englewood Cliffs, N.J.: Prentice-Hall, Inc. Page 69.)*
>
> *In the article that follows the poem, Dr. Thomas Jukes, an ardent seeker out of heresies, lays out somewhat more fully the argument that organic agriculture is all muck and mystery, and that only modern chemical agriculture can guarantee us a future food supply.*

SILENT FALL*

Man learned to feed, clothe, protect, and transport himself more efficiently so he might enjoy life.
He built cars, houses on top of each other, and nylon.
And life was more enjoyable.
The men called Farmers became efficient.
A single farmer grew food for 41 Industrialists, Artists, and Doctors,
And Writers, Engineers, and Teachers as well.
To protect his crops and animals, the Farmer produced substances to repel or destroy Insects, Diseases, and Weeds.
These were called Pesticides.
Similar substances were made by Doctors to protect humans.
These were called Medicine.
The Age of Science had arrived and with it came better diet and longer, happier lives for more members of Society.

---

*"Silent Fall." National Live Stock and Meat Board. *Food & Nutrition News*, Volume 47, Number 2, December-January 1975–1976. Used with permission.

Soon it came to pass
That certain well-fed members of Society
Disapproved of the Farmer using Science.
They spoke harshly of his techniques for feeding, protecting, and
preserving plants and animals.
They longed for the Good Old Days.
And this had emotional appeal to the rest of Society.
By this time Farmers had become so efficient, Society gave them a
new title:
Unimportant Minority.
Because Society could not ever imagine a shortage of food,
Laws were passed abolishing Pesticides, Fertilizers, and Food Pre-
servatives.
Insects, Diseases, and Weeds flourished.
Crops and animals died.
Food became scarce.
To survive, Industrialists, Artists and Doctors were forced to grow
their own food.
They were not very efficient.
People and governments fought wars to gain more agricultural land.
Millions of people were exterminated.
The remaining few lived like animals.
Feeding themselves on creatures and plants around them.
And these were called Organic Foods.

SCIENTIFIC AGRICULTURE AT THE CROSSROADS*

Thomas H. Jukes, Ph.D.

What is the matter with farming? Why is the food supply being attacked and criticized? Why has the safest of all pesticides, DDT, been
banned? Why are so many people paying fancy food prices for off-
grade "organic" junk? What does all the hullabaloo about additives, residues and cancer mean? Why can a few sensation-seeking "scientists"
give a safe food-seasoning compound a black eye? Why does the public listen to scare stories about food told by people who simply don't
know what they are talking about? Who would have dreamed ten years

*"Scientific Agriculture at the Crossroads" by Thomas H. Jukes. *Agrichemical Age Mag-azine.* © 1972 California Farmer Publishing Company, San Francisco, CA. Used with per-mission.

ago, that the California State Department of Agriculture and Health would back a bill setting standards for "organic foods"? — instead of prosecuting the merchandisers who peddle this shabby fraud!

In A Fix

What is going to happen to California agriculture; the pride and wonder of the farm world; the provider of delicious fruits and vegetables to the USA?

Plenty, unless some sense is brought into the situation. Don't look for any help from the so-called "environmentalist movement," run by city lads and lasses who live in automobiles and air-conditioned apartments, and who blandly tell you that "modern agriculture is an ecological disaster!" When is someone going to tell *them* that the farmer is a professional environmentalist who understands and cares for his patch of Mother Earth better than any ecoactivist? . . .

Where We Are

How did we get where we are in agriculture?

Two hundred years ago, the average family in the western world, just as in many of the disadvantaged countries today, had to spend most of its time grubbing a meager living from the soil. The lack of fertilizer, the presence of pests that demolished crops, and the absence of knowledge about plant-breeding all combined to keep most people hungry. Then chemists discovered that plants were actually nourished by chemical, or inorganic, fertilizers. Phosphate, potash, nitrate and ammonia were needed, and they could come either from the breakdown of manure by soil bacteria, or from rock phosphate, inorganic potash, nitrates and salts of ammonia. The agricultural revolution was on. With it started the industrial revolution and the waves of migration to the cities. As the years went by, the farmers fed more and more "city folk." You would not be reading this if it were not for the fact that one farmer in the USA now produces, on the average, enough food for more than forty non-farmers! Chances are you would be out hoeing weeds.

But one thing was missing a century ago — pesticides. This lack resulted in the Irish potato famine, in which a fungus blight turned the potato crop into a stinking black slime. One million people starved to death. Many of the survivors fled to the New World. They and their descendants worked hard and gave many great citizens to our country. And chemists solved the problem of the potato blight. It is still in the fields, but it is controlled by pesticides.

As agricultural knowledge increased by leaps and bounds, farming became increasingly scientific. Plant and animal breeding gave us fine

241

new strains of grains, vegetables, fruits, poultry, pigs and cattle. Delicacies that the average family could buy only once or twice a year are now in every supermarket, everyday. The new methods required careful regulation to see that the chemical tools for the farmers were properly used. Pure food laws were passed to make sure that only insignificant traces of unwanted residues were present in foods. As a result, millions of tons of food have been eaten by millions of people without a single case of illness in America being attributable to an approved procedure in scientific agriculture. In contrast, in countries where "organic" fertilizers, such as human waste, are used, food poisoning often results from intestinal disease organisms. For Nature is not kind to us. Deadly bacteria can lurk in putrid food and in the soil. Molds can produce cancer-causing substances in food.

A major part in solving the problem of food protection was played by acceptance of the principle of *comparative toxicity*. This says that if a chemical, such as a pesticide or a food additive, is used, the residues in food should be such that a daily portion of the food will contain no more than one-hundredth of a dose toxic to human beings. The toxic dose is often measured on two species of laboratory animals through a complete generation. In other words, we are trading off a large benefit — an abundant and cheap food supply — for a very small risk — the risk that one-hundredth of a toxic dose may be harmful. The trade-off has been a colossal success; so successful that an entire generation of healthy young people have been raised on food produced with the aid of pesticides and additives. As a direct result of the modern agricultural revolution, life is so easy that many people have nothing better to do than nit-pick. The voice of the prophet of Doomsday is heard in the land, proclaiming that bacon will cause mutations, that sex hormones will lead to cancer, and that antioxidants and mold preventives will keep food fresh beyond the time when it, by all rights, should be rancid and moldly, so therefore preservatives are bad. An article in an Eastern magazine said that the crops of the San Joaquin Valley were "poisoned," and that the "green landscape" was "lifeless." What nonsense!

Bugged Out

How did the big chemical companies oppose the campaign against DDT? They had a perfect answer. They bugged out. They quit making DDT. This is what the eco-activists would like to see happen to scientific agriculture in California. Quit using fertilizers, pesticides and big machinery! Back to dung heap, the fly swatter and the hoe! The Santa Cruz campus of the University of California has bought some horses to do the farm work. The Sierra Club advocates taking livestock out of feed lots and putting them back on the land, only sixty years after John Muir won his fight to drive the sheep out of Yosemite. If the critters in feed lots are to be sent back to the land, they won't be put in the peach orchards, vineyards and lettuce fields:

They will be turned out to graze in the National and State Parks. . . .

Without chemical fertilizers, pesticides, food additives and medicines for farm animals, it would be impossible to feed the people in the USA or in the world. Any legal measures to counteract the practice of scientific agriculture are against the public interest.

Well, says Biologist Barry Commoner, there may be some mystery, but in fact organic agriculture is different, and has different impacts on the soil, and the economics of farming.

A ROSE (NATURAL) IS A ROSE (ORGANIC) IS A ROSE?*

Barry Commoner, Ph.D.

The words "natural" and "organic" are troublesome new entries into the lexicon of everyday life. They turn up frequently to describe items ranging from breakfast food to cosmetics. The trouble arises with any effort to discover what these words mean when applied to any given item.

Take, for example, a well-known cereal, heavily advertised as "natural" because it contains no artificial preservatives. Fair enough. After all, it is surely true that in nature an artificial preservative — let us say butylated hydroxytoluene — does not occur as a constituent of grain. One can readily agree, therefore, that in contrast with the virgin grain a product containing BHT ought to be regarded as unnatural. Nor is this argument merely a matter of terminology, for there are good reasons to suspect that organic compounds that are not ordinarily synthesized by living things may often be incompatible with normal biochemical processes and therefore likely to disrupt some of them.

However, a serious natural food buff is not likely to be satisfied with the claim that a cereal is merely free of artificially added synthetics. What about the grain itself? Does it already contain artificial synthetic compounds when it arrives at the cereal packaging plant? After all, numerous synthetic organic compounds, many of them suspected of biologic effects, have been dispersed into the environment and are therefore likely to find their way into a crop. A great variety of pesticides, for example, are applied directly to the crop or the soil to control the ravages of unwanted forms of life. Traces of these substances, and sometimes more formidable amounts of them, occur in food crops either in their original form or as some metabolic product of equal or greater danger to the delicate balance of cellular chemistry. While the Food and Drug Administration does monitor foods for undue concentrations of pesticide residues and is supposed to keep such foods off the market, the serious health food fan is likely to find small comfort in this assurance.

244 *"A Rose (Natural) Is a Rose (Organic) Is a Rose?," by Barry Commoner. *Hospital Practice*, 10:147–148, April 1975. Edited portions used with permission.

And so, let us follow our fan to a health food store to find a sack of cereal, usually priced somewhat higher than the well-advertised "natural" one, this time labeled "organic." And let us suppose that the organic product is conscientiously labelled to show that the cereal crop from which it was made was grown without application of offending pesticides.

Will the organic food fans find this satisfactory? Some will not, asking in turn whether the grain was grown with artificial (sometimes called "chemical") fertlizers or with natural, organic ones. Now we enter a fascinating and confused realm, in which both lay zealots and scientific experts can become equally lost.

To begin with, let us recall some basic facts about plant nutrition. Green plants obtain raw materials for their biosynthetic processes in rather simple forms: carbon dioxide, water, nitrate, phosphate, and ionic forms of potassium, calcium, and other essential elements. Nitrogen, to choose a particularly contentious example, almost always enters the roots as nitrate, becoming assimilated by the plant's biochemistry into organic compounds such as amino acids and nucleotides. There is no doubt, then, that nitrate is a "natural" plant nutrient. Nevertheless, a strict organic farmer does not wittingly fertilize his crops with nitrate — or with ammonium salts, which are quickly converted to nitrate by soil bacteria.

Why should a natural plant nutrient such as nitrate be regarded as unnatural when added to the soil as fertilizer? To appreciate this argument we need to go back into soil ecology beyond the immediate entry of nitrogen into the roots. In a natural system, nitrate in the soil is derived from the gradual breakdown of humus, the dark, complex, polymeric material that gives the soil its "tilth." Nitrogen is integrally bound to the carbon atoms that make up the organic structure of humus, which is itself the end product of a complex chain of events that carries nitrogen into the soil. The main path of entry begins with the deposition of organic nitrogenous compounds on the soil in the form of animal feces and urine and the dead remains of animals and plants. These largely organic materials are subjected to hydrolytic and oxidative degradation by decay microorganisms, yielding organic low-molecular-weight products that support the growth of soil microbial flora. These processes finally yield a mass of microbial cells, which, on their death, together with some other remains, become humus. The other source of soil nitrogen is nitrogen-fixation, which also delivers the element to the soil system in organic form. Thus, in a natural soil system, untouched by human technology, nitrogen enters into the system in organic combination with carbon, largely as the nutrient for microorganisms that eventually produce humus.

Now a farmer who wishes to add nitrogen fertilizer to the soil to support crop nutrition has two main alternatives. Nitrogen can be added in a natural, organic form — as plant residues, manure, sewage, food wastes, or, for that matter, in the form of *any* nitrogenous or-

245

ganic compound that can be metabolized by the soil's microbial flora and thereby yield humus. Alternatively, nitrogen can be added in an equally natural, but *inorganic* form, such as nitrate or ammonia. The first choice is the one made by the organic farmer; the second is the conventional route of modern agricultural technology. The strict devotee of natural foods is likely to reject grain grown with inorganic fertilizer in favor of that grown "organically" with manure or compost, claiming that the nutritional value and keeping qualities are superior — a claim that at this point can neither be confirmed nor denied.

Is there, then, any point in differentiating between the two ways of supplying fertilizer nitrogen? Indeed there is. Considering the soil as an integrated system, there is a vast difference in the outcomes of the two methods. Because nutrient uptake is a work-requiring process, it must be driven by the root's oxygen-dependent energetic metabolism. Humus is much more than a store of nutrients; it is also the chief source of the soil's porosity, hence of its oxygen content, and therefore of the efficiency with which nutrients, such as nitrate, are taken up by the crop.

Thus, the critical difference between the alternative means of supplying nitrogen fertilizer is that the organic form leads to the production of humus, while the inorganic form does not. The use of synthetic urea as a fertilizer provides an informative test of this distinction. Urea is, of course, an authentic organic compound and is, in fact, an ordinary constituent of a clearly natural source of nitrogen — urine. The scientific agronomist may often cite the organic farmer's objection to pure urea as a fertilizer — it is a fairly common one in modern agriculture — as evidence of the irrational basis of organic farming. But is it?

While urea is, indeed, an organic compound, it will not support the bacterial growth that is essential for the formation of humus. When urea is metabolized, the products are ammonia and carbon dioxide. Thus, urea yields carbon in a form that will not support the oxidative metabolism of soil bacteria. To accomplish that, carbon must be in the reduced state, combined with hydrogen, as it is in nearly all more complex organic compounds. Although urea is an organic compound, by failing to support the growth of soil bacteria, and therefore the formation of humus, it does not qualify as an "organic fertilizer."

The intensive use of inorganic nitrogen fertilizer (or urea) may so overload a humus-depleted soil with nitrate as to cause it to leach into surface waters where nitrate levels may readily exceed public health standards. Leached nitrate also wastes expensive fertilizer synthesized from an increasingly diminished supply of natural gas. Apart from any other possible and yet to be established virtues, the use of organic fertilizer (as defined above) avoids these difficulties and holds the promise of restoring the natural source of soil fertility — humus. While it remains to be seen whether food grown in such naturally fertile soil contributes distinctively to the health of people, the practice can, it seems to me, contribute significantly to the health of the soil and the economy.

Is organic agriculture an invitation to starvation? Is it a nostalgic return to a pre-industrial lifestyle, incompatible with modern food needs? Or is it a way of growing food whose virtues have been lost sight of in our arguments over the quality of the food it produces? The article excerpted here was originally written in response to Dr. Juke's article included earlier. (We cannot, in this case, conceal our own views — but you still must decide for yourself where you come out on this issue.)

THE ORGANIC ALTERNATIVE*

Joan Dye Gussow, Ed.D.

With the passing years, the subject of "organic agriculture" appears to generate progressively more heat and less light in the nutrition literature. While those who sang the praises of compost-based fertilizers and crushed-garlic insect sprays were once viewed as relatively harmless cranks, the burgeoning environmental movement has both increased their numbers and, apparently, enlarged their menace potential. Here is a method of farming which, according to its critics, produces relatively expensive food and offers no advantages except emotional and sentimental ones; yet, if its many attackers are to be believed, it is now threatening to emerge from its Pennsylvania stronghold to displace a government-fostered agricultural system long recognized as the world's most "efficient" and productive.

In fact, more food is undoubtedly being "organically-grown" today than five years ago; moreover, for a variety of reasons, concern over the viability of certain modern farming practices may well be warranted. Nevertheless, the rapid displacement of "Scientific Agriculture" by "Organic Agriculture" seems, to put it mildly, unlikely.

Careless Arguments

As nutrition professionals, we have long been taught to view organic agriculture and the food it produces as one of the more extreme of the "fads" with which we must regularly contend. Harried by a growing swarm of ardent amateurs, and disturbed by the deceptions and excesses of some "health food" purveyors, we have understandably felt the need to mount a strong counterattack. Unfortunately, we have sometimes allowed ourselves to become careless in our arguments,

*"The Organic Alternative," by Joan Dye Gussow. *Nutrition Today Magazine*, 9:31–32, March/April 1974. Williams & Wilkins, Baltimore, MD. Used with permission.

turning to conventional wisdoms rather than available new information to buttress our long-held positions. This is especially true in regard to the "organic movement."

Conditioned to view anything preceded by the word "organic" as "faddist," most of us have failed to see what the proponents of "organic" agriculture have come to recognize — that the merits, if any, of the "organic" approach to agriculture must be evaluated separately from the merits, if any, of the food produced by such methods.

Not only is the usefulness of "organic" agriculture not dependent upon whether it produces more nutritious food (and at this point there is no *convincing* scientific evidence that it does, or does not), neither should our judgment of organic agriculture depend upon the nutritional beliefs of some of its supporters. We must not allow ourselves to be misled into believing that modern agriculture is unassailable simply because some of the people who attack it also recommend (however unwisely) apricot kernels and bone meal. Guilt by association is an unscientific principle.

Despite widespread evidence that ideas (and facts) can be wrong even when they are put forward by well-trained scientists, we continue to resist the notion that some ideas (and facts) may turn out to be right even though they were first put forward by "faddists." The recent discovery of the probable importance of fiber in the diet, a clear case of our having overlooked the forest for the trees, might stand as a reminder of our fallibility. Despite our prolonged attack on the intelligence and morals of those who questioned the healthfulness of the "refined" Western diet, those "faddists" may turn out in the end to have been somewhat more than half right all along.

Organic farming is not a fraud. Despite the fact that money has lured a number of cheaters into the "organic food market," farmers growing by the organic method often are not receiving premium prices for what they produce. Many of them sell their "organic" produce on the open market, for the going open market price. Considering this fact, it seems extraordinary how much hostility this relatively small band of growers and those who buy their produce have generated. Here is a group of farmers who choose to produce food by a variety of energy-conserving and non-polluting agriculture techniques. They are not breaking any laws; their food is safe and no less nutritious than food produced by farmers using other methods. Surely in this vast, free country we ought to be able to tolerate such independence of mind. Surely those who choose to experiment with "organic" agriculture ought to be allowed to do so without being harassed as faddists.

Needed Certification

The people who choose to buy the food these farmers produce ought to be told that we have no evidence that there is more or "better" nutrition in "organically grown" foods. However, unless we are willing to conduct the long-term intergenerational feeding studies that would be required to *prove* that there are no differences in total nutritional value, that is all that can be said to discourage would-be "organic food" purchasers. Therefore, if people choose to buy organically grown foods, whether they do so in an attempt to live a more "natural" life, as a way of supporting organic agriculture, or because, despite our educational efforts, they still wish to believe such foods to be more nutritious, they ought to be allowed to buy them, as long as some form of certification can guarantee that the food they are buying was, in fact, grown by a farmer using organic methods.

Though many people in nutrition find it surprising, the fact is that a growing number of thoughtful people concerned with ecology, agriculture and the world food supply, support, or at least take seriously, the experiments being conducted by organic agriculturists. For it is becoming increasingly clear that in our understandable enthusiasm for the spectacular yields achievable through heavy applications of pesticides, herbicides, and N-P-K fertilizers (as well as through confinement feeding of livestock), we have failed to take into account a number of "costs" of such an approach to food production, costs that will, with time, become increasingly intolerable. Some of these costs are social, *e.g.*, the destruction of rural life (and of the central cities) caused by the industrialization of farming; and some of them are ecological.

The distinguished agriculturist, Lester Brown, a Senior Fellow of the Overseas Development Council in Washington, D.C., has pointed out that the four technologies responsible for modern agricultural productivity, mechanization, irrigation, fertilization, and chemical control of weeds and insects, are producing — in his words — "ominous alterations in the biosphere, not just on a local scale, but for the first time in history on a global scale as well." It is no secret to anyone interested in the world environment that on a global scale, some of man's interventions have had unanticipated side effects. At a recent meeting on the world food situation, for example, one speaker pointed out that a significant portion of the electricity being generated by the Aswan Dam was being used to produce nitrogen fertilizer that is being used to replace the fertility of the Nile delta which has been lost because of the Aswan Dam.

Abundant Waste

In this country, three decades of agricultural progress also have produced some rather remarkable side effects. Agriculture is now the largest single source of solid waste in the United States, producing *half* of the more than four billion tons of solid waste produced annually. (For comparison, all mining wastes account for one-third, and all municipal, industrial, commercial and residential wastes for one-tenth

249

of the total.) Half of all agricultural waste, one-billion-plus tons a year, is manure, much of which does not go back into the soil to increase tilth and fertility as it used to twenty years ago, but has become part (a large part) of our solid waste problem. One advantage of organic agriculture, at a time when waste disposal is becoming a national obsession, is that instead of producing waste, it attempts to make use of it.

To add humus to his soil, one of the principal things organic farmers do to maintain fertility, the organic grower makes use of all kinds of waste organic material — everything from feed-lot manure to spent coffee grounds generated by the manufacture of instant coffee. Moreover, the organic method not only attempts to utilize some of our unused agricultural waste, it also offers us a way to get rid of some other end products of civilization which are threatening to get out of hand, such things as municipal garbage, and treated sewage sludge which we are now dumping into the oceans in such quantities that it is killing off marine life. It is interesting, and novel, to see the U.S. Department of Agriculture at its Beltsville, Md., research station celebrating the agricultural virtues of composted municipal sewage sludge, a concept derided for years when it was put forward by the "organic crowd."

Another increasingly troubling aspect of modern farming is its enormous energetic cost. The huge "fossil fuel subsidy" represented by nitrogen fertilizers, pesticides, herbicides, tractors, gasoline, irrigation and so forth, was acceptable as long as energy was abundant and cheap. Now that it is not, the most energy intensive agriculture is inevitably going to produce the most expensive food. It is interesting to note in this regard that already last summer one California "organic food store" was selling its labor-intensive "organic" produce for less than energy-intensive "conventional produce" was bringing at local markets. American agriculture is only "efficient" in terms of reducing human labor.

It is my understanding that those who are experimenting with what is called "organic farming" (I prefer the broader term "ecologically-sound agriculture"), are attempting to develop a modern *high-yielding* food production system which will be socially, ecologically and energetically more sustainable than the system we have developed over the last 30 years. Many different people here and abroad are engaged in this attempt. The people at Rodale Press, publishers of *Organic Gardening and Farming*, who are most identified with the movement in this country, do not have *the* answer any more than the Department of Agriculture has *the* answer, though the former have sometimes tended to be more open-minded about such a possibility than the latter.

"Heartless Alternative"

Finally, it is necessary to deal with the widespread notion that anyone who raises questions about the long-range effects of current agricultural methods is willing to cold-heartedly condemn most of the world to starvation; it is part of the Conventional Wisdom of the nutrition profession that "organic" farming is not only an absurd, but a heartless alternative. The accusation is, of course, absurd. To begin with, even those most strongly critical of "chemical farming" have not proposed its immediate wholesale abandonment. Rather what is proposed is a gradual phasing in of a number of good farming practices which can make the farmer less dependent on biocides and other petrochemical products. Second, as most ecologically oriented agriculturists have recognized, the ultimate solution, namely the maximization of *sustainable* yield, may well involve some combination of "chemical" and "organic" methods. And third, contrary to rumor, the "organic method" does not consist merely of throwing a little cow manure on the soil and praying. It is a complex and varied response to local conditions. Therefore, the Conventional Wisdom that says present crop yields are only obtainable through an extension of present methods, like the Conventional Wisdom regarding the nutritional value of "organic foods," has yet to be proved out experimentally. . . .

> *The next articles address questions we raised in the chapter prologue. Do organic foods always cost more? If so, why? These selections are intended to show that even where something as apparently objective as price is concerned, it is well to be skeptical — and open-minded.*

EATING NATURAL GAINS POPULARITY*

Charlene Price

Prices for Organic and Nonorganic Products Differ[1]

Item	*Size*	*Supermarket (nonorganic)* Dollars	*Store (organic)* Dollars	*Price difference* Percent
Unprocessed foods:				
Eggs		1.11	1.40	27
Fresh fruits & veg.	Doz.			
Apples		.59	.64	9
Brussel sprouts	Lb.	1.57	1.17	−25
Cabbage, green	Lb.	.29	.35	40
Cabbage, red	Lb.	.59	.36	−39
Carrots	Lb.	.49	.39	−20
Cucumbers	Lb.	.57	.67	17
Garlic	Lb.	1.69	1.60	−5
Green beans	Lb.	.89	.56	−37
Green peppers	Lb.	1.00	.78	−22
Greens, collards, kale	Lb.	.35	.87	149
Lettuce, head	Lb.	.69	.78	13
Lettuce, romaine	Lb.	.89	.56	−37
Mushrooms	Lb.	1.09	2.22	104
Onions	Lb.	.45	.42	−6
Potatoes	Lb.	.45	.30	−33
Squash	Lb.	.79	.64	−19
Tomatoes	Lb.	.89	.59	−22
Subtotal	Lb.	14.39	14.40	0

---

*"Eating "Natural" Gains Popularity", by Charlene C. Price. *National Food Review.* NFR−28, 1985, pp. 14–18.

[1]Based on a survey of Washington, D.C. Metropolitan Area, October, 1980

Item	Size	Supermarket (nonorganic)	Store (organic)	Price difference
		Dollars	Dollars	Percent
Processed foods:				
Canned fruits and veg.				
Apple juice	Qt.	.83	1.92	131
Apple sauce	Qt.	.73	.92	26
Tomatoes	Lb.	.55	.92	68
Dried fruits and veg.				
Lentils	Lb.	.89	1.28	44
Raisins	Lb.	1.91	1.68	- 12
Flour, cereal, pastas, and bread				
Corn meal, yellow	Lb.	.33	.30	- 9
Grits	Lb.	.53	.75	41
Oats, rolled (not quick cooked)	Lb.	.80	.57	- 28
Wheat cereal	Lb.	.80	.50	- 37
Whole wheat bread	Lb.	.50	.92	84
Whole wheat flour	Lb.	.50	.47	57
Other				
Honey	Lb.	1.55	2.21	43
Peanut butter	Lb.	1.29	1.92	49
Vinegar, cider	Qt.	.34	.73	115
Subtotal		11.35	15.09	33
Total		25.74	29.49	15

HEALTH FOOD STORES INVESTIGATION*

Simon P. Gourdine, Warren W. Traiger, and David S. Cohen

The only simple definition of a health food store is tautological: Health food stores sell "health foods" and other "health" products. The liberal use of the adjective "health" by these stores is apparently intended to distinguish their merchandise from that of other establishments, which is presumably "unhealthy" or at least not as beneficial to the consumer's health.

In 1981 nationwide retail sales for health food stores totaled nearly two billion dollars. Of total health food store sales, "food products"

*Simon P. Gourdine, Warren W. Traiger and David S. Cohen: "Health Food Stores Investigation." Copyright The American Dietetic Association. Reprinted by permission from *Journal of the American Dietetic Association,* Vol. 83: 285, 1983.

account for 50.2%, "vitamins and supplements" account for 36%, and "appliances, body care items, books, and other non-ingestible items" account for the remaining 13.8%. As evidenced by their allotment of display space, the New York City health food stores visited by the [New York City Department of Consumer Affairs] in September through November 1982 conform with the national norm by predominantly selling: (a) food products and (b) vitamins, supplements, diet aids, and other items in pill, capsule, or powder form.

The Department focused its investigation on these two categories of health food stores' merchandise. The Department noted that, in the case of both categories, much of the merchandise sold by health food stores was *at least superficially* similar to items sold by conventional food markets and pharmacies. For example, every item found in the Department's biweekly "Market Basket" report on current food market prices, with the exception of some meats, soft drinks, and beer, had a counterpart sold in at least one of the health food stores visited. Likewise, nearly every food item sold by health food stores, with exceptions such as loose grains, nuts, and beans and herbal teas and other beverages, had a counterpart that could be found in a large supermarket. In the case of non-food items, health food stores were found to be selling various vitamin types which are also sold in most pharmacies. . . .

Having established the parameters of the merchandise to be investigated, the Department proceeded to compare the current cost of this merchandise with that of its conventional counterparts and to examine the validity of the claims made for the physical benefits of health food store products.

Methodology

Table 1 summarizes the results of a health and conventional foods price survey, in which the Department noted the cost for consumers of various health foods at 23 health food stores and of conventional foods at 10 conventional food markets. The Department also made use of the Market Basket Survey to obtain average prices for some conventional food items. The Department tried to match conventional food items as closely as possible with their health food store correlatives in terms of weight and composition. For example, the Department compared a frozen 9-oz. package of Bird's Eye Cut Green Beans (ingredients: "cut green beans") with a 9-oz. package of Health Valley Green Beans (ingredients: "organically grown green beans"). The Department was not able to find every item surveyed in every health food store visited, but the health food store price listed is the average of at least eight stores. Where a specific brand name is not listed for an item in Table 1, the Department priced the least expensive brand of that item found in a store.

Results

The results of the health food and conventional food price comparison survey, as shown in Table 1, demonstrate that health foods are generally much more expensive than their conventional counterparts. Often they cost twice as much or more. Only in the case of tofu was the health food store variety cheaper than its conventional counterpart; in the most extreme case, that of beef liver, the health food variety cost 438% more than its conventional counterpart. (Not all foods covered in the survey are listed in Table 1, as some were sold in only a few stores.). . .

Table 1. Price comparisons of health foods and conventional foods

food items	conventional food prices*	health food prices†	% difference
	$		%
grains			
brown rice, long grain (16 oz.)	0.80	1.42	+ 77.5
whole wheat flour (5 lb.)	1.44 (Gold Medal)	2.85	+ 97.9
barley (raw) (1-lb. package)	0.48 (Jack Rabbit)	1.10	+ 129.2
meats/fish			
tuna fish (albacore, solid white, packaged in water, 6.5 oz.)	1.13‡ (Star-Kist)	3.27 (Health Valley)	+ 189.3
whole chicken (1 lb.)	0.75	2.58	+ 244.0
leg of lamb (1 lb.)	1.79	5.38	+ 200.1
haddock, fillet (1 lb.)	2.59	4.43	+ 71.0
dairy			
eggs, extra large (1 doz.)	1.09	1.92	+ 76.1
butter, stick (1 lb.)	2.33‡	4.18	+ 79.4
cream cheese (8 oz.)	1.08	2.21	+ 104.0

*Average of at least 10 stores.
†Average of at least 8 stores.
‡Prices from Market Basket Survey, September 13 to September 24, 1982.
#Average of four stores.

255

food items	conventional food prices*	health food prices†	% difference
fruits/vegetables —fresh			
apples, Macintosh			
(1 lb.)	0.69‡	1.10	+ 59.4
bananas			
(1 lb.)	0.36‡	0.89	+147.2
broccoli			
(1 lb.)	0.66	1.39	+110.6
cabbage, green			
(1 lb.)	0.23	0.77	+234.8
carrots			
(1 lb.)	0.32‡	0.58	+ 81.3
eggplant			
(1 lb.)	0.62	0.84	+ 35.5
potatoes, white			
loose (1 lb.)	0.41	0.84	+104.9
tomatoes			
(1 lb.)	0.91	1.21	+ 33.0
zucchini			
(1 lb.)	0.85	1.36	+ 60.0
lemons			
(1 lb.)	0.54	1.13	+109.3
grapes, green			
(1 lb.)	0.93	1.89	+103.2
fruits/vegetables — processed			
orange juice	1.01	1.94	+ 92.1
(1 qt.)	(Tropicana)		
tofu			
(1 lb.)	1.59#	1.57	− 1.3
green beans, frozen	0.64‡	1.10	+ 71.9
(9 oz.)	(Bird's Eye)	(Health Valley)	
corn, frozen	0.73	1.20	+ 64.4
(10 oz.)		(Health Valley)	
raisins			
(1 lb.)	1.82	2.64	+ 45.1
chick-peas, dried	0.90	1.79	+ 98.9
(1 lb.)	(Jack Rabbit)		
red kidney beans,	0.60	1.41	+135.0
dried (1 lb.)	(Jack Rabbit)		
Lima beans, dried			
(1 lb.)	0.79	1.43	+ 81.0
other			
clover honey			
(1 lb.)	1.60	2.11	+ 24.2

Summary and Conclusions

Our survey of comparative prices at health food stores and conventional food markets determined that health foods are generally much more expensive than their conventional food counterparts. Often they cost two times as much or more.

Yet in most cases, health foods are in no way demonstrably superior to their cheaper conventional counterparts. The weight of scientific evidence suggests that health foods grown without the use of pesticides or chemical fertilizers (i.e., "organic foods") are indistinguishable from conventional foods in terms of nutritional composition, appearance, and taste. To compare pesticide residue levels in health and conventional foods, the Department commissioned a food laboratory to conduct an analysis of six items; there were no pesticides detected in either the conventional or the health foods.

Our conclusion is that most "health" foods are no healthier than conventional foods unlabeled with the adjective; in fact, they are often indistinguishable. Consumers should be wary of paying premium prices for the nonexistent advantages of health foods. . . .

WHY HEALTH FOODS COST SO MUCH*

Paul Obis

You go into your health food store and pick up a 10-oz. box of whole grain cereal that sells for $2.00. Across the street at the supermarket, they're selling 10 ounces of cornflakes for $1.20. You ask yourself: "How come cereal at the health food store costs almost twice as much? Since whole grain cereal requires less processing, shouldn't it really cost less? Can the efficiencies of size really be so great that smaller companies have to charge so much more to cover their costs?" Good questions.

I asked Jim Rosen, owner of Fantastic Foods, about this. Rosen's company manufactures tofu burger mix, falafel mix and other healthful convenience foods which are sold widely in natural food stores.

"It's basically due to the distribution process and slower turnover of goods at health food stores," he explained.

"In the supermarkets, products are geared to a mass market and sell very quickly. With this high volume, supermarkets can price things just pennies above their cost.

"In comparison, health food stores are more specialized and smaller. The turnover of merchandise is much slower, so the stores buy less."

Because of their high volume, supermarkets can buy many of their goods directly from the manufacturer. The big chains buy Cheerios and paper towels by the truckload. But the average health food store operator can't sell a truck load of tofu burger mix over the weekend. In fact, the store may sell only 12 boxes of burger mix all month.

This is where the distributor comes in. Distributors act as a liaison between manufacturers and retailers. A distributor in a large city might be able to buy 100 cases of tofu burger mix in a month. The distributor will also buy natural toothpaste, carob brownies and a thousand other items that you may find in your local health food store.

Companies like Fantastic Foods would rather sell 100 cases of their product to one company than one case each to 100 companies. It makes doing business a whole lot easier. And most health food stores would rather buy from one distributor than 100 manufacturers. It makes the paperwork easier on both sides.

But distributors have costs to cover, so they mark up the price they pay to the manufacturer by about one-third. If a distributor pays $1.00 for a box of tofu burger mix, they sell it to the store for about $1.33. The store, with its own costs to cover, will mark up the price about 50%, so the consumer will end up paying $2.00 for something

---

*"Why Health Foods Cost So Much," by Paul Obis. *Vegetarian Times*, April 1985, page 6. Used with permission.

the manufacturer sold to the distributor for $1.00. Every time the health food store sells a box of mix, it makes 67 cents (before overhead costs are figured in). Maybe they sell three boxes in a week.

Meanwhile, the supermarket just purchased 100 cases of cornflakes from the manufacturer for $1.00 a box. At this level, the supermarket doesn't need a distributor. The supermarket marks up the price 20% and sells the cornflakes to the consumer for $1.19. The supermarket makes 19 cents on each box (before costs), but it sells 50 boxes on Saturday morning.

To some people, the higher price of natural foods (especially natural convenience foods) is worth the cost, but in most places, there aren't enough natural food consumers to support a store large enough to compete with supermarkets in price. And even when supermarkets sell natural food items, the prices are still high.

"Health foods are like any other specialty item," says Rosen. "Even supermarkets charge more for slow moving goods. The markup on chutney or capers is higher than it is on toilet paper."

Consider maple syrup. You can buy Log Cabin or Mrs. Butterworth's (which contains 2% maple syrup and 98% corn syrup) for about half the price of real maple syrup, which sells for the same price in both the supermarket and the health food store. The same is true of bread. You can buy Wonder for half the price of whole grain and it doesn't matter where you buy it.

In some parts of the country supermarkets are adding health food sections to their stores to grab customers away from health food stores. But are the supermarkets pricing their health food products like they price cornflakes and coffee? No way. They're charging just as much as the specialty stores, because the products don't turn over as fast as mass-market items. The supermarkets always charge a higher percentage for slower-moving merchandise.

Better quality adds something to the price of natural foods items, and so does the fact that natural foods are basically a specialty market (not unlike gourmet foods). Finally, convenience is always more expensive. It costs less to make potato pancakes from potatoes than it does to make them from potato pancake mix, but it also involves more work. Time is money.

When enough people start buying tofu burger mix and tempeh lasagna, lower prices will follow. In the meantime, those of us who want such things are going to have to pay a little extra.

Afterword

So here we are. Aside from agreeing that we'd rather not eat "unnatural" foods, what can we agree about?

A useful first step would be to calm down and talk respectfully with one another. Nothing is resolved by calling names. People who take bone meal are not necessarily irrational, as Packard seems to imply they are, simply because they object to your putting bone particles in their meat without telling them. Being able to buy bone when we want bone and meat when we want meat seem simple consumer rights, not signs of madness or stupidity.

Moreover, guilt by association is not a scientific principle, and while there is no disputing that much of what is sold at health food stores is silly and overpriced, much that is sold in supermarkets and drugstores is also silly and overpriced. We do not for that reason condemn those who shop there. It's unreasonable to criticize everyone who sells or buys food labeled as *healthy, natural* or *organic* simply because we disapprove of some products that carry such a label. As our initial excerpt intended to suggest, we cannot afford to lose our sense of humor or our perspective. Sometimes humans should be allowed to be foolish.

What are the issues? The most serious of them, of course, is medical fraud. Medical fraud is clearly distressing to everyone (except presumably those who profit from it). People who take advantage of the fear and despair of very sick people by offering them false hope and useless treatments are to be condemned, whether they are overenthusiastic members of the medical profession offering experimental drugs and unnecessary surgery, or entirely untrained laypeople offering foods and herbs.

But leaving aside the sub-group of those who buy "health foods" as medicine, what about people who buy them because they want to remain healthy? Max Huberman's customers, for example. What is wrong with their doing some of their shopping at a natural or health food store? What makes the nutrition profession so angry?

Three kinds of objections are generally expressed: first, that the terms *health, natural* and *organic* are undefinable when applied to food and therefore meaningless; second, that the claims made or implied for such foods, even if the words could be defined, are untrue; and finally that the foods are overpriced so that people are induced to waste money buying them.

Let's begin, then, with definitions. As for "so-called natural, organic, or health foods," Packard says, "you must first be able to define them, to know precisely what they are. Then and only then can you make judgment of their relative worth." His own conviction, expressed at the beginning of his article, is that "today as never before" these terms defy definition, although he ultimately admits that it would be useful to define *natural* and then to require that natural foods be *organically* grown according to something like the definition described in the Federal Trade Commission (FTC) record included in this chapter.

He is absolutely correct that, at the moment, the label tells you little or nothing. And although he exaggerates for emphasis — talking about the naturalness of the cleaning compounds used on the containers in which the "natural" milk is stored — his points are valid demonstrations of the difficulty of making any definition truly "scientific."

It may well be that nothing worth much thinking about can have a really "scientific" definition. Most words eventually get defined by public consensus. It is in the nature of words that they come to mean what a majority of those using them has decided that they mean — to try to stop a word from meeting public demand is a losing battle.

So what does *natural* mean? Fifteen years or so ago, the natural food phenomenon was still part of the counterculture, and natural foods were sold at little run-down stores in the unfashionable part of town. Now such foods have moved out into the supermarket boutiques and it is possible to find "natural" margarine, "natural" instant bouillon, "natural" yoghurt chips, "natural" dog food, "natural" lemon flavored creme pie (that's not "cream" — a clue to its naturalness), and even "natural" cigarettes.

The FTC hearing excerpt made clear what must be taken into account in assessing the usefulness of the term *natural* — scientific definitions, public perception, and the misbehavior of food processors and advertisers.

It is worth noting that scientists and food technologists "who considered the term undefinable" were in "reluctant agreement" that *natural* referred to treatment after harvest and that it had something to do with "minimal processing and the absence of artificial or synthetic ingredients or additives."

Their particular problem was in defining the term "minimal processing." Dickinson worried that if *natural* weren't defined, ordinary food would disappear, so she outlined some of the decisions that would have to be made to determine what sorts of processing would be permitted a "natural food."

Most of us would agree that cream would not be unnatural just because it has been separated from whole milk. Most of us would also agree that non-dairy creamer, made up of a mass of ingredients generally unrelated to cream was probably an unnatural product. But where between those two extremes "unnaturalness" begins is — like much else we have talked about in this book — a judgment, not a scientific decision.

Should the government make such judgments and spend money regulating which products are allowed to call themselves

261

natural? Or would you rather have full ingredient labeling and make the decision for yourself? Right now the word *natural* on the label won't help you, because the Federal Trade Commission never acted on the recommendations of its own staff. So you are just as likely to be deceived in the supermarket as in the health food store, unless you read the ingredient label carefully and decide for yourself what *natural* means to you.

A bit further on, we will discuss the question of whether "natural foods" are healthier. For the moment we wish simply to make clear the fact that *natural* can be defined, either by the government or by the consumer who makes his or her own decision about what it ought to mean.

As for the term *organic*, the FTC testimony revealed a conflict between what the scientists strongly believed and what they would admit to knowing. "All foods are 'organic' in the only sense in which that term is scientifically meaningful," as one of them testified — meaning, of course, that they are all composed of carbon-containing chemicals. And the FTC staff reported that "most scientists" would only reluctantly admit that the term *organic* could have any other legitimate meaning.

However, most of the scientific witnesses recognized "that the designation of a food as 'organic' or 'organically grown' had come to be used, generally outside the scientific community, to refer to the method by which the food has been grown." In other words they were aware of the popular meaning even though they were "largely unwilling to accept this use of the term as scientifically meaningful."

In short, just as *natural* was recognized by scientists as referring to post-harvest treatment of food, *organic* was acknowledged, "albeit often reluctantly," to have a popularly agreed-upon meaning having to do with how the food was produced.

As for the term "health food," it is the least specific (or specifiable) of the terms. The FTC could find virtually no one of scientific repute to defend the term; it tends to cover such a variety of items — presumably everything edible sold in a health food store — that it is definitionally useless. Yet as Denise Foley's *Prevention* article shows, even "health foods" can have a popular meaning. Health foods are, she implies, merely highly nutritious foods, a definition most nutritionists would find it hard to fault, even though they are, as a group, reluctant to describe single foods as healthy.

So much for definitions. The second major concern is that when applied to foods, these words are misunderstood in a very specific way. In the FTC hearing, what obviously offended many of the scientists was not only that the public had given to a set of words a meaning these scientists believed to be scientifically indefensible, but that part of this same public seemed convinced that these foods were nutritionally superior. This is a major theme throughout the chapter — namely that the words *health, natural* and *organic* used with food impart an undeserved halo of superiority.

This then, relates to the second major concern of nutrition professionals — that the claims, spoken or implied, are untrue. There are three separate issues here, of which the first is public perception of the meanings of words. If words like *natural* or *organic* can be defined in regard to food, and the public generally understands these definitions but also thinks the words mean or imply something they do not (e.g., superiority), is that fraud?

Should terms be banned if they create inappropriate or inaccurate impressions? Even to state the problem in that way is to make clear that such an argument is silly. We are always fighting over the meanings of words, especially in politics, but we do not for that reason propose to ban the words.

Nor can the issue be that we put a special demand for accuracy on terms used in the marketplace since they lure consumers into spending money for implied (but not necessarily real) benefits. Consumers regularly buy products, including foods, because they believe those products will provide benefits not provided by other products. Many of these supposed attributes, e.g., that a product will make you loveable or popular, are imaginary.

Indeed, a recent Chairman of the Federal Trade Commission has argued that these kinds of deceptions, especially in regard to small items like food products, should not be prosecuted because the deception causes so little material harm to the consumer. So it is surely unfair to argue against the words *natural, organic* and *health* simply because they seem to some consumers to imply more than their definitions guarantee.

The second part of the truthfulness issue has to do with *what* the words imply. For much of the public, it is clear, the terms convey a special aura of goodness. "Natural" and "organic" foods seem on the whole better than foods which are unnatural and non-organic. And health foods seem . . . healthy. As far as most nutritionists are concerned, this is precisely the problem. They argue that the cachet of "betterness" is undeserved, that there is nothing intrinsically better about such foods where nutrition and health are concerned.

In that regard these terms are, however, not different from terms like *new, improved, doctor tested, scientifically formulated* and the like. Those terms also imply various kinds of superiority, and are quite common in American life. If the products they are used to describe are not actually superior, should those terms be banned? Or is the public not misled by those terms because they know they are dealing with what sociologist Jules Henry once called "pecuniary truth" — the knowledge that this product is not **263** literally what it says it is? Is the problem, then, that the terms *organic, natural* and *health* retain consumer trust while the implications of terms like *improved* and *doctor tested* are discounted?

Once again we are led into an absurdity. Clearly one cannot condemn the terms *organic, natural* and *health* foods simply because the public may believe that such words misleadingly imply superiority. The better solution to such misunderstanding would seem to be to define the terms and then educate the public to know what they actually mean. (We might want to do the same with terms like *new and improved, doctor tested* and so on.)

The third part of the "deceptive claim" issue is the only real one — are "organic," "natural" or "health" foods really superior? Health foods can be disposed of rather easily. The term is really meaningless when applied to that multitude of objects sold in health food stores. It is impossible to ask whether such foods have nutritional superiority, since it is not even clear what the term includes.

As for the question, "Are natural foods healthy?", the answer to that has to be, "It depends on what you mean by natural." If natural means minimally processed foods ("whole foods" as the British call them), then such foods are likely to be more nutritious and to have their nutrients better balanced than do foods which are extensively processed or fabricated from a few highly refined ingredients. "Natural" beef *may* have been raised without antibiotics or steroid hormones because many people are wary of these growth promoters; not using them may thus allow a producer to sell his animals at a higher price.

But the operative phrase is *may have.* "Natural" eggs may come from chickens whose feet have touched the earth — what are called free range chickens — but you can't be sure unless someone who saw them walking around assures you it is true. The issue is, however, whether the question is even worth asking. Is it worth the trouble to read labels and hunt for such foods?

It is easiest to address this question by talking first about foods called *organic,* simply because, as we have seen, we can begin with a clear definition. There are several legal definitions of "organic foods," meaning in the broadest sense foods produced on humus rich soil whose fertility has been maintained with organic materials and natural mineral fertilizers, using no pesticides, artificial fertilizers or synthetic additives.

Are foods produced in such a manner better for your health? The answer at the moment has to be that we simply don't know. We have no convincing evidence that they are, but on the other hand we really haven't tried to find out.

The most thorough review of this question to appear in the U.S. was published by a food scientist, Deitrich Knorr, in 1982.

(Deitrich Knorr. "Natural and organic foods: Definitions, quality, and problems." *Cereal Foods World.* 27:163 – 168, April 1982.) Despite his obvious interest in finding significant differences between organically grown foods and their conventionally grown counterparts, he was able to report only that there were "certain compositional differences" between these products — meaning that sometimes organic foods had higher levels of certain vitamins or minerals than conventionally grown foods, or lower levels of moisture.

Often organic produce has lower levels of pesticide residues — it should have since it is supposed to be produced without synthetic pesticides. But when organic food is tested for such residues (usually by someone trying to prove such produce is a fraud), small amounts of such residues are usually found. This may, of course, reflect cheating on the part of the farmer; on the other hand it may reflect the general pollution of the planet, or — more likely than either — it may simply reflect the fact that sprays travel and the farmer next door is probably not an organic one.

Findings of more vitamins or minerals or less water or pesticides in organically grown foods, even if they were consistent, are a long way from proof that those who eat the organic foods are healthier than those consuming foods grown in more conventional ways. The difficulty in making a valid comparison starts long before the food is actually harvested. Many studies that claim to compare the influence of organic and conventional farming practices on the nutritional qualities of foods are poorly designed and too short-term to show differences even if there were any.

In order to demonstrate that there were or were not marked differences in nutritional quality related entirely to the method of growing, one would have to carry out a very carefully controlled long-term experiment, an experiment in which all variables other than management practices — site, seed, water availability, soil type and so on — were identical to begin with. Then, since the differences between soils managed organically and conventionally may take years to emerge, the plots would have to be farmed, with their different treatments, over a long enough period of time to permit each of them to acquire the characteristics of their respective management techniques. Only then would it be possible to begin a definitive experiment comparing nutritive values.

At this point a diet composed of identical foods, grown in the one case organically and in the other case conventionally, would have to be fed to someone, or something. The surrogate of choice in experiments is usually a rat, not because it's so much like a human in its biochemical reactions or temperament but because it's cheap, small and has a fairly short lifespan, so that intergenerational studies can be done within a reasonable period of time. But a rat does best on lab chow, which illustrates only one of the ma-

265

jor differences between rats and humans — namely that you can keep rats on monotonous controlled diets over long periods of time, which is a tough thing to do with people.

So the requisite experiments have simply not been done. They would be long and expensive. The people who grow organically don't have the money to spend, and the Department of Agriculture which might have the money to spend seems to think that organic growing is a bit of a fraud anyway and so is unlikely to carry out the experiments. (Since there is a tendency for both sides in this dispute to think they're right, there isn't a lot of motivation to carry out the needed studies.)

Now there are anecdotal accounts of slow and sickly children brought to a farm to eat fresh organic vegetables who have grown into healthy, brilliant teenagers, etc. There is nothing wrong with such accounts; they may well be true. But they are simply not proof of the superiority of organically grown food because there are too many other uncontrolled variables — things happening which can't be taken into account. Perhaps the fresh air and country life alone would have done it, even if the vegetables were not organically grown.

What we do know about organically-grown crops, from a variety of interesting observations and experiments over the last half-century, is what Commoner points out, that soils treated organically behave differently than soils not so treated. There is also evidence that animals fed on forage crops raised on organically-fertilized soils show certain differences, e.g., in total fertility and in feed efficiency. Whether the ability to produce extended fertility or more weight gain on less food are desirable qualities in human diets is at least questionable; but what is most important is that we simply don't know whether those findings mean anything in terms of human health and longevity.

Which brings us to our last question — price. Are "natural," "health" and "organic" foods always more expensive? Since natural and health foods remain vague terms in the marketplace, we have offered two selections that deal with these questions in regard to organic foods. As the tables show, some organic produce was *less* expensive in Washington, D.C. in 1980, although processed organic foods cost more. In New York in 1982, on the other hand, foods sold in health food stores were considerably more expensive than the same foods sold in supermarkets (note that it was not possible to judge which of these foods was "organic"). Thus prices vary store by store, year by year, and food item by food item. Taken as a whole, what are generically called "health foods" are probably more expensive.

Much of the price differential comes from the fact that we are comparing a supermarket (economies of scale, remember?) to a much smaller store with (as Paul Obis points out) a much smaller

266

turnover. What is more important are the underlying questions: Why go to such a store? Is there any good reason at all for paying such higher prices?

To enquire whether organic foods are more nutritious or safer may be the wrong questions. Some people believe they taste better. Commoner points out that organic growing contributes to the health of the soil and the economy, even if its contribution to the health of people is unclear. Gussow suggests that some people might want to support organic growing because it is an ecologically responsible method of raising food. It may be as rational to pay more to support a sustainable way of growing food as it is to pay more (as many people do) for convenience.

Implicit in all that has been said, however, is the assumption that you should get what you pay for. If you mean to support a particular form of agriculture with your food purchases, you are just as deceived if the produce you are buying is not really "organic" as you would be if you were buying that produce because you hoped it might make you healthier. Since there are no legal meanings for any of these terms, except in the few states where "organic" has been defined, anyone who wants such products needs to understand that it will require substantial research and very careful shopping to know what you are getting, and to get what you are paying for.

6 Nutritional Supplements: To Pill or Not to Pill, Is That the Question?

W e come now to another topic that reliably generates more heat than light among nutritionists. Who, if anyone, needs nutritional supplements? Thoughtful discussion of this issue is almost non-existent among professional nutritionists, as if there were a tacit agreement throughout the nutrition community to avoid real inquiry. Yet even as nutrition professionals seek to teach Americans to "eat well" and avoid "pills," they themselves are swallowing supplementary nutrients (as a study included in this chapter shows). "Do as I say," nutritionists seem to be telling the public, "not as I do"; and few of them dare to defend their own pill practices before their fellows.

Yet whatever professionals may urge, the public use of nutritional supplements is growing. According to a recent report by the Stanford Research Institute, supplement sales rose from $500 million in 1972 to $1.2 billion in 1980 with projected sales of $3.5 billion by 1988. (The booming U.S. vitamins and minerals business — changes and challenges. *Nutrition Today.* 16:26, November/December 1981.)

What are the implications of this trend for health professionals? The report notes that "the medical-scientific establishment, the pharmaceutical industry and the consumer foods and health products industry at large are now being challenged to become more relevant to consumers by a health counter-culture that is no longer a fringe in society but . . . is moving rapidly toward the center. These consumers are willing to pay for wellness and disease prevention."

But even if consumers are willing to pay for health through supplementation, are they getting it? Clearly many of them believe they are — with a fervor that is reflected in their consistent defeat of attempts by the Food and Drug Administration (FDA) to limit sale of many supplements to a prescription basis. Consumer outrage — fueled, critics would argue, by a concerted campaign by "faddist" pressure groups — propelled the Congress to pass legislation which effectively prevents the FDA from regulating these "food products."

This chapter, like the others, tries to give you some sense of the debate — in this case, the debate about whether nutritional supplement use by millions of Americans can be justified. As each side presents its arguments, you'll learn that intelligent decisions depend upon coming to terms with some vague, value-laden terms, like "nutritional insurance," "optimal nutrient intakes" and the like.

When you finish reading these selections, you may conclude that there is no simple answer to the question, "Who needs vitamin pills?" We hope, however, that you will also have acquired an information base broad enough to stand on comfortably while you make a considered decision for yourself.

Because it is a topic few nutrition texts ever explore, we have also included in this chapter some information on how supplements (and the ingredients in supplements) are actually manufactured, what "natural" really means when applied to supplements, and whether particular products might be better than others. These are matters you may want to consider in deciding whether it's a good idea to take, or recommend, any supplements at all.

A final word. Since all the answers are not yet in (we may not even have asked all the right questions yet), we encourage you to keep reading, keep asking questions, and keep thinking about this issue.

All of us need to eat just to stay alive. Since our ancestors lived without them, it is clear that we do not need to take supplements to survive. Yet increasingly we seem to be doing so. It is important that we keep asking ourselves why.

- Webster's New World Dictionary, 2nd College Edition:

VI-TA-MIN [. . . L. vita, life . . . + AMINE: from the orig. mistaken idea that these substances all contain amino acids] any of a number of unrelated, complex organic substances found variously in most foods, or sometimes synthesized in the body, and essential, in small amounts, for the regulation of the metabolism and normal growth and functioning of the body.

- Samuel Vaisrub, M.D.:

The physician must be repeatedly reminded that if vita *in vitamin stands for life,* min *is short for minimum.** *

- Victor Herbert, M.D., J.D.:

*'More is better' is slogan, not science. More is sometimes better, sometimes worse, and always costlier.** *

- Bonnie Liebman, M.S.:

*The making of a multi-vitamin and mineral supplement: Take one part science, two parts Madison Avenue, and then take a look at the competition.*** *

---

*Samuel Vaisrub. Editorial: "Vitamin abuse." *Journal of the American Medical Association.* 238:1762, October 17, 1977.

**Victor Herbert. "The vitamin craze." *Archives of Internal Medicine.* 140:173 - 176, February 1980.

***Bonnie Liebman. "Supplements: Which one's for you?" *Nutrition Action.* 13:8 - 11, March 1986.

> *Who uses nutrient supplements anyway? Many people apparently — and they are not all "cranks" — not unless you define "cranks" as adults leading health-oriented lives who are well educated and hold white collar jobs. That is the profile of the "typical" supplement user that emerges from a news sheet put out by the world's largest supplement manufacturer, Hoffmann-LaRoche.*

VITAMIN USAGE: RAMPANT OR REASONABLE?*

Reviewed by John L. Stanton, Ph.D.

I. Who Takes Vitamin Supplements?

In 1982, 37% of American adults took vitamin supplements. Based on an adult population estimate of 165 million, the number of adult vitamin users is approximately 60.8 million.

Vitamin supplement usage is greater among women than men (especially fulltime working women); among college graduates than high school graduates or non-graduates; and among professional, clerical and sales people than manual laborers or those not in the work force at all. There is greater usage in the $10,000+ income groups and in households without children living at home. Finally, vitamin supplement usage is more common in the West than in any other area of the country.

. . . Of the total U.S. vitamin market, more than half of all vitamin users are either under 18 (growth years) or over 59 years of age (years of declining caloric intakes).

About 41% of women surveyed in 1982 said they give vitamin supplements regularly to one or more of their children. Among children, vitamin usage is highest among 3- to 5-year-olds and decreases continuously as children age (37% of children under age 3; 47% of children aged 3 to 5; 36% of children aged 6 to 12; 30% of teenagers).

II. How Often Are Supplements Taken?

According to the 1982 Gallup survey, the vast majority of adults (85%) took vitamins every day or nearly every day. Another series of studies tracking vitamin usage over the past four years has separated

---

*"Vitamin Usage: Rampant or Reasonable," by John L. Stanton, Ph.D. *Vitamin Issues*, Volume 3, No. 2. Vitamin Nutrition Information Service. Used with permission.

consumers into three categories — "light users" (those who take vitamins less than once per day), "medium users" (take vitamins once per day) and "heavy users" (take vitamins more than once per day). By these criteria, 28% of vitamin consumers in 1982 were light users, 62% were medium users and 10% were heavy users.

Vitamin User Demographics

Characteristic	% of group who use vitamins	
Sex:	Female	42%
	Male	31%
Education:	College	46%
	High school	39%
	Grade school	27%
Occupation:	Professional/business	43%
	Clerical/sales	45%
	Manual worker	33%
	Non-labor force	35%
Annual household income:	$30,000 or more	41%
	$20-$30,000	37%
	$10-$20,000	39%
	Under $10,000	31%
Region:	West	45%
	Midwest	36%
	East	35%
	South	34%
Children at home:	Yes	35%
	No	38%

III. What Vitamins Do People Take?

Vitamin product sales are led by multivitamin formulations (47% of sales volume; 68% of adult users), followed by vitamin C, B vitamins and vitamin E, in descending order of popularity. Multivitamin users most commonly take a product containing iron and/or minerals (58% of adult users), and most multivitamin users take the product once a day.

In 1981 about 21 million adults, or 31% of adult vitamin product consumers, purchased vitamin C as a single supplement. The majority (82%) selected 500 mg or less, and 50% also bought multivitamins. About 16 million adults, or 24% of adult vitamin users purchased vitamin E, and about half of these also purchased a multivitamin. The vast majority (89%) selected a vitamin E potency of 400/IU or less.

272

B vitamins are taken by 27% of adult vitamin users, and roughly 45% of these people also take a multivitamin. About 19% of adult consumers take straight mineral supplements, with iron, zinc and calcium being the most popular single mineral products.

Only a few minor variations are revealed in the specific vitamins taken among different demographic groups. For example, a slightly higher percentage of men than women take vitamins C and E, whereas the reverse is true with multivitamins. The incidence of taking specific supplements such as C, B, E and minerals is higher among whites than nonwhites, while the use of multivitamins is more prevalent among nonwhites.

About a third of regular vitamin users describe the supplement they take as "high potency," although levels were not specified. This percentage has not increased significantly over the past years. About half of regular vitamin users are aware of the Recommended Dietary Allowances (RDAs). Awareness of the RDAs correlates positively with age (younger groups more aware), education (college), income (upper levels) and sex (women).

When asked how they determine the proper dosage of vitamins to take, most people said they rely on the supplement label (48%), while another 29% of adult users said they rely on their doctor for the information. No other category of information — books, catalogs, friends/relatives, pharmacists, clerks, commercials, electronic or print media — was mentioned by more than seven percent of respondents in this study.

Current Vitamin/Mineral Supplement Usage Among the Adult Population

Product	% of Adult Supplement Users*	# of Adult Supplement Users	Most Common Form Taken**
Multivitamins	68%	40 million	With minerals/iron (83%)
Vitamin C	32%	19 million	500 mg or less (82%)
B Vitamins	27%	16 million	With vitamin C (37%)
Vitamin E	20%	12 million	400 IU or less (89%)
Minerals	19%	11 million	Calcium (45%) and iron (41%)
Vitamin A	6%	2 million	(not asked in survey)
Vitamin D	2%	1 million	(not asked in survey)
Vitamins A + D	3%	2 million	(not asked in survey)

*According to 1982 Gallup usage data
**According to 1981 product sales data

IV. Why Do People Take Vitamin Supplements?

Reasons for taking vitamin supplements were assessed in two ways in this survey. In one section, respondents (current users only) were asked to give in their own words the most important reason they had for taking vitamins; their answers were then clustered into general categories. In a second section, different reasons adults might take vitamins were listed on a card, and all respondents were asked to check those reasons which they felt were most important.

In the first instance, the majority of people gave general answers such as "to supplement the diet," "to be healthy" or "to make me feel better." Among multivitamin users, responses clustered in the following major categories:

To supplement diet: 31%
(Don't get a balanced diet at all times; don't eat right; don't get enough vitamins during the day; I'm an irregular eater.)

Healthy/Make me feel better: 30%
(To be healthy; health supplement; good for you; for general health reasons.)

For energy/strength: 12%
(Gives me pep; to keep going; I am run down; pick-me-up.)

Doctor recommended/prescribed: 7%

Pregnant: 5%

Among single supplement users, major reasons for taking a given vitamin included some more specific expectations such as "to fight colds" (36% of vitamin C users), "to help eyesight" (14% of vitamin A/D users), "for stress" (14% of B vitamin users), "builds blood" (13% of mineral users), "for skin problems" (11% of vitamin A/D users and 11% of vitamin E users), in addition to the general health/dietary supplement categories.

When given a list of reasons for taking vitamins (both multivitamins and single supplements), adults responded as follows:

Reasons for Taking Vitamins	% of Adults
To stay healthy	45
When feeling run down	45
When there's not enough time for proper meals	41
During illness	40
When exposed to colds/flu	38
Being on a diet	33
In times of stress/worry	20
When you have a heavy work schedule	17
If you smoke heavily	13
Other	3

These findings appear to support earlier survey findings wherein vitamin supplements have been perceived as nutritional insurance, particularly when food intakes are curtailed or eating habits are haphazard. For example, in a 1980 *Woman's Day*/FMI survey, 43% of adults agreed that "even if you eat a good diet, you should still take a vitamin supplement." In a 1978 A. C. Nielsen survey, 51% said they took vitamin supplements, predominantly multivitamins, while dieting to lose weight.

The vast majority of people do not, however, perceive supplements as meal or food replacements. In a 1978 survey of consumer attitudes and practices, 97% of the respondents *disagreed* with the statement, "It is okay to skip meals as long as you take a vitamin supplement."

Risk factors other than dieting/poor eating habits — such as smoking, heavy consumption of alcohol, chronic use of certain drugs, surgery/wound healing or chronic exposure to heavy air pollution — appear to be less well understood and/or accepted by consumers as reasons for taking vitamins. . . .

> *Supporters of supplement use see those who practice it as reasonable (and exceptionally health-conscious) people. Critics decry the ignorance and misinformation on which pill-popping behavior is based. This first survey of supplement usage by nutrition professionals, published originally in 1984, raises some unsettling questions for those who assume that more knowledge of nutrition will stamp out supplementation.*

SUPPLEMENTATION PATTERNS OF WASHINGTON STATE DIETITIANS*

Bonnie Worthington-Roberts, Ph.D., and Maryann Breskin, M.S., R.D.

. . . Methods

All known dietitians in the state of Washington were contacted by mail and asked to complete a 1-page questionnaire. Nine hundred and thirty individuals were identified; each was provided with 1 questionnaire and a return envelope with postage affixed. The questionnaire sought

*Bonnie Worthington-Roberts, and Maryann Breskin: "Supplementation Patterns of Washington State Dietitians." Copyright The American Dietetic Association. Reprinted by permission from *Journal of the American Dietetic Association*, Vol. 84:795, 1984.

information related to sex, age, place of residence, and body weight status. It also provided a listing of nutritional supplements, with directions to identify those supplements taken and frequency of use (daily, alternate days, twice each week, weekly, irregularly). . . .

The survey was initiated in the autumn of 1981 and completed by December 15 of that year. Of 930 questionnaires delivered, 40 were returned unopened; 665 were completed and returned as requested. Data were evaluated for the 665 responders, or 74.7% of the available population.

Results

More than 96% of the subjects were women; of them, 4.5% were pregnant or lactating. Three percent of the respondents were men; the others did not indicate their sex. With regard to age, nearly half (47.5%) were 30 to 50 years old, with 25.6% indicating an age less than 30 years and 26.6% an age over 50 years. Most subjects resided in urban or suburban areas, with 39.1% and 46.8%, respectively, falling into these categories; only 13.7% of the subjects lived in rural regions. The vast majority of the respondents (74.6%) defined their body weight as normal; underweight subjects represented 2.9% of the population, while overweight ones accounted for 22.3% of the group.

. . . Nearly 60% of the total population used some nutritional supplement, some daily and some infrequently. Men did not differ significantly from women in this regard; 52.6% of the men and 56.8% of the women indicated that they supplemented their diets. The sub-group of pregnant and lactating women was clearly an exception, as 100% of them used some nutritional supplement. Place of residence did not markedly affect supplementation patterns, with 58.1% of the urban, 55% of the suburban, and 60% of the rural responders indicating supplement use. Body weight status appeared to be most influential in affecting supplementation use; 73.7% of the underweight subjects used some supplement, while only 57.3% and 53.1% of the normal weight and overweight subjects, respectively, supplemented their diets.

With regard to use of specific supplements, responses were grouped into 7 different categories. The categories selected included the following: multivitamins (no minerals), multivitamins plus minerals, vitamin C only, iron only or iron with vitamin C, calcium only or calcium plus vitamin D, protein only, and extra calories only. . . .

Two categories of supplements were most frequently used, with 20.9% of the total population choosing multivitamins plus minerals and 19.1% electing to take vitamin C only. Multivitamins (no minerals) and iron only or with vitamin C were each chosen by 6.9% of the population. Other supplement categories were used less often: calcium with or without vitamin D (2.7%), protein only (3%), and extra calories only (0%).

Since a space was provided on the questionnaire for "other" supplements to be listed, some (less than 1%) respondents indicated use of specific nutrients or products not accounted for in the previously mentioned categories. Among the other supplements chosen by respondents were potassium (N = 6), fluoride (N = 4), lysine (N = 2), lecithin (N = 2), selenium (N = 2), inositol (N = 1), choline (N = 1), dessicated liver with alfalfa, garlic, rutin, and kelp (N = 1), thymus tissue (N = 1), and thiamin (N = 1). . . .

Frequency of use of specific supplements was also evaluated from questionnaire responses. Of individuals using supplements, approximately 60% did so on a daily basis; thus 37% of the entire sample population took supplements daily. This was especially true for users of protein supplements (80% daily use). Those using some supplement on a less than daily basis did so most often on alternate days or twice each week. Thirteen percent of individuals taking vitamin C only did so weekly and 8% less than once per week. Fifteen percent of users of iron took iron supplements weekly, and 3% at less than weekly intervals. . . .

> *Why do people use supplements? "Simple," reply physicians Victor Herbert and Stephen Barrett. "They're sold on them" by self-appointed experts and by questionable advice and information coming out of health food stores.*

PROMISES EVERYWHERE*

Victor Herbert, M.D., J.D. and Stephen Barrett, M.D.

Suggestions to take vitamins seem to be everywhere. Advertisements on radio and television and in magazines and newspapers warn against deficiencies. Self-appointed "experts," echoed by a chorus of believers, praise the "miracles" of nutrition. Colorful bottles line the shelves — not only in health food stores but also in pharmacies, supermarkets and department stores. Doctors even prescribe vitamins as placebos. The great vitamin hustle now costs consumers more than two *billion* dollars a year. . . .

---

*Chapter 4: "Promises Everywhere," from Victor Herbert, M.D., J.D. and Stephen Barrett, M.D. *Vitamins and "Health" Foods: The Great American Hustle.* George F. Stickley Co., Philadelphia, PA. Used with permission.

Industry Guidelines

A close look at food supplement bottles will show that almost none of them contains *therapeutic* claims on their labels. The reason for this is obvious. Unless a claim is backed by proof acceptable to the FDA (which simply means that there is reasonable evidence that it is true), it is illegal to make that claim on a label. Misbranded products can be seized and ultimately destroyed by government agencies. This means, incidentally, that if a health claim does not appear on a product's label or accompanying literature from its manufacturer, you can be sure the product won't do what is claimed.

It is also illegal for health food store operators to practice medicine without a license by diagnosing ailments or recommending that specific foods or food supplements be taken at specific times for specific ailments.

The National Nutritional Foods Association (NNFA), an organization of health food retailers, producers and distributors, has issued guidelines that provide "a reasonable and acceptable way to give nutritional advice to customers without prescribing." NNFA suggests that if a customer asks for advice about a specific ailment, the retailer should respond with a disclaimer. He should say that the store sells items for the building of health, rather than for the treatment of disease, and if the customer has a definite problem in mind, he should consult a physician. After doing this, the retailer can then redirect the discussion to "the relationship of better nutrition and a better state of health." (Do you think any such discussion will ever fail to recommend a product sold in the store?) If a customer asks about the efficacy of a particular item, the recommended answer is, "Yes, I have heard this, and many of our publications are available for your information." NNFA also warns retailers not to diagnose disease or advise customers to abandon their current medical care.

Similar advice is given from time to time in the trade magazine, *Health Foods Business*. A 1977 issue, for example, describes how a proprietor "keeps a couple of nutrition textbooks handy under the sales counter and when a question arises about the function or use of a product, he looks it up. He's very careful to stress that he is not a physician and that what he says should be taken as informative rather than authoritative." In a more recent issue, another storekeeper states: "We can avoid prescribing through the use of books . . .

In our stores we provide an area near the book display where people can sit and look at the books . . . Sometimes they will then purchase one or more of the books, but even if they don't, they have usually found a suggestion of at least one product they will buy before leaving . . .

Any time we sell a book, we know that it will help to generate sales of other items within our stores. . . ."

278

Other Promotional Activities

Many retailers appear on local radio or TV shows where it is legally safe to give advice as long as specific products are not recommended. "Getting on a talk show is not difficult," says an article in *Health Foods Business*, entitled *From Store to Star.* "Nutrition is a popular and controversial subject these days, and you, a health food store owner, are — by definition — an expert on the subject . . . Chances are good that a station in your area would like to do a talk show on the subject, particularly if the guest is an area businessperson". . . .

Some retailers publish newsletters and many give lectures in their own communities. One has even formed a "separate" educational society which imports guest speakers for public appearances, but most who sponsor prominent guests do so directly. A recent article in *Health Foods Retailing* describes the selling power of prominent lecturers. According to a Nebraska health food store owner, "When Dale Alexander explained the nutritional benefits of cod liver oil, we sold 75 cases of it. I tell you, cod liver oil was going like flowing water." (Alexander claims that cod liver oil reduces the pain of arthritis by lubricating people's joints!) . . .

In *Natural Foods Merchandiser,* a Florida retailer describes how a restaurant can help to "create customers that otherwise would never come into a health food store." The first stop is to attract customers by offering low-priced salads and sandwiches. Inside, a large sign near the dining area announces in-store health lectures by a local osteopath who also appears on a daily 5-minute radio show sponsored by the store. Prominent lecturers are imported from time-to-time, and the store also sponsors radio programs by Carlton Fredericks. Vitamin manufacturers who help finance the radio programs are also plugged during the programs. . . .

Oral Claims

Although industry leaders have devised "safe" ways to convey advice "indirectly," retailers actually risk little by making direct oral claims in the relative privacy of a store. Government enforcement efforts, which are quite limited, are directed primarily against manufacturers and distributors of a small number of the more notorious quack remedies such as laetrile. Retailers are generally quite willing to give advice about supplements to their customers. . . .

"Nutrition Consultants"

People who sell food supplements typically acquire their knowledge of nutrition by reading popular "nutrition" books and magazines, attend-

279

ing seminars sponsored by supplement manufacturers and distributors, and possibly self-experimentation. Industry leaders, anxious to upgrade their image, have been devising ways for their salespeople to acquire "credentials."

The most active individual working in this direction is probably Kurt Donsbach, a former health food store operator who was prosecuted 10 years ago for practicing medicine without a license. His many projects include Donsbach University (which awards mail-order diplomas in nutrition); the International Academy of Nutrition Consultants (which *anyone* can join for $12); a journal which discusses nutrition topics and carries ads for questionable health products; the International Institute of Natural Health Sciences (which sells publications and provides computerized analysis of "The Nutrient Deficiency Test," a 266-item dietary questionnaire developed by Donsbach); and Health Education Products (a firm that sells publications and food supplement products). According to a Nutri-Books catalogue, *Dr. Donsbach's Nutritional Tape Cassettes*, intended for sale through health food stores, are "like having Dr. Donsbach as your personal physician right in your own home. Each . . . gives pertinent information and direction to aid in diagnosis and remedial action". . . .

A recent article in *Health Foods Business* suggests that health food stores should work toward achieving professional status. "It's likely that the health food store of the future will have a certified nutritionist on its staff — the equivalent of a pharmacist in a drug store," the article states. "Health food store owners — and the whole industry — should begin thinking about how such a system of accreditation from a recognized and respected institution might work". . . .

Nutrition Roulette

The health food industry has a huge number of "treatment" methods. Thousands of food supplement products are being produced by hundreds of manufacturers, and a wide variety of foods are also being promoted for their supposedly special health-giving properties. The overall industry philosophy seems to be that anything is worth trying for anything and that "more is better" when it comes to dosage. Its salespeople may not understand biochemistry, but they do understand how to sell.

The degree of danger in following advice from a popular publication, a health food store clerk or a "nutrition consultant," varies with the degree of customer belief and the presence or absence of significant illness. Reliance upon an unproven method can endanger your health or your life in addition to your pocketbook. But it is clear that on a person-to-person basis, anyone can get away with recommending almost any type of "treatment" for almost any health problem.

It is not only the blandishments of health food stores and their "experts" who are promoting supplement usage. Popular publications too carry advertisements that link vitamins to much more than health. The ads on the following pages link supplement taking to athletic performance and fears of eating inadequately.

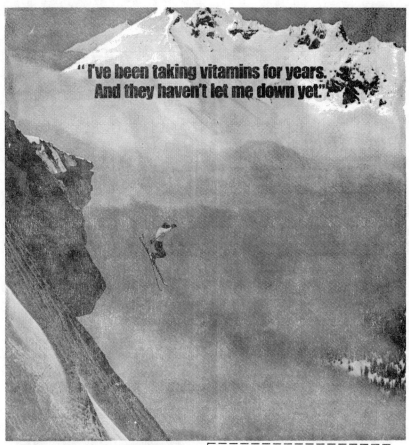

Advertisement. "I've been taking vitamins for years. And they haven't let me down yet." *Roche.* Hoffmann-LaRoche, Inc., Nutley, NJ. Used with permission.

Sure a well-balanced diet is a key to good health, but...

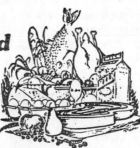

what about the millions of food-faddists, daffy-dieters, junk-food kids and gulp-&-dash execs?

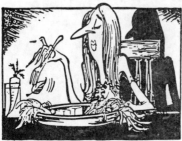

Food-faddist

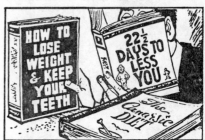

Daffy-dieter

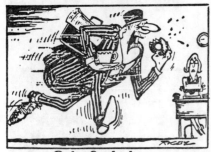

Gulp-&-dash exec.

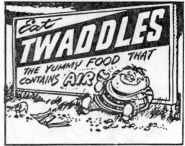

Junk-food kid

Maybe they need the additional support of a balanced nutritional supplement.

For information on diet quackery vs. nutritional supplements, call or write:
Public Affairs Department, Lederle Laboratories
Wayne, New Jersey 0 √0, 201/831-4684

> *Will vitamins improve athletic performance, make up for care-less eating or make you a better person? Don't count on the advertisers to tell you, says nutritionist Denise Hatfield. You'd better learn to read between the lines, since there are few federal or state laws to protect you.*

TRUTH IN ADVERTISING: DOES IT APPLY TO VITAMIN SUPPLEMENTS?*

Denise Hatfield, Ph.D., R.D.

. . . Implied Message Quite Clear

In a great number of existing ads, the potential to mislead is more a matter of what is implied than what is actually said. However, the message is usually quite clear; i.e., we are all on the verge of deficiency as a result of stress, environmental pollutants, and a nutrient-poor food supply, and the best solution is the regular use of supplements. None of this is founded on scientific facts.

The current most popular theme is related to stress and its effects on vitamin requirements. As a result, drugstore shelves are filled to overflowing with "stress formula" vitamins. The catch is that "stress" is never consistently defined, and whether vitamin requirements are affected by stress depends on how it is defined. Although stress that is defined as injury, infection, fever, shock, illness, surgery or bone frac-tures can increase nutrient requirements, there is no scientific evi-dence to back up advertising claims that we are placing ourselves under immediate risk of vitamin deficiencies due to the emotional stresses of everyday life; unless, of course, that "stress" causes you to eat improperly for an extended period of time.

It is true that there are periods in everyone's life in which good nutrition takes a low priority due to mounting pressures and responsi-bilities, and if these periods are prolonged, vitamin supplementation may be indicated. However, contrary to what most of the ads imply, receiving less than the recommended allowance for a vitamin for a few days does not result in a vitamin deficiency. Since even the water-soluble B vitamins and vitamin C are stored in the body to some extent, the risk of vitamin deficiency from an occasional less than adequate vitamin intake is virtually nil.

*"Truth in Advertising: Does It Apply to Vitamin Supplements?", by Denise Hatfield. *ACSH News & Views*, 5:1, 13–14, January/February 1984. American Council on Science and Health.

Accuracy of Ads

What do these ads actually say to convey their message? . . .

Among the superabundance of ads for supplements are those that have been brought to the attention of the National Advertising Division (NAD) of the Better Business Bureau for their misleading and/or false claims. The National Advertising Division initiates inquiries, determines the issues, collects and evaluates data, and negotiates agreements in regard to advertising claims. This procedure is part of a self-regulatory system established in 1971 by the advertising community and is sponsored in part by the Council of Better Business Bureaus. . . .

The American Council on Science and Health (ACSH) reviewed NAD case reports and several recent issues of popular magazines for vitamin advertisements and found the following misleading statements:

Claim: ". . . a librarian might exercise regularly after work, for example, not realizing the added activity may increase the need for vitamins and minerals." (Ayerst Laboratories for Beminal Stress Plus.)

Fact: Although some research has indicated that there may be *slight* variations in some vitamin requirements with caloric intake and energy expenditure, a wisely chosen varied diet can compensate for these minor fluctuations in vitamin needs. It is not implicit that librarians, or anyone else for that matter, need to take supplemental vitamins just because they attend an exercise class two or three times a week.

Claim: "Heavy consumption of alcohol can rob your body because it interferes with the body's utilization of vitamins. What's more, alcohol consumption can lead to poor eating habits and a consistently poor diet." (Hoffmann-LaRoche Inc. for Vitamin Information Service.)

Fact: Although it is true that alcoholics are prone to vitamin deficiencies, there are many more pressing problems for the alcoholic to deal with. In addition, by omitting the adjective "heavy" when referring to alcohol consumption in the second sentence, one comes away with the impression that *any* drinking can induce vitamin deficiencies.

Claim: "Overwork, exercising, dieting, cold and flu . . . may burn up essential vitamins you need for balanced nutrition every day. That's vitamin burnout." (A. H. Robins Company Inc. for Albee.)

Fact: There is simply no medically recognized condition of vitamin burnout.

Claim: ". . . Zinc is an essential for every man who wants to maintain good physical condition." (A. H. Robins Company Inc. for Z-BEC.)

Fact: While this statement is essentially accurate, the implication from the ad is that zinc *supplements* are essential to good physical condition. That implication is not valid.

Claim: "No matter how hard you try, though, in our fast food society, it's often difficult to make sure you're getting enough essential vitamins and minerals in the food you eat." (Safeway Brand for Safeway vitamins.)

Fact: Although a diet that consists exclusively of fast foods will not meet the recommended allowances for all vitamins without greatly exceeding caloric allowances, occasional fast food meals are definitely not cause for vitamin supplementation. . . .

The following claims, marked by asterisks, were brought to the attention of the NAD at an earlier date by . . . concerned groups and were judged to be unsubstantiated or were voluntarily discontinued by the company following the inquiry.

*Claim: "Up tight or up in smoke — With both acute stress and heavy cigarette smoking, the plasma levels of vitamin C in your blood may be lowered." (Hoffmann-LaRoche Inc. for Vitamin C.)

Fact: Although some research has indicated that people who smoke may have lower vitamin C levels in their blood than those who don't, the levels are still within the normal range. If your goal is to improve your health, quit smoking. In addition it is not scientifically accepted that emotional stress lowers vitamin C levels in the blood.

*Claim: "The B-complex and C vitamins you take today probably won't do anything for you tomorrow. Because they're water-soluble and are eliminated daily." (A. H. Robins Company Inc. for Z-BEC.)

Fact: This is simply not true. Vitamin C stores in the body are sufficient to protect against 20 – 45 days of deprivation in man. The B vitamins are also stored in significant amounts, making it impossible to develop deficiencies overnight as the ad implies.

*Claim: "The aspirin you take for pain can lower your vitamin C by up to 75 percent." (J. B. Williams Company, Inc. for Femiron Multi-Vitamins.)

Fact: Someone who takes aspirin regularly and in large doses (an individual with arthritis, for example) may indeed have problems with vitamin C absorption. However this does not apply to someone taking aspirin for occasional aches and pains. The ad does not make that distinction and is misleading. . . .

ACSH's primary objection to these ads is the impression left with consumers that vitamin supplements will prevent or alleviate any problems or symptoms associated with smoking, drinking, stress, and/or exercise. With this concept firmly ingrained via advertising, consumers are being cajoled into throwing away good money on unnecessary vitamin/mineral supplements. They may also be lured into thinking that by taking vitamin supplements, they have counteracted all the ill-effects that smoking or abuse of alcohol would otherwise have on their health. This is a dangerous misconception.

Who Has Responsibility?

The answer to this question seems to be everyone and yet no one. Everyone, in this case, refers to the Bureau of Foods of the Food and

285

Drug Administration (FDA), the Metabolism and Endocrine Drug Products Division of the FDA, the Over-the-Counter (OTC) Drug Division of the FDA, the Federal Trade Commission (FTC), and even to some degree, the National Advertising Division (NAD) of the Better Business Bureau (BBB). . . .

Yet, although these organizations have the responsibility, there are no effective regulations for their respective groups to apply to vitamin/mineral supplements. Developing reasonable regulations has been difficult because there are no standard definitions to determine into what regulatory category, i.e., food or drug, vitamin supplements should fall. Without any such regulations there is a blatant lack of standards for potency, labeling and advertising of these supplements. . . .

Unless more specific regulations are developed and put into effect, advertisements will continue to be the siren call for those in search of a panacea for good health and well-being. Until that time, however, consumers should beware of cleverly worded advertisements that are devised to sell their products and be aware that "truth in advertising" often gets somewhat stretched.

> *The public enthusiasm for supplements occasionally puts sci-*
> *entists themselves in a bind. Research showing that diets con-*
> *taining large amounts of certain fish oils (EPA and DHA)*
> *might reduce the risks of heart disease led almost instantly to*
> *the availability of products containing these fats in concen-*
> *trated form, and to promotions in consumer magazines sug-*
> *gesting that using these supplements was an "easy to swallow"*
> *way to get the "nutritional benefits of fish." When the National*
> *Academy of Sciences Committee on Diet, Nutrition, and Can-*
> *cer concluded that vegetables like broccoli, cauliflower and*
> *cabbage might be good for you, what purported to be concen-*
> *trates of these vegetables quickly appeared on the market with*
> *ads implying they would help you avoid cancer. In the follow-*
> *ing selections the question seems to be: Would you rather eat*
> *lots of mackerel and broccoli or take your MaxEPA and Daily*
> *Greens?*

FISHING FOR HEALTH*

Bonnie Liebman, M.S.

... Black and Blue Eskimos

The clue to another heart-protecting effect of seafood, especially the fattier varieties, was found in the far North — Greenland to be exact. The Eskimos there, who live on a diet loaded with whale, fish, and seal, rarely suffer from heart disease. Among one population of 1800, only three heart attacks occurred between the years 1950 and 1974, a rate about 100 times lower than that of Americans.

Eskimo cholesterol levels are relatively low, but not low enough to explain their minimal heart attack rate. Rather, there is an additional factor, one linked to a characteristic that at first glance would hardly seem relevant — Eskimos bruise easily.

When compared to blood from a Scandinavian, an Eskimo's blood contains fewer platelets, the blood components that help to initiate the clotting process. Not surprisingly, their blood also takes longer to coagulate. That accounts for the Eskimos' quickness to bruise, which is caused by minor bleeding under the skin. But this slowness to clot is linked to their cardiovascular health as well. In the U.S., most heart

---

*"Fishing for Health," by Bonnie Liebman. *Nutrition Action*, 11:8–11, September 1984. Edited portions used with permission by Center for Science in the Public Interest.

attacks and strokes occur when blood clots get stuck in arteries narrowed by a buildup of cholesterol. Blood that's less likely to clot could certainly reduce the risk that a blood vessel will suddenly get blocked.

The key to the Eskimos' clot-resistant blood is their fishy diet. Between 5 and 40 percent of the fat in seafood consists of omega-3 fatty acids, specifically eicosapentaenoic acid (EPA) and docosahexaenoic acid (DHA). Fatty fishes, such as salmon and mackerel, are the richest sources of EPA and DHA. In contrast, polyunsaturated vegetable oils are rich in omega-6 fatty acids such as linoleic acid. (The number refers to the location of the first unsaturated bond in the fat. In the omega-3 fats, the bond occurs between the third and fourth carbon; in the omega-6 variety, it occurs between the sixth and seventh.)

Researchers now suspect that omega-6 fatty acids are precursors of substances that encourage platelets to stick together. But, in Eskimos, omega-3 fatty acids replace some of the omega-6 variety normally found in platelets, thus reducing their tendency to congeal. What excites researchers is that by feeding non-Eskimos diets high in omega-3 fatty acids, it is possible to produce slow-to-clot platelets like those of the Eskimos.

The question, of course, is how much fish fat in the diet is needed to make platelets less sticky. Three British and Scandinavian studies on small numbers of people suggest that about three to six grams of omega-3 fatty acids per day are needed to slow clotting time.

Further research in this fascinating new field may show that smaller amounts are beneficial. But if three to six grams per day represent a minimum amount, we're talking about eating a lot of fish. Three grams of omega-3 fatty acids translates to about half a pound of canned sockeye salmon or mackerel, roughly three-quarters of a pound of herring or whitefish, one-and-a-half pounds of shrimp or white tuna, two-and-a-half pounds of cod, flounder, or sole, or about four pounds of haddock or light tuna per day. By comparison, the average Greenland Eskimo eats nearly one pound of whale and seal meat a day, while the average American consumes 15 pounds of fish per *year*.

Needless to say, most people would have trouble downing that much fish (or seal) on a regular basis. . . .

Fish in a Pill

Is there an alternative? MaxEPA is a fish oil supplement used in most scientific studies on omega-3 fatty acids. Each one-gram capsule contains 0.3 grams of EPA and DHA. In addition, the capsules contain a mixture of other oils from fish flesh, not from fish liver which in large quantities contains toxic amounts of vitamins A and D.

While a handy bottle of pills might sound more practical than fish for breakfast, lunch, and supper, MaxEPA also has its problems. The first is cost. To get those three to six grams, you'd have to take between 10 and 20 capsules a day. . . . Another is nutritional. That dose of MaxEPA adds up to the small but significant total of 90 to 180 fat calories.

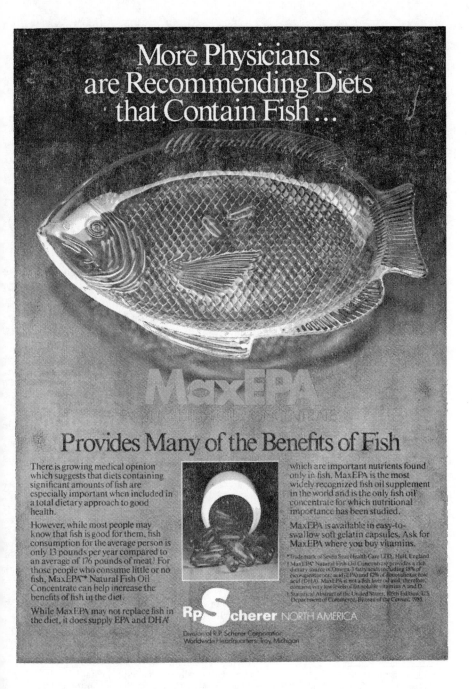

More Physicians are Recommending Diets that Contain Fish ...

MaxEPA

Provides Many of the Benefits of Fish

There is growing medical opinion which suggests that diets containing significant amounts of fish are especially important when included in a total dietary approach to good health.

However, while most people may know that fish is good for them, fish consumption for the average person is only 13 pounds per year compared to an average of 176 pounds of meat.[1] For those people who consume little or no fish, MaxEPA™ Natural Fish Oil Concentrate can help increase the benefits of fish in the diet.

While MaxEPA may not replace fish in the diet, it does supply EPA and DHA[2]

which are important nutrients found only in fish. MaxEPA is the most widely recognized fish oil supplement in the world and is the only fish oil concentrate for which nutritional importance has been studied.

MaxEPA is available in easy-to-swallow soft gelatin capsules. Ask for MaxEPA where you buy vitamins.

* Trademark of Seven Seas Health Care LTD., Hull, England.
† MaxEPA™ Natural Fish Oil Concentrate provides a rich dietary source of Omega-3 fatty acids including 18% of eicosapentaenoic acid (EPA) and 12% of docosahexaenoic acid (DHA). MaxEPA is not a fish liver oil and, therefore, contains very low levels of fat-soluble vitamins A and D.
‡ Statistical Abstract of the United States, 109th Edition, U.S. Department of Commerce, Bureau of the Census, 1988.

Rp Scherer NORTH AMERICA

Division of R.P. Scherer Corporation
Worldwide Headquarters: Troy, Michigan

More importantly, some researchers are not convinced that there is enough evidence yet to write a nationwide prescription for fish oil capsules. Says Dr. William Connor of the Oregon Health Sciences University in Portland, "MaxEPA certainly isn't going to hurt anyone, but we simply don't have the evidence that such small quantities will help, and we don't know the long-term effects. More subjects have to be studied."

Among other concerns, the Greenland Eskimos seem to have an especially high incidence of strokes, probably caused by burst blood vessels. Whether the strokes are related to the omega-3 fatty acids needs to be studied. Though the blood of most Americans could probably benefit from reduced stickiness, the stroke question needs to be answered before we rush to stock up on fish oil capsules. However, people who know they have trouble with blood clots may want to consider taking supplements, after discussing the matter with a nutritionally aware physician.

Nevertheless, Connor has no trouble urging people to eat more seafood in general. "My advice to the public is to eat fish in preference to red meat. In coronary prevention diets, we stress foods low in cholesterol and saturated fat. But we don't have the evidence to advise the public to consume [high-fat] mackerel over [low-fat] codfish or [high-fat] salmon over [low-fat] flounder." . . .

LETTER TO THE FEDERAL TRADE COMMISSION ABOUT THE DAILY GREENS SUPPLEMENT*

Michael F. Jacobson, Ph.D. and Bonnie F. Liebman, M.S.

Hearing Clerk
Federal Trade Commission
6th and Pennsylvania Ave., N.W.
Washington, DC 20850

Dear Hearing Clerk:

In 1982, the Diet, Nutrition and Cancer Committee of the National Academy of Sciences issued a set of dietary guidelines to help consumers reduce their risk of cancer. One of these recommendations encouraged people to include fruits (especially citrus fruits), vegetables

*Letter to the Federal Trade Commission about the Daily Greens Supplement, by Michael F. Jacobson, Ph.D. and Bonnie F. Liebman, M.S., Center for Science in the Public Interest, July 19, 1983. Used with permission.

(especially carotene-rich and cruciferous vegetables) and whole grain cereal products in their daily diets. The Committee specifically noted that "these recommendations apply only to foods as sources of nutrients — not to dietary supplements of individual nutrients."

In recent months, an advertisement for a product called Daily Greens has appeared in several magazines and newspapers. Daily Greens is a supplement containing dehydrated vegetables as well as vitamins A, C, E, and beta-carotene. We believe the advertisement, which relies heavily on the 1982 NAS report, misleads consumers by suggesting (a) that the Academy endorses Daily Greens or similar supplements, and (b) that the pills contain substantial amounts of the vegetables pictured in the ad and on the box. Below we elaborate on each of these deceptive claims.

I. The National Academy of Sciences Has Not Endorsed Daily Greens

The advertisement for Daily Greens implies in several ways that the National Academy of Sciences has recommended consumption of such supplements. . . .

In fact, the Academy specifically cautioned against the use of "dietary supplements of individual nutrients," such as vitamins A, C, E, and beta-carotene. While the Academy did not specifically warn against the use of dietary supplements of vegetables (which had not yet been marketed), the Academy never recommended the use of such pills.

Moreover, in stating that ". . . you may not cook [these vegetables] quite right," the ad also implies that PharmTech prepared the vegetables in Daily Greens according to a procedure specified by the NAS. In fact, the NAS specified no such procedure and certainly made no statement endorsing the dehydration procedure used by PharmTech.

II. Daily Greens Contain A Limited Quantity of Vegetables

In stating that Daily Greens are concentrated servings of cruciferous and carotene-rich vegetables, the ad suggests that these tablets contain the equivalent of a typical "serving" of vegetables. Indeed, some consumers may infer that the pills contain even more than a typical serving because these servings are "concentrated" and because the ad and package picture large amounts of vegetables.

In fact, *if these pills were comprised of one vegetable only*, each tablet would contain only about one-half of a raw brussels sprout, one-tenth of a cup of raw shredded or chopped cabbage, one-tenth of a cup of raw cauliflower buds, one-tenth of a medium stalk of broccoli, one-fifth of a cup of raw spinach, or one-tenth of a carrot. This information was not obtained from PharmTech, which has not disclosed

291

Cabbage, Brussels Sprouts, Carrots, Cauliflower, Spinach and Broccoli vs. Cancer.

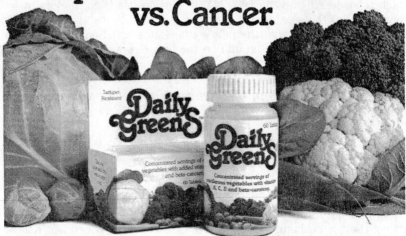

Your grandmother was right.

Eating vegetables is good for you. According to the National Academy of Sciences, a regular diet of cruciferous (cabbage, brussels sprouts, broccoli, cauliflower) and carotene-rich (carrots and spinach) vegetables is associated with a reduction in the incidence of certain cancers.*

Of course you may not really like these vegetables. Or you may not cook them quite right. And even if you have all that worked out, you still have to contend with seasonal availability.

That's why there are Daily Greens.™

Daily Greens are concentrated servings of cruciferous and carotene-rich vegetables. Picked ripe. Carefully washed. And quickly dehydrated without cooking. Then they're fortified with vitamins A, C, E, beta-carotene and selenium.

Finally, the ingredients are shaped into tablets and given a protective vegetable coating, freeing Daily Greens from the need for any preservatives.

The National Academy of Sciences thinks a balanced diet may reduce your risk of cancer. Daily

Greens were designed to be a part of that balanced diet: Decrease your intake of all fats by one-fourth; drink alcohol only in moderation; try to avoid pickled, smoked or salt-cured foods; eat plenty of fruits, whole grains and vegetables. And of course, don't smoke.

Daily Greens are not a cure for cancer, and there are no guarantees against cancer. But substantial evidence exists that regular consumption of cruciferous vegetables is associated with a reduction in the incidence of certain cancers.

Thanks to the process of dehydration, Daily Greens allow you to eat cruciferous vegetables regularly, with the convenience of a food supplement. Ask your doctor.

Even if you already take vitamins, Daily Greens are one more step toward a complete daily health program.

One of the simplest steps you can take.

*Diet, Nutrition and Cancer. Committee on Diet, Nutrition and Cancer. National Academy Press, 1982. Not all doctors agree with the National Academy of Sciences Study.

A food supplement from PharmTech Research. Daily Greens and Help your body defend itself are trademarks of PharmTech Research, Inc.
© 1982 PharmTech Research, Inc.
1750 Montgomery St.
San Francisco, CA 94111

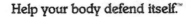

Help your body defend itself.™

the quantity of vegetables its product contains. It was calculated by weighing the tablets and correcting for water lost through dehydration.

The ad misinterprets the Academy's recommendations by suggesting that pills containing such small quantities of vegetables are associated with a reduced risk of cancer. In fact, the NAS stated that "in epidemiological studies, frequent consumption of these foods has been correlated with the incidence of various cancers." Surely, someone who eats one half of a brussels sprout or one-tenth of a broccoli stalk per day would ingest much smaller amounts of these vegetables than individuals characterized as "frequent" consumers of these foods.

Furthermore, the ad implies that the pills contain an assortment of vegetables in roughly the same proportion as pictured in the ad and on the box. Yet according to an individual who has been involved with PharmTech and has asked not to be identified, Daily Greens are 95% cabbage, the least expensive of the vegetables pictured.

In short, the ad suggests that Daily Greens reflect the Academy's dietary guidelines, but the Academy did not recommend that people consume very small amounts of cabbage and even tinier amounts of other cruciferous and beta-carotene rich vegetables. No scientific evidence suggests that such minute quantities of vegetables can reduce the risk of cancer.

We urge the FTC to halt PharmTech's exceedingly misleading ads for Daily Greens. We also call on the Commission to monitor carefully ads for similar supplements marketed by other companies.

Sincerely,

Michael F. Jacobson, Ph.D.
Executive Director [Center for Science in the Public Interest]

Bonnie F. Liebman, M.S.
Staff Nutritionist

> *When it comes to vitamins (and other supplements as well),*
> *you hear a lot of health claims that sound (and probably are)*
> *too good to be true. The next three selections try to make a*
> *case for regular supplement use, beginning with the point of*
> *view of physician Willard Krehl, who says that his patients*
> *can, but don't, eat properly.*

VITAMIN SUPPLEMENTATION — A PRACTICAL VIEW*

Willard A. Krehl, M.D.

My own bias on the value of nutrient supplementation has developed over the years through my experience in clinical practice. One of the standard procedures at our clinic is to take a dietary history of each patient. Reviewing these, I continually see that in spite of the fact that our clients are generally in the executive category and can therefore easily purchase an excellent diet, most of them do not eat properly. For whatever reasons, a large percent either skip breakfast or eat the wrong things for breakfast; they have a fast food lunch high in fat and often low in micronutrients; they consume a good deal of sugar, sweets and alcoholic beverages. In short, my search for the individuals who consistently eat a well-balanced, varied and nutritionally adequate diet has merely impressed me with the fact that millions of people do not.

Thus it comes as no surprise to me that national surveys reflect the nutritional imbalances and micronutrient shortages they do. It's not that the food supply is deficient; the "deficiency" lies in people's ability or motivation to use food properly.

I strongly favor multivitamin supplementation and recommend it to my patients because I believe it is a simple, economical and highly practical way to insure they receive 100% of the RDA for essential micronutrients, and because I believe these intakes are important to health and well being.

Some of the standard arguments against supplementation are that it encourages poor food habits, that marginal vitamin intakes are not really significant, and that people spend too much money on supplements. Let us consider each of these points.

Does supplementation encourage poor eating habits? I know of no

*"Vitamin Supplementation — A Practical View," by Willard A. Krehl, M.D. *Vitamin Issues*, Volume 4, No. 1, pp. 8–11. Hoffmann-LaRoche, Inc., Nutley, NJ. Vitamin Nutrition Information Service. Used with permission.

evidence to support the notion that the diets of people who take supplements are worse than those of people who do not. In fact, the opposite seems to be true: supplement users tend to be more health- and nutrition-conscious than non-users. Perhaps the reason there is no support for this "logic" is that it is, upon closer examination, illogical. What comes first? — food habits, of course. Eating habits are in place long before people consider supplementation. People consider supplementation when they learn why their eating habits need improvement. Something usually prompts this realization. It may be pregnancy, when supplements are prescribed, or dieting, which requires education about foods, or some medical crisis requiring nutritional support. In any case, supplementation seems to occur as part of the first stage of nutrition "consciousness-raising", when maintaining good nutrition becomes a matter of personal importance. As people attempt to make some positive changes in their habits, supplementation is *one* of the things they may do. Saying that supplementation encourages us to eat poorly is like saying antiseptics encourage us to cut ourselves more frequently.

This argument usually goes on to say that nutrition education can correct poor eating habits and eliminate the need for supplementation. It usually positions supplementation *versus* nutrition education. I think that is a mixture of wishful thinking and misinformation. More in tune with reality and therefore more useful would be nutrition education which encompasses the proper role of supplementation. Eating habits are deeply engrained and are often a function of lifestyle, divorced from nutritional considerations altogether. This makes them quite difficult to change. Change requires a willingness to undergo some inconvenience (there are no salads in the office candy machine), deprivation (cutting down on favorite sweets, alcohol, snacks, etc.) and rescheduling of activities (setting aside time for exercise and proper meals). Such changes do not come easily. They require time, patience and commitment, in addition to education/knowledge.

Moreover, even with the best nutrition planning and knowledge, there is no guarantee that all nutritional guidelines and recommendations can be met, notably when caloric intakes fall below about 1600 calories. Consider the menus published by the U.S. Department of Agriculture in "Ideas for Better Eating." Even with thorough and careful nutritional planning by competent professionals, these diets fall short of recommended levels of some essential nutrients at the 1600 calorie level. If nutritionists have trouble devising menus to meet nutrient recommendations at the 1600 calorie level, we should not be surprised at consumers' inability to do so. As it happens, the average caloric intakes of women in the United States hover around this level or lower. Other groups, such as the elderly and dieters, also consume low calorie diets that may put them at risk for some micronutrients.

Preliminary data from the National Health and Nutrition Survey

(N-HANES II) indicate the median caloric intake of the general population is 1,831 calories. (For women, the median is even lower, at 1,493 calories.) Median means that 50% of the population take in higher amounts and 50% take in lower amounts. So these data are telling us that the caloric intakes of half of American women are lower than 1,493 calories — a level where even trained nutritionists have trouble creating meals to provide RDA levels of vitamins and minerals!

. . . Indeed, the data from these surveys have shown shortages of vitamins and minerals among numerous sex-age groups, and the shortages were more prevalent among those who consumed lower calorie diets.

Are these micronutrient shortages significant? Most nutrition professionals agree that intakes below the RDA do not necessarily indicate serious nutritional risk, because the RDA are set higher than average requirements. . . . For this reason, nutritionists generally look at the percent of population groups with intakes lower than 70% – 80% of the RDA, rather than the percentages below 100%, as indicative of nutritional risk. The Food and Nutrition Board has noted in the 1980 edition of the Recommended Dietary Allowances:

"In assessing dietary surveys of populations, if the amounts of nutrients consumed fall below the RDA for a particular age-sex group, some individuals can be assumed to be at nutritional risk. When the proportion of individuals with such low intakes is extensive, the risk of deficiency in the population is increased."

What is "extensive"? Ten percent? Twenty? If one projects the numbers, ten percent of our present population would include more than 23 million people — an "extensive" group by any standards. According to the 1977 – 78 Nationwide Food Consumption Survey, significant percentages of the population were consuming less than 70% of the RDA for the nutrients listed:

Nutrient	% of Individuals with Intakes less than 70% RDA
Vitamin B_6	51%
Calcium	42%
Magnesium	39%
Iron	32%
Vitamin A	31%
Vitamin C	26%
Thiamin	17%
Vitamin B_{12}	15%
Riboflavin	12%

Since at 70% of the RDA or lower we can no longer be certain about an ample margin of safety, these data should alert us to an astonishing prevalence of potential nutritional risk. Furthermore, factors such as smoking, the use of alcohol, oral contraceptives or other drugs may increase risk among individuals whose diets are inadequate.

Among the strongest evidence illustrating wide-spread nutritional inadequacies are studies of our hospitalized population. Marginal or deficient levels of vitamins have been found in at least 30% of hospital patients, and protein-calorie malnutrition has been seen in some 44%. These individuals are in "double jeopardy," so to speak. Their disease or injury dramatically increases nutritional needs, even to the point of precipitating malnutrition which in turn impairs the immune response and the ability to heal.

In healthy people, suboptimal nutrition may result in vague symptoms such as depression, loss of appetite, irritability and so forth. These everyday complaints may be tolerable; however, serious problems can arise when illness, injury and/or surgery are superimposed upon preexisting marginal status.

The wisdom of maintaining the best nutritional health possible is self-evident. From my perspective, it certainly makes sense to err on the side of caution and insure adequate micronutrient intakes with a well-balanced multivitamin supplement, especially among populations known to be at nutritional risk — dieters, pregnant and lactating women, adolescent girls, smokers, alcoholics, the elderly, low income groups and others. When one considers the number of people potentially involved, the 60 million or so currently taking supplements probably far undershoots the number who could benefit from them.

I think it also makes sense for physicians to make this recommendation, since we can at the same time deter our patients from self-medicating or using supplements irresponsibly. I do not believe anyone should take therapeutic amounts of nutrients without medical supervision, but unless doctors are willing to give strong counsel on the proper use of supplements, I doubt if anyone will listen to our warnings about improper use.

Some people believe Americans are spending huge sums of money on vitamin supplements. Actually the average cost is about 8 – 9¢ per day, which is within the economic reach of just about everyone. The total vitamin supplement market was under $2 billion last year; I should think that those who are concerned with "unnecessary" expenditures might better target their efforts toward the $40 billion alcoholic beverage market or the $20 billion tobacco market.

One of the areas that concerns me most is the cost of health care in general — some 320 billion dollars in 1982. This cost has been increasing at a rate of 12 – 15% per year, about three times the general rate of inflation. It is breaking the back of American industry, which supplies much of the health care, and it is overwhelming the taxpayer

297

who has to foot the bill for Medicare, Medicaid and other government insurance programs. I believe that improved nutrition, in which vitamin supplementation can play an important role, might help to reduce this problem.

In sum, the high incidence of below-RDA micronutrient intakes, resulting from multiple factors including poor food choices, decreased caloric intakes and personal/environmental/lifestyle factors, presents a situation in which multivitamin supplementation is both a rational and beneficial choice. Supplementation provides a practical and economical means of insuring adequate nutrient intakes and is of particular importance for risk groups such as dieters, the elderly, heavy drinkers, chronic drug users and others whose diets are insufficient or whose ability to utilize food is impaired. Therapeutic amounts of micronutrients should not be used without medical supervision. In addition to education about food, consumers need nutrition education that teaches the proper role and value of rational supplementation and cautions against improper use. I see absolutely no reason to tolerate nutrient inadequacies when such a simple and sensible alternative as a multivitamin exists.

> *Paavo Airola, the recently deceased popular naturopath and writer, was typical of the self-appointed expert many nutritionists denounce. Here he makes his case for why everyone should supplement.*

VITAMINS AND SUPPLEMENTS: ARE THEY REALLY NEEDED?*

Paavo Airola

Q: I eat what I think is a very good diet, mostly in line with your writings. I'm only 29, and I feel great. Must I also take vitamins and supplements? Somehow, I have an aversion to pills and, frankly, I don't think I need them. Can't I get everything I need from the foods I eat? — C. K., Boston, Massachusetts

A: Although your idea of getting all the vitamins and minerals you need from the foods you eat seems logical — and would have been

*Letter: "Vitamins and Supplements: Are They Really Needed?" by Paavo Airola, N.D., Ph.D. *Vegetarian Times*, October 1981, Issue #50, page 89. Used with permission.

correct and sensible 100 or even 50 years ago — today, in our polluted, chemicalized and very unnatural environment, vitamins and supplements, in "pill" form, are imperative and can be lifesaving, even at your age.

Keep in mind the following facts:

1. You are most likely breathing polluted air.
2. You are subjected, perhaps unknowingly, to a great toxic insult of chemicals in clothing, cosmetics, bedding materials and a whole array of household chemicals.
3. You may drink city water, which is polluted and treated with chemicals.
4. No matter how hard you try, it is not very likely that *all* foods you eat are organically grown. Regular supermarket foods contain toxic chemical residues and additives.
5. Even most organically grown foods are now grown in depleted soils, are watered by polluted waters, and are subjected to air pollution and fallout.
6. You may be subjected to severe mental stress and anxieties — so common in our competitive society — and also lacking sufficient physical exercise due to a sedentary life.

To counteract all the above-mentioned negative influences in your environment, you must complement your diet with vitamins and supplements. They have a dual purpose: (1) to return to your diet the missing nutrients; (2) to protect your health from the health-destroying factors in our modern, toxic environment. Many vitamins and minerals possess specific protective and detoxifying properties against most environmental poisons in our food, water, air and environment.

> *Another perspective on the pill story comes from the Council*
> *for Responsible Nutrition, a trade group composed of supple-*
> *ment manufacturers and sellers. In this 1983 position paper,*
> *they approach the supplement issue as a problem of helping*
> *individuals whose lives seem to require more nutrients than*
> *their diets provide.*

WHO MAY BENEFIT FROM SUPPLEMENTATION?*

The Council for Responsible Nutrition

. . . Diets may fall short in nutrients when people do not eat enough,
when eating habits are poor, or when nutritional status is compromised by factors such as heavy smoking, drinking or medications. In
addition, nutritional needs are increased by infection, surgery, injury
and disease and during special life periods such as pregnancy and
lactation.

How many people are affected by one or more of these factors?
Let's look at the size of some potential risk groups:

People Who Do Not Eat Enough Food . . .

- 50 million dieters. Every year, some 20 to 40% of the population is
  dieting to lose weight, often involving "crash" or fad diets.
- 10 million alcoholics. Approximately 90 million Americans consume
  alcoholic beverages and of these, an estimated 9 to 10 million are
  problem drinkers or alcoholics.
- 25 million elderly citizens. The elderly may not be eating enough
  food to get all the nutrients they need. Poor teeth, inefficient diges-
  tion, low economic status and medications may compound the dietary problems of the aging.
- Women. Recent surveys show that women in the U.S. are consuming an average of 1600 calories daily. At these low calorie levels,
  nutrient intakes will be low unless food selections are made with
  extreme care.

People Whose Nutritional Status Is Compromised by Lifestyle/Habits . . .

- 50 million regular cigarette smokers may have reduced blood levels
  of vitamin C.

- 80 million "moderate" drinkers may be at risk for B complex vitamins.
- Up to 10 million women taking oral contraceptives may be at risk for some B vitamins.
- People who live in highly polluted areas may have increased needs for Vitamin E to help protect against the effects of ozone and other environmental contaminants.

People Whose Nutritional Status Is Compromised by Disease or Surgery . . .

- 36 million people in hospitals in a typical year may not receive appropriate nutritional monitoring and support.
- Commonly used medications may interfere with nutrient absorption or utilization or deplete body stores of nutrients.

People Passing Through Special Life Periods . . .

- 3.3 million new mothers. Physicians recognize the special nutritional needs of pregnant or nursing women, and a vitamin/mineral supplement is almost always recommended. For some nutrients, especially iron and folic acid, the increased needs of pregnant or lactating women cannot practically be achieved by eating more food or changing food patterns.
- 17 million adolescents. Many teenagers are undergoing the typical "growth spurt" during which nutrient needs are extremely important. Teenagers often do not eat properly, and some may be nutritionally at risk, particularly the girls who are also dieting to lose weight during these critical years.
- 25 million elderly citizens may not eat properly for a variety of reasons and may not be able to fully absorb the nutrients in the foods they eat, and thus may be at nutritional risk.

> *Before we hear from the other side, we offer a piece of objective information. Both proponents and critics of nutrient supplementation agree that "too much" can be harmful. But how much is too much? Just what is the margin of safety between the amount of certain nutrients we require and the amount that could be toxic? The tables of nutritionist John N. Hathcock provide some answers.*

QUANTITATIVE EVALUATION OF VITAMIN SAFETY*

John N. Hathcock, Ph.D.

Table 1: Vitamin Safety Indexes

Vitamin	Recommended Adult Intake[a]	Estimated Adult Oral MTD	VSI
Vitamin A	5,000 IU	25 to 50,000 IU	5 to 10
Vitamin D	400 IU	50,000 IU[b]	125
		1 to 2,000 IU	2.5 to 5
Vitamin E	30 IU	1,200 IU	40
Vitamin C	30 mg	2 to 5,000 mg[c]	33 to 83
		1,000 mg	17
Thiamin (B$_1$)	1.5 mg	300 mg	200
Riboflavin	1.7 mg	1,000 mg	588
Niacin (niacinamide)	20 mg	1,000 mg	50
Pyridoxine (B$_6$)	2.2 mg	2,000 mg[d]	900
		200 mg	90
Folacin	0.4 mg	400 mg[e]	1,000
		15 mg	37
Biotin	0.3 mg	50 mg	167
Pantothenic Acid	10 mg	10,000 mg	1,000

[a]The highest of the individual RDA (except those for pregnancy and lactation) or the U. S. RDA, whichever is higher
[b]For infants and also for adults with certain infections or metabolic diseases; 50,000 IU for most adults
[c]To produce slightly altered mineral excretion patterns
[d]For antagonism of some drugs; 2,000 mg for most adults
[e]For antagonism of anticonvulsants in epileptics; 400 mg or more for most adults

*"Quantitative Evaluation of Vitamin Safety", by John N. Hathcock, Ph.D. *Pharmacy Times*, May 1985, Pgs. 104–113. Romaine Pierson Publishers, Inc., Port Washington, N Y Used with permission.

Table 2: Mineral Safety Indexes

Mineral	*Recommended Adult Intake*[a]	*Estimated Adult Oral MTD*	*MSI*
Calcium	1,200 mg	12,000 mg	10
Phosphorus[b]	1,200 mg	12,000 mg	10
Magnesium	400 mg	6,000 mg	15
Iron	18 mg	100 mg	5.5
Zinc	15 mg	500 mg	33
Copper	3 mg	100 mg	33
		< 3 mg[c]	< 1
Fluoride[d]	4 mg	20 mg	5
		4 mg[e]	1
Iodine	0.15 mg	2 mg	13
Selenium	0.2 mg	1 mg	5

[a]The highest of the individual RDA (except those for pregnancy and lactation) or the U. S. RDA, whichever is higher
[b]As the orthophosphate ion
[c]For people with Wilson's disease
[d]As fluoride ion
[e]Level producing slight fluorosis of dental enamel

Editor's Note:

MTD — Minimum Toxic Dose. Generally, the smallest dose of a nutrient that has been shown to be harmful when swallowed over a period of time.

VSI (Vitamin Safety Index) and MSI (Mineral Safety Index) — These are the ratios between the Minimum Toxic Dose and the Recommended Intake for any nutrient. They indicate what multiple of the recommendation is likely to lead to toxic effects for a given vitamin or mineral. For example, the MSI for calcium is 10. This means that a calcium intake (through foods and supplements) at a level of 10 or more times the amount recommended over a period of time could be dangerous to your health. The lower the VSI or MSI, the greater the risk of overdosing.

And now the view of Dr. Alfred Harper from whom we have heard several times earlier on the subject of the RDAs and in opposition to dietary goals. There is little evidence, he argues, that any substantial portion of the U.S. population is short of vitamins and minerals. Therefore, why supplement?

VITAMIN SUPPLEMENTATION — A SKEPTICAL VIEW*

Alfred E. Harper, Ph.D.

Vitamin deficiency diseases have not been encountered in the major health and nutrition surveys done recently in the United States; in fact, such diseases occur so rarely now in this country as to be medical curiosities. Large numbers of apparently healthy people, nonetheless, take vitamin supplements. The reasons they give for this are: the belief that they are not getting enough vitamins from their diets and the belief that they will be less healthy without them. There is obviously a widespread popular perception that health is at risk when food is the only source of nutrients and that taking vitamin supplements will ensure a better state of health. Is this popular perception accurate? What type of evidence can be marshalled to support it? Is the available evidence reliable?

Probably the main evidence used to support recommendations for vitamin supplements is that, in health and nutrition surveys, intakes of some vitamins by some segments of the population are found to be below the recommended dietary allowances (RDA). To evaluate evidence of this type critically requires knowledge of how the RDA are established and how dietary surveys are done. . . .

Because people differ in size and genetic makeup, their nutrient requirements vary; requirements of individuals for essential nutrients range from about 50% below to 50% above the population average. The RDA, therefore, were set high enough to ensure that, if the quantities of nutrients in the food being served met this standard, they would meet the needs of individuals with the highest requirements. Thus, the amounts of nutrients required by most people will be below the RDA and about half the population should require from 40–75% of the RDA. Obviously a dietary standard of this type cannot be used to determine if the intakes of people who are consuming less than the

*"Vitamin Supplementation — A Skeptical View", by Alfred E. Harper, Ph.D. *Vitamin Issues*, Volume 4, No. 1, pp. 5–8, 11. Hoffmann-LaRoche, Inc., Nutley, NJ. The Vitamin Nutrition Information Service. Used with permission.

RDA are inadequate. Using the RDA as standards for evaluating the adequacy of nutrient intakes is like setting the standard for height at 7 feet and assuming that all of those under 7 feet have suffered growth retardation.

Even then, when the estimates of nutrient intakes obtained during dietary surveys are compared with the RDA, we find that only two vitamins, A and C, are identified consistently as "problem" nutrients. In interpreting these observations, we encounter two additional problems. The RDA for vitamin C is twice as high as that used by the World Health Organization. It is high enough to ensure that a person who is consuming an amount of vitamin C equal to the RDA will have a store of the vitamin sufficient to prevent signs of deficiency from occurring even if he/she consumes no vitamin C for about two months. With a standard such as this, which is disproportionately high, one would expect to find problems of inadequate intake where none exist, and that is exactly what happens. With vitamin A, a different problem is encountered. The main sources of vitamin A in the diet are carotenoids in dark green and yellow to orange vegetables. These foods are not usually eaten every day so, when the results of dietary surveys are based on measurements of nutrient intakes for a single day, as they ordinarily are, many people will have low intakes of vitamin A on that day. Others will have unusually high intakes. As vitamin A is stored efficiently in the liver, a surplus of vitamin A consumed on one day will provide a store that will be available on subsequent days. Intakes of vitamin A can probably be estimated accurately only by averaging daily intakes over at least a week.

Because of the nature of the RDA and of dietary surveys, it is not possible to assess nutritional status by comparing estimates of nutrient intakes with the RDA. The only way that vitamin status can be determined reliably is from clinical observations and measurements of blood or tissue concentrations or the rates of metabolic reactions for which the vitamins are needed. When this is done, a very small proportion of the population surveyed is found to have low, but seldom deficient, values. With such a high proportion of the population showing no evidence of inadequate vitamin intakes, the low values cannot be attributed to inadequacies of the food supply.

Estimates of the nutrient content of the food supply indicate that amounts of nutrients available to the consumer have increased during this century. Consumption of fruits, vegetables, cheese, fish, poultry and pork, all excellent sources of essential nutrients, have increased during the past 10 years more than enough to compensate for declines in the consumption of beef, dairy products and eggs. Of low income families studied by USDA, 42% were consuming a diet that met the RDA for 11 nutrients. This is incontrovertible evidence that the food supply contains adequate amounts of essential nutrients. Families that were dependent on food stamp allotments were consuming less adequate diets, indicating that as income falls, food choices become more

305

limited and intakes of some essential nutrients decrease. Inadequate intakes of food, and hence usually of nutrients, occur because of neglect, illness, alcoholism and ignorance. These are not problems that can be solved by the use of vitamin or other dietary supplements.

Another reason given for the use of vitamin supplements is deteriorating or haphazard eating habits. That eating habits have changed is undeniable but whether or not this represents deterioration is certainly debatable. A pattern of eating three or more substantial meals a day is common in agricultural communities and others in which energy expenditure is high. This was accepted as the most desirable pattern when our population was largely rural and when mechanization was much less in both the home and the workplace than it is today. One might well ask if, in a society in which energy expenditure is low, it may not be preferable to eat several small meals throughout the day and to eat when hungry rather than when the clock says it is meal-time. There is much speculation but little evidence that unusual eating patterns result in consumption of inadequate amounts of essential nutrients except when total calorie (food) intake is low. . . .

There is little evidence that will stand up to scrutiny to suggest that any substantial proportion of the U.S. population is consuming a nutritionally inadequate diet for any length of time. There is, thus, little reason to assume that vitamin supplements will be beneficial for a substantial portion of the population. Foods contain many nutrients besides those provided in vitamin supplements; they also contain many constituents whose significance for health is unknown. Learning how to select foods properly to meet nutritional needs, regardless of changing eating patterns or changes in the food supply is the only reliable way to ensure lifelong nutritional health. Encouraging the use of vitamin supplements as a corrective for poor eating habits defeats the entire purpose of nutrition education, i.e., to learn the nutritional principles needed to select a healthful diet instead of accepting nutritional advice on faith.

In recent years there have been suggestions that larger than usual amounts of vitamins are needed to counteract the effects of environmental hazards and practices that increase risk to health. The suggestion that smokers need high doses of vitamin C seems incongruous when one considers that most of the subjects used in the major experiments that served as the basis for present vitamin C allowances were smokers. It would seem much more appropriate to suggest that non-smokers need less. For heavy consumers of alcohol, vitamin supplements may prevent the development of some nutritional inadequacies. They may also encourage further consumption of alcohol to the point where toxicity becomes more severe than it otherwise might. Minor infections or stresses may increase nutritional needs modestly for a short time. As the human subjects used in experiments which provided the information on which requirements are based were not

protected from usual environmental stresses or infections, it is doubtful that vitamin supplements are needed in these conditions. During
illness, recovery from illness and during periods of drug therapy, food
intake may be so low that it becomes difficult or even impossible to
meet nutritional needs from foods. RDA are not therapeutic recommendations. Nutritional supplements are often appropriate under such
conditions but as part of a comprehensive program of treatment under
the guidance of a physician.

There have been a variety of observations suggesting that certain
vitamins, A, E and C in particular, may have some unique value in preventing or reducing adverse effects from environmental hazards. Some
of these observations are tantalizing, e.g., that these vitamins may act
in some way to protect against certain cancer-inducing agents; and,
that vitamins E and C, as antioxidants, may protect against ill effects
from certain chemical contaminants. These studies are suggestive, not
conclusive. They are the subject of much current research. They suggest that vitamin deficiencies often increase susceptibility to toxic
agents, but the assumption that large doses of nutrients — larger than
the usual recommended intakes — are uniquely beneficial is controversial. Promotion of vitamin supplements as therapeutic agents tends to
encourage self-medication with large quantities of specific vitamins.
Such practices create the risk of people delaying or not accepting
appropriate medical treatment for illnesses and taking doses of vitamins that create risks of toxicity. With the advent of the widespread
use of large doses of vitamins the incidence of vitamin toxicity has increased.

The most appropriate use of vitamin supplements is in conditions
in which caloric intake is low, below 1200 Kcal per day, and particularly if, at the same time, requirements are increased, say as the result of
illness. An appropriately balanced multivitamin supplement for the pregnant woman and supplements of vitamins A and D of appropriate
potency for the young infant can be justified as insurance against nutritional inadequacy. Evaluation of the nutrition literature on vitamin
requirements and intakes and claims for the use of vitamins as therapeutic and pharmacologic agents, however, provides no evidence to
convince me that the population generally requires vitamin supplements but much to convince me that the nutritional knowledge of the
public generally is inadequate and inaccurate. The assumed nutritional
problems of most people are best solved by providing them with accurate nutrition information about food and health and countering the
nutrition misinformation to which so many of them are constantly exposed.

307

> *In this long and thoughtful piece, medical doctor Arthur J.*
> *Vander describes the research problems inherent in attempt-*
> *ing to determine what an "optimal" intake of each nutrient*
> *would be. Alert readers will recall that some of the issues he*
> *raises — about appropriate goals for nutrition — were dis-*
> *cussed in the Introduction and in Chapter 1 on the RDAs.*

THE TASK OF NUTRITIONAL SCIENCE*

Arthur J. Vander, M.D.

. . . For many years, we viewed most essential nutrients as bearing
one-to-one relationships with specific diseases; vitamin D prevented
rickets, vitamin C scurvy, and so on. Then came a radical reorientation
of our thinking as it became obvious that, in addition to these quite
specific effects, any particular essential nutrient often exerted widespread actions on a host of bodily functions; for example, vitamin C, in
amounts larger than those specified by its RDA, enhances the activity
of the liver enzymes which catabolize environmental pollutants, and
vitamin D interferes with the transformation of cholesterol to other
molecules. The inference from this knowledge (as well as the simul-
taneous recognition that virtually all diseases are multicausal) was
that each nutrient might influence the development of a variety of diseases, perhaps with very different dose-responses. Thus, evaluation of
the optimal intake of the nutrient requires the taking into account of
all these different interactions and dose-responses.

If we look at the entire potential spectrum of nutrient effects, we
can make several generalizations. At the opposite ends of the spectrum are the known beneficial actions (prevention of clear-cut specific
disease) and the toxic effects. There is no question that, at high
enough doses, many nutrients begin to cause damage; for example,
iodine, which is essential for normal thyroid function, actually causes
thyroid malfunction at high enough doses (this was first recognized
when, soon after discovery of its physiological role, iodine became
such a food fad that it was often carried by persons in little vials
from which drinks were taken whenever the person felt sluggish or
"down").

Between these two ends of the spectrum lies most of the dose-
range over which most persons can maintain nutrient balance without
obvious deficiency or toxicity. In this physiological range, the body's

---

*Excerpted from Chapter 3: "The Task of Nutritional Science," by Arthur J. Vander, M.D.
Nutrition, Stress, and Toxic Chemicals. Copyright 1981 by the University of Michigan,
pp. 99 – 110. Used with permission of the University of Michigan Press.

homeostatic mechanisms tend to minimize changes in total body content of the nutrient as intake changes, but . . . some change must occur, and this leads to the crucial question: Do these differences over the physiological midrange of the spectrum of bodily nutrient concentrations really matter? Is it better (or worse) to have a few percent more sodium in the body (the range of change of body sodium over the entire range of intakes compatible with the absence of frank disease)? A few percent more or less protein? 10 to 20 percent more zinc? 1,000 percent more vitamin C?

For such questions to have meaning, we must specify precisely those end points we will use in answering them: longevity, enhanced resistance to cancer or heart disease, increased ability to run marathons, and so on. The list is infinite as is the sister list for potentially harmful effects, and the experiments required to answer them are, for the most part, far more difficult to perform and analyze than those for setting RDAs. Just to perform such experiments for a single nutrient — say vitamin C — requires a massive outlay of funds and scientific personnel, and so we must choose carefully our priorities. Let us now use vitamin C as an example illustrating certain of these points.

Many studies have demonstrated, in human subjects, that 10 mg of vitamin C per day is adequate to prevent almost all signs or symptoms of scurvy. Only maintenance of gum health seems to require more, and even here, 30 mg/day is adequate in virtually all cases. Studies using balance methods and measurements of pool size also document that 30 mg/day is more than adequate to maintain body stores of vitamin C at levels which prevent all the signs and symptoms of scurvy. Accordingly, the most recent National Research Council RDA for vitamin C has been set at 60 mg/day, the extra 30 mg/day being a safety factor added on to cover individual variation, losses in cooking, and other environmental factors.

There is unanimous agreement about the facts concerning vitamin C and scurvy; why then the controversy, led by Linus Pauling and Irwin Stone, who argue that the optimum intake of ascorbic acid — that is, the daily amount of this food that leads to the best of health — is somewhere between 250 mg and 10 g? Pauling and Stone are emphasizing "optimum intake" and "best of health," not the amount adequate to prevent scurvy. They and their followers argue that scientists have been misguided in allowing scurvy — a dramatic, clear-cut disease — to dominate thinking about the role of vitamin C in bodily function. They believe that this vitamin, which is present in all body tissues, is a central substance in the functioning of these tissues and, as such, may be involved in a host of phenomena, including defenses against a wide variety of diseases. If all this is true, then basing our estimates of vitamin C "requirements" on experiments having only to do with scurvy is foolish. In short, they argue that scientists have been using the wrong end points in establishing recommendations for daily intakes of vitamin C.

309

There is no doubt that the furor over vitamin C and the fact that it has stimulated a large and rapidly growing number of studies is due mainly to the brilliance and achievements of Linus Pauling. The type of claims he has made for the efficacy of large doses of vitamin C in reducing the frequency of colds had previously been made by many others (and ignored) as Pauling was to emphasize. In addition to citing what he felt to be strong clinical data supporting the curative powers of vitamin C, Pauling buttressed his views with purely theoretical considerations of what was known about the normal physiology and biochemistry of vitamin C. . . . This is a perfectly sound way of pursuing a possible connection between an environmental factor and a disease.

Pauling particularly emphasized the intriguing metabolism of vitamin C. Almost all mammals except primates, the guinea pig, and the Indian fruit-eating bats are capable of synthesizing (in the liver) their own vitamin C, so that this substance is not an essential nutrient for them. Importantly, the amounts that they synthesize are usually considerably larger than those needed to prevent scurvy. Second, vitamin C is an example of a nutrient the plasma concentration and total body content of which changes markedly (compared, say, to sodium or protein) as intake is increased. This relation is at first almost a linear one. At an intake of 10 mg/day, plasma concentration is 1.4 mg/L and the pool size is about 300 mg; when intake is 100 mg/day, plasma concentration is 12 mg/L and pool size is 3,000 mg. So a tenfold increase in vitamin C intake produces close to a tenfold increase in its body content and plasma concentration.

How different this is from the case of sodium, the intake of which can be increased over a fiftyfold range with a resulting change in body sodium content of only a few percent. The major homeostatically controlled pathway for both sodium and vitamin C is urinary excretion, but obviously the control of sodium excretion is much more precise than that of vitamin C over the usual range of intakes. Within forty-eight to seventy-two hours after sodium intake has been doubled the kidneys have adjusted their handling of this mineral so as to double its excretion, because only a tiny increase in body sodium is required to trigger these sodium-losing reflexes. In contrast, a doubling of vitamin C intake does not lead to a doubling of urinary vitamin C until many days have elapsed and until body content has slowly built up until it is virtually doubled. In other words, a 1 to 2 percent change in body sodium can effect a 100 percent change in urinary sodium excretion, whereas a 100 percent increase in body content of vitamin C is required to drive a 100 percent increase in urinary excretion of this vitamin.

In terms of evolution, a possible inference is that there must be a strong selection pressure (survival value) for keeping the body's sodium content within very narrow limits but relatively little for keeping vitamin C unchanged over the almost tenfold range of plasma concentrations from 1.4 mg/L to 12 mg/L. Pauling, of course, draws a very different inference (with just as much justification), namely that the body is trying to conserve as much vitamin C as possible even at levels ten times greater than those needed to prevent scurvy.

But the pattern changes dramatically when vitamin C intake goes beyond approximately 100 to 150 mg/day, for then the concentration of vitamin C in the blood and the total amount in the body increase very little with increasing intake. For example, an intake of 2 g/day fails to produce a sustained rise in plasma concentration of vitamin C of more than a few percent over that seen at intakes of 250 mg (there is a rise of 20 to 30 percent during the first days after one goes on such an intake, but the plasma concentration soon is adjusted back toward its original values; this is probably also the case for body stores of the vitamin). There are two reasons for this. For one thing, absorption of vitamin C from the gut, close to 100 percent at low intakes, begins to decrease; only about 50 percent is absorbed when the intake is 2 g and still smaller at larger doses. Far more important, the kidneys resist the ability of large intakes of vitamin C to raise plasma concentration because they increase excretion very rapidly to match intake. Thus, the excretion of vitamin C in large amounts looks very much like that of sodium, in that no amount of ingestion (short of quantities so huge as to overwhelm the kidneys) can raise the plasma concentration or pool size of the nutrient by more than a few percent; the body is said to be "fully saturated."

Most nutritionists argue that it is logical (but not necessarily correct) to postulate two conclusions from these facts: (1) it makes little sense to ingest daily more than 100 to 150 mg of vitamin C since only a small sustained change in bodily concentration is achieved by so doing; (2) the presence of mechanisms which strongly resist elevations of plasma and pool vitamin C beyond intakes of 100 to 150 mg/day raise the suspicion that further increases might be harmful, i.e., that we have evolved protective mechanisms against large intakes.

Yet, flying in the face of these hypotheses, Linus Pauling and his followers have advocated daily intakes of 400 to 10,000 mg (0.4 to 10 g). It is this "megavitamin" approach which probably most upsets nutritionists and other scientists, who argue that such huge doses have nothing to do with nutrition, that human beings do not naturally consume these amounts, that Pauling is really advocating the use of vitamin C as a "medicine" not a nutrient, and that the likelihood of undesirable side effects at this dose is every bit as likely as that of beneficial effects. The distinction between "medicine" (or "drug") on the one hand and "nutrient" on the other is not trivial, for the label "nutrient" somehow connotes a beneficial "natural" substance (which explains the intense effort on the part of those who favor the use of laetrile to dignify it with the completely undeserved appellation, vitamin B_{17}). Moreover, a drug, unlike a nutrient, must be validated in carefully controlled animal and human experiments before it is advo-

311

cated or allowed for widespread use by the public.

Pauling disagrees that his recommended doses are completely counteracted by decreased gastrointestinal absorption and increased kidney excretion or that they are really large and unphysiological, and he offers a variety of theoretical arguments to back up his position. For one thing, there is no question that the plasma concentration of vitamin C is quite elevated transiently after each ingestion of the recommended dose, and it is quite possible that the concentration of this vitamin in critical cells remains permanently elevated. Second, it is known that the utilization of vitamin C increases in a variety of stress situations, and it may be that large doses are required to maintain a high blood concentration of the vitamin at such times. Third, echoing Dr. Williams, Pauling believes that individual variation in nutrient requirements is so great that what seem to be extremely large amounts are required by many people (of course, by the same token, there ought to be the same degree of individual variation vis-à-vis toxicity so that some people might be highly susceptible to any toxic effects). Finally, and most important, Pauling argues that his recommendations are not large at all, when compared to the amounts synthesized or ingested by other mammalian species. When weight differences are taken into account, most of the animals which have retained the capacity to produce vitamin C do so in amounts equivalent to 2 to 15 g/day for human beings. The gorilla, only twice our weight, ingests 4 to 5 g of the vitamin each day, and, based on the amounts of vitamin C in purely vegetarian diets, our evolutionary predecessors were probably ingesting, Pauling believes, more than 2 g of vitamin C each day. Indeed, he reasons that it was this ample intake of vitamin C that permitted our distant ancestors to do without the machinery of synthesizing vitamin C. In this view the gene mutation resulting in loss of the enzymes needed for making vitamin C was selected because it saved the body the energy required to make a substance which the diet was already supplying in large quantities. Of course, this evolutionary guessing game is a double-edged sword, for one might argue a quite different view, that our ancestors never did ingest such large amounts of vitamin C, that these amounts are more harmful than beneficial, and that this accounts for the success of the mutation which prevented manufacture of vitamin C. Such games are great fun to play, but solve nothing. Nor do any of the other theoretical arguments, either pro or con. . . . Theory alone can never by itself provide answers to questions of benefit and toxicity. The answer must come from research designed to answer the specific questions at hand. Do such doses of vitamin C really protect against the common cold (or cancer, arthritis, and mental disease, among others)? Do such doses exert harmful effects which would outweigh any beneficial effects?

Pauling felt, at the time he wrote the first edition of his book *Vitamin C and the Common Cold* (1970), that the existing human experiments were already adequate to answer those questions, that vitamin C definitely had been shown to be effective against the common cold.

312

However, of the five major studies he cited, only two meet even some of the criteria required for trustworthy human experimentation. . . .

So far as the other much more serious diseases that vitamin C is hypothesized to be effective against, the data are far too few to permit any conclusions.

What about the other side of the coin — toxicity? Pauling has emphasized over and over again that vitamin C "is known to have extremely low toxicity," and it is certainly true that, other than diarrhea, no diseases have been proven to result from the use of large doses. But the fact is that we have not yet looked very hard, and if we have learned anything about toxicology in the past ten years, it is that subtle long-term toxicity is extremely difficult to determine without appropriate extensive testing, not merely the gross observation that people seem able to tolerate large doses without obvious harm. Such studies expressly designed to test long-term toxicity in experimental animals are in their infancy but are already yielding enough suggestive data to warrant caution.

Perhaps the single most important effects to test for are those on the fetus, since so many pregnant women are now taking large amounts of vitamin C. In one fascinating but very inconclusive study, it was found that two infants born to such women developed scurvy postnatally despite normal intakes of vitamin C; the researchers hypothesized that the presence of high blood concentrations of vitamin C *in utero* had "imprinted" on the fetus an increased requirement for this vitamin.

I would like now to return to the issue I raised earlier about priorities. There are approximately fifty essential nutrients and testing all of them at supra-RDA intakes for specific beneficial (and harmful) effects to obtain data pertaining to "optimal" rather than merely "acceptable" intakes will be a massive, perhaps unachievable, but nonetheless worthwhile task. In the particular case of vitamin C, it seems to me a matter of high priority to investigate possible beneficial effects against serious diseases over the range of 45 to 150 mg (the "saturation" intake) daily intake. So far as higher intakes are concerned, I share the opinion of T. W. Anderson, a professor of epidemiology and a person quite friendly to Pauling's argument that the RDA is not the "optimal" intake for vitamin C:

"Higher intakes than those necessary to produce saturation may eventually prove to be desirable in certain situations, but until we have a clearer idea of the benefit/risk ratios involved, such "mega-vitamin" dosages should only be used on a short-term or experimental basis, or where the potential risk is far outweighed by the nature of the disease being treated [cancer, for example]."

These guidelines are probably appropriate for the search for optimal levels of most other nutrients as well, and it is important that

313

such guidelines be set, since the controversy over "meganutrient" therapy is by no means limited to vitamin C. Nor did it really begin with vitamin C; the concept, now termed orthomolecular therapy, began about twenty-five years ago with the idea that massive doses of vitamin B_3 (niacin) might be effective in the therapy of schizophrenia. The concept has been, over the years, extended to many other nutrients and a host of diseases. Results claimed by its advocates were initially modest but, more and more, have become broad categorical statements and calls to action offered usually without much evidence; typical is the recommendation by Dr. A. Hoffer that "enrichment of our food with vitamin B_3 will prevent most cases of . . . schizophrenia from becoming manifest. I estimate that one gram per day started early in life will protect most of us." The RDA for vitamin B_3, based mainly on the amount needed to prevent pellagra, is only 20 mg/day, and this vitamin is known to produce toxic effects at doses of 3 to 6 g/day. What makes this recommendation triply irresponsible is the lack of evidence that vitamin B_3 is effective at all in the therapy of schizophrenia, the good chances of toxicity in some people at the doses suggested, and the request that everyone in the population, not just patients with schizophrenia, be exposed to these amounts through the vehicle of enriching the food supply. . . .

Unfortunately, the claims and recommendations made by disciples of orthomolecular therapy (including Pauling) have been so numerous, so varied, and so little supported in most cases by solid evidence that it is easy for nutritionists and other scientists to become exasperated and dismiss the whole subject of "optimal" intakes as nonsense. This would be throwing out the baby with the bath water. The problem could be minimized if a clear distinction were made between the levels of nutrient intakes achievable through normal dietary habits (i.e., by the ingestion of ordinary foods) and those which can be accomplished only by ingesting extremely large quantities of nutrient supplements. Studying potential beneficial effects of nutrients in the first instance really represents the pursuit of "ideal" or "optimal" nutrition, whereas the second instance (a perfectly legitimate one) is using nutrients as medication and should be subject to the usual constraints which apply to such research.

In conclusion, the quest for better means of determining RDAs and altered needs due to environmental factors, particularly disease, along with the just-beginning quest for optimal or ideal intakes as well as toxic effects of nutrients, establish nutrition as one of the most important areas of human health for future research efforts. . . .

314

In the face of a highly skeptical questioner, Professor David R. Roll asserts the necessity to be thoughtful in our critique of nutritional supplementation. No one should take useless or harmful drugs, he agrees, but supplements should not be singled out for criticism.

VITAMINS: IS THE PUBLIC SWALLOWING A NECESSARY PILL?*

David B. Roll, Ph.D.

. . . We asked Dr. Stephen Barrett, co-author of *Vitamins and "Health" Foods: The Great American Hustle* and consulting editor to *ACSH News & Views*, to prepare some questions on vitamin use, vitamin marketing, and the role of the pharmacy profession. We presented these questions to . . . David B. Roll, Ph.D., Professor of Medicinal Chemistry and Associate Dean for Academic Affairs at the University of Utah College of Pharmacy. . . .

Dr. Roll: Before discussing the individual questions, I believe it is important to emphasize that in the area of vitamin supplementation there is a great deal of subjective opinion. There is not a lot of agreement, just as there is little agreement among psychiatrists as to what constitutes criminal insanity. The fact is that we do not know all we wish we did about the vitamin requirements of man. This due in part to the fact that the definitive studies have not been done in humans and in fact will not be done due to the nature of the required experiments and the time required to conduct them. Our imperfect knowledge is illustrated by the fact that the National Research Council has repeatedly made changes in the Recommended Dietary Allowances for many vitamins over the years as new knowledge has become available.

Unfortunately, some advertising for vitamin supplements plays on the uncertainty of our knowledge. Just as unfortunate is the belief perpetuated by some that we know everything there is to know about the nutrition of man and that supplementation is of no value to anyone, a view that is reflected in the tenor of some of the questions below. . . .

ACSH: How many . . . people don't need the supplements they are taking because they are getting adequate amounts of vitamins in the food they eat?

Dr. Roll: I have no way of knowing, nor does anyone else. We do

---

*"Vitamins: Is the Public Swallowing a Necessary Pill?." *ACSH News & Views*, 5:1, 11–14, May/June 1984. American Council on Science and Health.

know, however, that the results of four major national nutrition surveys have revealed that some segments of our population have vitamin intakes below the recommended levels.

ACSH: Then you would agree that millions of Americans are taking unnecessary vitamins?

Dr. Roll: I agree that we need to better identify the segments of the population who would most benefit from supplementation and then do what we can to improve their nutrition. In other words, there is a large body of the population who might benefit from supplementation just as there are those who are probably receiving no physiological benefit from taking supplements. . . .

ACSH: Do you think that the pharmaceutical profession has any ethical obligation to conduct public educational campaigns to discourage people from taking vitamins that are not needed?

Dr. Roll: The pharmaceutical profession has an ethical responsibility to encourage the rational use of medication whether prescribed or over-the-counter. In all cases the stress should be on risks versus benefits. In my opinion, there has been a tendency to emphasize the former. We must realize that some people will feel better simply as the result of taking *something.* This placebo effect can be beneficial and the risk from taking a low-dose multi-vitamin supplement is negligible. The public must also be educated not to treat the symptoms of serious disease with vitamins, or with their neighbor's prescribed medication.

I am sure that the pharmaceutical profession does not have an ethical obligation to scare the hell out of people by publicizing isolated reports of vitamin toxicity.

ACSH: Do you think that "unnecessary vitamins" should be an ethical issue of concern to pharmacy school educators?

Dr. Roll: Unnecessary and improper use of all medication is an ethical issue to pharmacy educators. Frankly, we spend more of our efforts in identifying the unnecessary and improper use of prescription medications than in doing the same for nonprescription products, since there are many physicians who know little about the pharmacology of the drugs they prescribe. The potential for harm from these drugs and their interactions with each other is much greater than that from the daily ingestion of a low-dose multi-vitamin supplement. . . .

ACSH: On the whole, do you think that ads promoting vitamin supplements tend to be truthful or misleading?

Dr. Roll: I believe that much of the advertising is misleading, particularly as we seem to be in a "horsepower" race with more manufacturers trying to cram higher levels of vitamins (and in some cases non-nutrients) into single dosage units. I am not sure that the level of misinformation is any greater than it is in any other area of advertising, and I question the motivation of those who seem to be singling out advertising of vitamins in some sort of personal vendetta.

316

ACSH: Do you believe that advertising for "stress vitamins" has been misleading?

Dr. Roll: . . . This is an unfortunate development in the marketing of vitamins. I believe that manufacturers should be required to more rigorously document their advertising claims. However, in fairness, it is difficult to prove that these products, when taken as directed, cause physical harm to the user.

ACSH: You . . . agree that some vitamin advertising is misleading. It is obvious that the advertisers involved will continue to mislead unless stopped by some powerful legal or political force. The Federal Trade Commission (FTC) can provide sufficient legal force. Perhaps some component of the pharmaceutical profession could create sufficient political force. What do you think can be done to stop misleading vitamin advertising? What do you think should be done?

Dr. Roll: I am not at all sure that we can depend on regulatory agencies to prevent misleading advertising whether it is for vitamins, food, automobiles, or cigarettes. With the limited manpower available, we must do the best we can to regulate that misleading advertising which poses the greatest health threat, and I doubt that vitamin advertising is the most serious problem in this regard. . . .

> *While the experts argue, many people continue to take (or start taking) supplements. The very existence of heated controversy has induced many people to make their own decisions about their need for nutritional supplementation. In light of this fact, dietitian Susan Male Smith argues that professionals may be alienating their audience when, instead of intelligent and informed advice, they offer lectures against pill-popping.*

A NEW APPROACH TO VITAMIN SUPPLEMENTATION*

Susan Male Smith, M.A., R.D.

As reputable nutritionists, we spend much time counteracting the claims of mega-vitamin promoters, citing cases of vitamin overdoses and the resulting deleterious effects. But how common are these cases of toxicity? Is every vitamin user a potential abuser? . . .

Who Needs Them?

Current research and USDA Food Consumption Surveys indicate that a significant segment of the population ingests sub-optimal levels of particular nutrients (especially vitamin A, vitamin C, vitamin B6, calcium and iron). Those who are at risk, include individuals who:

- are in a particular demographic category: infants, adolescents, menstruating women, pregnant and lactating women, and elderly.
- *do* something to negatively affect vitamin levels: alcoholics, smokers, chronic users of certain medications.
- *don't* do something they *should*, to maintain adequate levels: dieters, strict vegetarians, food faddists.

It is apparent that these groups encompass nearly everyone except some adult males and some children. However, it is important to realize that vitamin deficiency — or even sub-optimal nutritional status — may not result unless an individual exhibits two or three of the above "risk factors."

*"A New Approach to Vitamin Supplementation", by Susan Male Smith, M.S., R.D. *Environmental Nutrition Newsletter,* 7:1 – 2, April 1984. Used with permission.

To Recommend or To Discourage?

Knowing this, and fearful of vitamin overdoses, we as nutritionists have traditionally downplayed the need for any vitamin supplementation, recommending food sources instead. Unwittingly, however, we may have cut ourselves off from the listener by seeming too conservative. What the public wants is *advice* on supplementation, not lectures.

In reality, some people will purchase and take vitamins, whether recommended by nutritionists or not. What they are looking for, and need, are guidelines to choosing a vitamin supplement, so risks can be minimized.

Guidelines for Choosing a Vitamin Supplement

The following guidelines can help consumers choose a safe and effective preparation for their money.

- Choose a balanced multi-vitamin, rather than one or two specific nutrients, unless it has been medically prescribed. (Excessive levels of one nutrient can disrupt the body's balance and actually alter nutrient requirements. In addition, one is rarely deficient or sub-optimal in one nutrient; usually several are involved.)
- Choose a preparation that provides approximately 100% of the RDA for *recognized* nutrients, in approximately equal proportions.
- Avoid preparations containing *un*recognized nutrients, or nutrients in minute amounts (this only increases the cost, but is of no real value).
- Avoid preparations that claim to be "natural," "organic," "therapeutic," "high-potency," or for "stress" (the extra cost is not worth any purported benefit; many unreputable firms use these claims, and thus may signal less effective preparations).
- Ignore "natural" versus "synthetic" claims; they are meaningless. In fact, certain synthetic vitamin preparations are *more* effective than their natural counterparts (e.g., folic acid and vitamin E).
- Choose a preparation with an expiration date on it. Certain nutrients interact with others (e.g., thiamin actually hastens the decomposition of both folate and vitamin B-12). As a result, vitamin preparations lose potency with time (and hot, humid environments, such as bathrooms, accelerate this process).

Positive vs. Negative Approach

While the potential for vitamin abuse is a real one, actual documented cases are not that common, and perhaps turn off the consumer more 319 than sound advice does. . . . Nutritionists should help discourage *unrealistic* expectations from supplementation, such as using vitamins to treat a disease.

For those individuals who may exhibit two or three of the "risk factors" listed above, sound guidelines in choosing a supplement are sorely needed, and can be positively perceived advice, rather than the often-used, if ineffective, negative "preaching."

What are *nutrient supplements anyway? Really. What are they made of? We wind down our discussion of the nutritional supplement controversy by focusing on the composition and manufacture of the products themselves. This first piece from the consumer-oriented* Tufts University Diet & Nutrition Letter *reports on research evaluating, for their content and potencies, specific nutritional supplement products on the market.*

ARE ALL VITAMIN/MINERAL SUPPLEMENTS THE SAME?*

When so many of her patients reported taking various vitamin and/or mineral supplements with which she was unfamiliar, Linda Schaffer Bell, RD, of Yale-New Haven Hospital, decided to take a close look at what these supplements really provided. We asked her about her findings on over-the-counter supplements. They surprised not only her but also a great many other people.

Of 41 adult multivitamin supplements studied, Bell found that only 7 had what she considered to be appropriate levels of vitamins. In assessing 41 other multivitamin/mineral combinations, she found that only 8 contained the RDA for iron, a most difficult nutrient to get from dietary sources, along with appropriate levels of vitamins. She considered a supplement to be "appropriate" if it supplied 50 to 200 percent of the RDA for 10 vitamins and for a variety of minerals.

There was a tendency for the "inappropriate" supplements to supply levels that were on the high side, meaning that they supplied more than 200 percent of the RDA for 1 nutrient or more. Bell was amazed at the lack of consistency in the mineral content of multivitamin/mineral supplements. For example, some had iodine or selenium but others did not.

*"Are All Vitamin/Mineral Supplements the Same?" Reprinted with permission, *Tufts University Diet and Nutrition Letter*, 475 Park Avenue South, 30th Floor, New York, NY 10016. (Vol. 2, p. 7, May, 1984)

Multivitamin/mineral supplements deemed appropriate for vitamins and iron

Unicap M (Upjohn)
One a Day + Iron (Miles)
Vigran + Iron (Squibb)
One Only + Iron (Prescott)
Vioday + Iron (Hudson)
Multivitamins + Iron (Foods Plus)
Daily Multivitamins + Iron (CVS)
Unitab M (Foods Plus)

Multivitamins deemed appropriate

Unicap (Upjohn)
One a Day (Miles)
Vigran (Squibb)
One Only (Prescott)
Vioday (Hudson)
All-Around (Foods Plus)
Daily Multivitamin (CVS)

Stress supplements were found to be inexpensive and inconsistent in content. Most had B vitamins and vitamin C, but only some had folic acid, iron, or vitamin E. Obviously, there is no standard of identity for a pill to be called a "stress" nutrient supplement.

After examining 6 over-the-counter prenatal supplements, Bell concluded that only 3 were appropriate. Two did not provide enough iron, and 1 did not meet the RDA for folic acid. All 6 had less than half the RDA for calcium — probably because a supplement that would meet this RDA would have to be the size of a horse pill!

Bell considered only about half of the 25 children's preparations she examined to be appropriate. Unlike the adult supplements, the children's tended to be low, rather than high, in certain nutrients. Of the more than half that listed ingredients, all contained sugar, artificial colors, and artificial flavors. She was surprised that supplements do not have to list ingredients other than vitamins and minerals.

The main point to be taken from all this, Bell believes, is that be- cause of the wide variation in supplement ingredients, "people don't know what they're taking or why — it's simply bad consumerism." Most people think vitamin and/or mineral supplements are created equal when, in fact, they are not.

Bell recommends supplements for people on low-calorie diets and for those who have certain medical conditions, but in such cases she suggests consulting a physician and a registered dietitian. She is not concerned about supplements that contain RDA levels — these should present no problem for most people. But problems can arise when RDA levels are exceeded, because some nutrients can be toxic and can interfere with drug metabolism if taken in large doses.

321

Finally, Bell's findings offer important information for pharmacists, nutritionists, and physicians. Because most multivitamin/mineral supplements are not considered drugs, pharmacists are often unfamiliar with them. And because vitamin/mineral supplements are not really food, nutritionists often shy away from recommending them. Physicians typically receive little nutrition education in their training and are not always well-versed in vitamin/mineral nutrition. . . .

The natural foods industry trade magazine Whole Foods *is often surprisingly candid about the truths of the trade. Here in an article on supplement manufacturing writer Jim Schreiber provides some surprising facts about "natural" vitamins.*

THE PILL PERPLEX*

Jim Schreiber

. . . Two Extremes

. . . Retail operations with most of their sales dollars in vitamins and minerals almost always describe themselves as *health* food stores. Those with less than half their sales dollars in these products almost always describe themselves as *natural* food stores. A far smaller number of stores in the middle show no particular preference, as a group, for one style of self-description or the other. Most shops tend either to deemphasize these items or to emphasize them strongly; the pattern is what statisticians call a "bi-modal distribution curve."

Various surveys indicate that between 30 and 40 percent of the annual retail sales dollars in the industry as a whole come from trade in vitamins, minerals and other nutritional supplements. Proprietors who reject this potential source of income usually base their decision on a conviction that such pills and powders are simply not natural, and therefore have no place in an authentic natural foods business. . . .

Unanswered Questions

For the many people in the industry who do not stand convinced that vitamin and mineral pills are unacceptable, but who have some doubts

*Chapter 53: "The Pill Perplex," by Jim Schreiber. *Whole Foods Natural Foods Guide,* © 1979, pp. 242–247. And/Or Press, Inc.: Berkeley, CA. Used with permission.

about them, the most usual questions are these: Just how "natural" are these products in our industry? How do they differ from the bottled vitamins and minerals usually displayed in supermarkets and drug stores? . . .

What is 'Natural'?

. . . Chemists in universities and in industry make clear-cut distinctions between natural and synthetic vitamins, giving them different names, and different descriptions of the molecules which comprise the vitamins. For example, a vitamin we call riboflavin or B2 as found in nature is called riboflavin mononucleotide, and a form made in the laboratory is known as 7-methyl-9-(D-1-ribityl)-isoxalloxazine. . . . The name alone does not reveal whether the chemical is beneficial or harmful, natural or synthetic. Natural vitamins, too, have imposing chemical names. . . .
In discussing the difference in natural and synthetic vitamins, Dr. James Hilbe of the Wm. T. Thompson Co. said, "First, in nature, *all* nutritional materials are accompanied by *other* nutritional materials. E.g., in plants, Vitamin C is accompanied by bioflavonoids, but this is not the situation in animals. When manufactured, Vitamin C is made as the pure, crystalline product with no other nutrients present unless they are added. Second, Vitamin E *can* be manufactured to be identical to the d-alpha tocopherol of nature. However, it can not be manufactured without also making the optical isomer, l-alpha tocopherol. As l-alpha tocopherol does not occur in nature (as far as is known), animals and man do not have the enzymes necessary to process this Vitamin E analog . . ."

Synthetic Distinction

When asked how much processing can be done to a vitamin derived from natural sources before it should be called synthetic, Dr. Hilbe replied, "This is apparently a subjective decision. For example, d-alpha tocopherol acetate is usually called 'natural E.' However, there has been a molecular change in the product. My opinion is that if the chemical optical qualities are changed, then it should no longer be called 'natural.' " . . .
A somewhat different view is offered by Harold Kutler, president of NuLife: "Synthetic vitamins are chemically the same as natural vitamins," he said, "and the difference has always been a nebulous one. Nebulous insofar as it is difficult to demonstrate the difference scientifically, unlike the example of synthetic seawater that will not support life." The NuLife Full Disclosure Book makes a distinction between nutrients from natural sources and those which are synthetic. It de-

fines as "from natural sources . . . any vitamin derived from a food source or any mineral derived from a food or geological source either by processing or synthesis. Thus Vitamin C synthesis from Corn Dextrose is from a natural source while Vitamin A Palmitate synthesized from acetylene or synthetic Beta Ionone would be classified as synthetic . . . so our definition of synthetic in regard to nutrition is any nutrient principally derived from chemicals."

On the same subject, Alfred Rechberger, president of Essential Organics, said, "It is believed that a synthetic vitamin is identical to an *isolated, purified* natural vitamin. Vitamins as they occur in nature are complexed with various compounds like synergistic factors, coenzymes, trace elements, etc. Laboratory-made vitamins are devoid of these factors. . . .

"A substance is not necessarily 'good' because it's 'Natural.' Many plants contain toxic substances or inhibitive factors like phytic acid in grains, oxalic acid in spinach and kale, etc. Special enzyme systems which humans don't have are required to digest these compounds and make them neutral. A genetic defect in humans is responsible for the fact that we do not synthesize Vitamin C like other mammals. Laboratory synthesis, in this case, can provide much good for man. On the other hand, there are also drawbacks with synthetics."

What Manufacturers Do

. . . In general, the companies specialize. An examination of the many lists and catalogs shows that specific components, such as inositol, thiamine hydrochloride, binders, and gelatin capsules each come from a small number of original sources. It is not a literal truth but is a significant metaphor that "All roads lead to Hoffman-LaRoche." The typical company in the health food trade buys its ingredients from these primary sources, purchasing the standardized — not tailor-made — chemicals offered by the primary-source firms. The food-grade chemicals available are of the highest quality of purity.

The vitamin manufacturer in the health foods trade takes these raw materials and decides what to do with them — how to combine them, whether to do the tablet-making in-house or farm it out, what quality-control measures will be taken, how the products will be tested and advertised, and how much information about their ingredients and processes to disclose to the public.

As a rule — regardless of arguments over the use of the word "natural" — the vitamin and mineral supplements offered by manufacturers in the health food industry differ greatly from those usually sold in drug stores and supermarkets. The mainstream commercial trade has no reason to avoid the total synthetics if they are cheaper than the isolates. The drug store brands can, and do, use artificial colors, preservatives, sugar, shellacs, and polyvinyl plastic fillers. Such things are within the laws governing foods. In our industry, the manufacturer,

324

with a prudent eye on the marketplace, will usually exclude some or all such ingredients. Some components are not required on labels.

Limits of Supply

Ironically, the manufacturers seem to have their own disclosure problems with their suppliers. This is illustrated by a disclaimer in NuLife's Full Disclosure Book. "The information contained here is limited by the data we have. We are not responsible for additives that may be present in raw materials we purchase unbeknown to us." Other limits are imposed by what is actually available from suppliers. Some vitamins are commercially available only in synthetic form because the cost of isolation is immense. Gelatin capsules are made from animal tissues and almost always contain a small amount of a preservative such as methylparaben. The smaller number of capsules without preservatives will, of course, not last as long. . . .

Doing The Possible

Imagine that you want to go into business as a manufacturer of vitamin and mineral supplements which are as natural as possible. No synthetics. You know that a provitamin A is in carrots, B's are in yeasts, C is in oranges, etc. All you have to do is get the vitamins from the foods into tablets and capsules in concentrations that make it worth doing. But how?

A little study shows that many vitamins can be isolated from natural sources. But a little more study shows that the only known methods of isolation involve a complicated series of chemical interactions using a variety of synthetic chemicals in the processing. To produce mineral nutrients which are chelated, as they are in nature, also involves a meticulous, tricky chemical procedure. You find the basic recipes, procedures and standards of purity in such references as the *US Pharmacopeia*, the *National Formulary*, and the *Food Chemicals Codex*. Patents on isolation methods are held by major pharmaceutical houses, and the chain of supply ultimately leads to firms like Hoffman-LaRoche, Merck & Co., Pfizer, Inc., and the Eastman — as in Kodak — Chemical Products Co.

In looking at equipment, you realize that, like all machinery, the punches that form the tablets come in standard sizes, so, to keep the dosage the same in each tablet, a filler will usually be needed. Some of the ingredients will not stick together to shape a pill, so a binder must be added, and some are so sticky that they won't pop out of the punch, which calls for a lubricant.

You decide to avoid all the ingredients and processes offered by the chemical industry, and do it yourself, naturally. Very few options are open at this point. Without the complex, high-powered processing,

325

few vitamins and minerals can be extracted in amounts that yield potencies normally called for in a pill. Without using the standardized chemicals and methods of the industry, there is no way to list the amounts of nutrients on the label: carrots and oranges naturally refuse to standardize themselves. The economics of the situation may require charging the consumer a few dollars for a pill that contains as much beta-carotene as a few cents worth of raw carrots—and the FDA may be eyeing your operation with questions about the purity of your non-standardized product.

We may dream about natural vitamins and minerals leaping in significant potencies from organically grown foods into vegetable gelatin capsules with no intervening chemical processes, but at present nobody has the remotest idea how that might be done in reality. . . .

> *To put a little vividness into the descriptions you have just read, we offer here a detailed account of the production of "natural" vitamin E. You will never again have trouble with questions about how "natural" vitamin pills (or for that matter oils) are.*

VITAMIN E: NATURAL? MIXED? SYNTHETIC?*

Paul Huff

. . . Source and Production

Vitamin E is obtained from numerous plant sources but soya bean is the most important source due to availability of adequate raw material. Wheat is the next most important source but this material is more expensive as well as quite limited in raw materials. There is but 20% enough wheat to supply the demand for vitamin E. Other sources are peanut oil, olive oil, corn oil, safflower oil and others.

Crude plant oils are generally prepared as follows:

1. Seeds or grains are placed in a hot solution of caustic soda. This breaks up the seed pod and separates the carbohydrate from the plant oils.
2. Hexane bath extracts the crude oil.

---

*"Vitamin E: Natural? Mixed? Synthetic?" by Paul Huff. *Journal of Applied Nutrition*, Volume 25 1 & 2 pp. 48–58. Used with permission.

3. Oils are filtered under about 50 lbs. pressure and insoluble materials are removed.
4. Hexane is evaporated and distilled for reuse.

The final product is crude "unprocessed" oil from "natural" sources.

Oils in the above stage are seldom sold for human consumption as the crude oil has an odor and taste that is not particularly pleasant. Also the oil lacks the clear crystalline appearance that is attractive to the eye. The following steps remove the odor, taste and materials causing the opaque appearance. Also shelf life is increased which is necessary under our present system of distribution.

The steps in processing are as follows: Unprocessed crude oil is boiled and infused with gases such as nitrogen. Hydrochloric acid, methanol (an alcohol) and other chemicals are added. This process is called "carrier gas deodorization." Animal oils as well as vegetable oils are treated in this manner or in similar processes depending on the type oils. The end product is the clear, odorless and tasteless oils you buy in your market or in your health food stores. All are "natural sources," etc. Thus all your cooking oils, salad oils, margarine and cooking fats undergo chemical treatment. Surprising, isn't it?

The above "deodorizing" process produces a thick sludge that floats to the surface of the oils. This sludge contains the ingredients in the crude unprocessed oils that supplies the cloudiness, odor and taste. This sludge is called "deodorizer sludge," "hot well scum," "clabber stock," "trap oil," "lighter than oil scum," "catch basin scum," etc.

One popularly used oil for a source of vitamin E is soya bean oil. The sludge from soya oil contains approximately 8% tocopherols, 20% sterols, sterol esters, glycerides, 20% free fatty acids, hydrocarbons and other material. In other words, the scum contains most of the food value in the original oil!

The following steps of chemical extraction separates the above materials from the hot well scum. This process is U.S. Patent #2,704,764 (3/22/55).

This shows one of many processes used to extract "natural mixed" tocopherols (vitamin E) from oils. You can readily see that your salad oils, cooking oils and fats have been pretty well stripped of most of their food value — something like refined sugar (which is another story). . . .

My apologies to the natural food and vitamin enthusiast. I have revealed some interesting facts about the presence of so many synthetic chemicals in your "natural" vitamins and basic foods. These facts may come as a surprise. If you think this story about natural vitamin E is a bit disillusioning, perhaps more articles are in order about rose hips, vitamin C, and other foods we consume daily. . . .

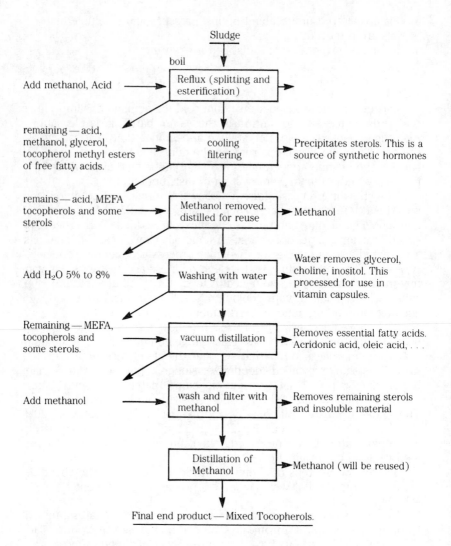

Sludge

boil

Add methanol, Acid → Reflux (splitting and esterification) →

remaining — acid, methanol, glycerol, tocopherol methyl esters of free fatty acids. → cooling filtering → Precipitates sterols. This is a source of synthetic hormones

remains — acid, MEFA tocopherols and some sterols → Methanol removed. distilled for reuse → Methanol

Add H_2O 5% to 8% → Washing with water → Water removes glycerol, choline, inositol. This processed for use in vitamin capsules.

Remaining — MEFA, tocopherols and some sterols. → vacuum distillation → Removes essential fatty acids. Acridonic acid, oleic acid, . . .

Add methanol → wash and filter with methanol → Removes remaining sterols and insoluble material

Distillation of Methanol → Methanol (will be reused)

Final end product — Mixed Tocopherols.

It is quite appropriate that we close a section on supplements with the words of nutritionist Walter Mertz. A scientist who never lost sight of wholes while he was investigating their smallest parts, Mertz reminds us that foods are more than collections of nutrients. The study of nutrition can never be reduced, he points out, to a study of those few chemicals we now identify as nutritionally essential.

FOODS AND NUTRIENTS*

Walter Mertz, M.D.

. . . Mankind has developed and persisted in eating foods for most of its history without knowledge of nutrients. We began to discover the latter only in our immediate past, during the last century. During the many centuries preceding those discoveries, vagaries of climate resulted in famine at times, and increasing population densities and poorly understood advances of technology led to isolated nutrient deficiencies. But, in general, mankind persisted. This incontrovertible fact proves that our food choices could not have been all bad. Apparently, the powerful regulators of hunger and satiety provided an adequate total food intake and an adequate balance of nutrients, except under catastrophic conditions.

Long before the discovery of nutrients, empirical observation and certain philosophical and religious beliefs attributed different health values to individual foods, some of which can be justified and explained on the basis of modern knowledge. The goiter-preventive effect of burned sponges is related to their iodine content, and the belief that apples pretreated with rusty nails are beneficial in anemia can be corroborated on the basis of our modern knowledge of iron bioavailability. The age-old belief that garlic and onions are good for the circulatory system is supported by modern experiments showing hypocholesterolemic and anticoagulating effects of extracts from those sources. The unproven association between consumption of yogurt and longevity is beginning to sound plausible on the basis of recent animal experiments demonstrating increased resistance against infections in yogurt-fed animals. The long-held belief in the healing quality of some waters that led to the establishment of hundreds of spas in many parts of the world is beginning to be scientifically investigated by epidemiological studies.

*Walter Mertz: "Foods and Nutrients." Reprinted from *Journal of the American Dietetic Association*, Vol. 84:769, 1984.

In addition to health-related beliefs, foods have in the past assumed symbolic and even religious connotations, often transcending by far their role as sources of nutrients.

The scientific era began with the discovery of the bulk nutrients during the 19th century. Progress accelerated with the identification of an increasing number of vitamins from about 1900 to 1948 and is now characterized by the rapid sequence of discoveries of new essential trace elements. These discoveries, followed by estimates of human nutrient requirements and by nutrient analysis in foods, have resulted in a substantial improvement in human health wherever the new knowledge could be applied. The latter was summarized in the first edition of the Recommended Dietary Allowances, which, appropriately, appeared during World War II, at a time when the adequacy of the population's food intake could not be taken for granted. From that first edition to the latest, the number of nutrients with a recommended intake has continuously increased and can be expected to increase further in the future.

Foods More Than Collections of Nutrients

The scientific approach, the dissection of foods into individual nutrients, and the study of their metabolism, health effects, and requirements, is necessary if the science of nutrition and its benefits to mankind are to grow. However, this approach presents the risk of substituting incomplete scientific knowledge of individual nutrients for the lessons learned from our historical experience with foods. Although much of the historical experience is not scientifically founded, we should not neglect that experience and thereby run the risk of losing important knowledge.

The experienced dietitian has recognized this risk and has long known how to avoid it. There remain, however, certain nutrition-related activities that are of special and practical concern. These include the design of new foods or substantial alterations of traditional foods, especially when they are designed for exclusive use, such as infant formulas or formulations for total parenteral nutrition. It has often been stated that a chemically pure food formulated to contain all nutrients as recommended in previous editions of the Recommended Dietary Allowances is not compatible with health. We recognize the truth of that statement for the 7th and 8th editions, in which no recommendations existed for the essential trace elements zinc and selenium, but we also must recognize the high probability that even our present recommendations are incomplete.

The sequence of reports during the past decade describing nutritional deficiencies induced in patients by exclusive feeding of intravenous formulas that were state of the art at their time of use is a powerful reminder. There is now a long list of nutrients recognized to be essential (or, at least, important for bioavailability) that await elucidation of their roles in human nutrition and application, such as the "new" trace elements, the meat factor, the garlic factor, the cruciferous vegetable factor, the yogurt factor, the zinc-binding ligand(s), the glucose tolerance factor, and many others.

The second danger arising from the nutrient-oriented approach lies in the undue emphasis on individual nutrients that happen to be popular at a given time. The 1930s and 1940s were the era of iron and iodine; the era of polyunsaturated fatty acids, which began in the late 1950s, is still continuing; and the zinc decade of the 1970s is now being supplemented by the selenium period of the 1980s. The exclusive concern with individual nutrients is not only unscientific but also potentially dangerous. It can result in pronounced changes of human exposure to these nutrients, either by public health measures or by self-supplementation, creating the risk of nutrient imbalances. Nutrient balance has become the subject of greatest concern to nutritionists, especially to those involved in trace element nutrition. That field of research has identified many dietary interactions that can affect nutritional status and health; many more can be predicted but have yet to be demonstrated.

Although we are only beginning to acknowledge the complexity of these interactions, we can summarize what we know by stating that the delicate balance of nutrients that is conducive to health can be disturbed not only by deficiencies but also by excesses of individual nutrients which, without being toxic by themselves, can adversely affect the bioavailability and function of others. Examples of at least theoretical concern are the changing ratio of iron to other essential elements, especially zinc, in our diet by way of iron-fortified products; the high exposure to iodine of large parts of our population; the impact of high intakes of polyunsaturated fatty acids on the requirement for the group of micronutrients protecting against oxidative damage; the copper-zinc interactions; and the effect of high intakes of simple carbohydrates on copper status.

Scientific research will eventually quantify many of those interactions and identify yet unidentified interacting factors, but at the present time our knowledge is not quite adequate as a basis for strong interventions and drastic changes. We have recognized the fallacy of treating "protein-energy malnutrition" with pure sources of protein and energy. Twenty years from now we may recognize that the selenium pill that may have reduced our risk for cancer may have created another risk by way of its interaction with arsenic, which, by then, may have become recognized as a very important element. Why not take care of the selenium requirement by more often eating seafood, in which nature has provided us with a reasonable balance of these two (and other) elements?

331

Implementation of Scientific Knowledge

What then can we use as guidelines on our way to implement what scientific knowledge we have? I believe it is necessary for all of us, but especially for the practicing dietitian, to complement our knowledge of nutrients with a knowledge of foods, not only as sources of the now known nutrients but also as potential carriers of substances that remain to be identified. We are beginning to realize that foods which may be nearly identical in their nutrient composition can have very different health effects. Some of these differences are beginning to be explored on a scientific basis, for example, those between yogurt and milk, while many others are still waiting for scientific treatment.

It would be wrong to state that nature has provided us with a perfect balance of all important nutrients in a mixed diet or to assign mysterious qualities to individual foods. Such attitudes have led to excessive and potentially dangerous nutrition practices in the past. It can be said, however, that societies have developed well whenever they have had access to adequate amounts of a variety of foods. Thus, the balance of nutrients offered by such varied diets can serve us as interim guidelines for implementing the RDAs.

The recognition by the Diet, Nutrition, Cancer Committee of a negative correlation between the consumption of cruciferous vegetables and cancer risk at several sites is the most recent example of an important health effect that cannot be totally explained on the basis of our present knowledge of nutrients. These considerations lead to the conclusion that foods are more than sources of the now known nutrients and that the choice of foods with which to implement the RDAs is as important as the implementation itself. . . .

Afterword

One fact is no doubt evident to any reader of this chapter: an awful lot of people are tired of waiting for nutritionists, and have decided on their own to take nutritional supplements. According to the Vitamin Information Service, more than a third of all adults supplement their diets, the percentage increasing for those who are educated, affluent and professional. The latest repor. d survey, one conducted by the Food and Drug Administration, confirms this (Michael L. Stewart, *et al.* Vitamin/mineral supplement use: a telephone survey of adults in the United States. *Journal of the American Dietetic Association* 85:1586–1590, December, 1985.) — which means that this is one of the areas of nutrition controversy most in need of discussion.

Unfortunately, such discussion seems rarely to occur. Instead serious questions are met with one of those unexamined standard truths: "Supplements are unnecessary if you eat a balanced diet, and can be dangerous if used." Case closed.

Now, however, confirmed supplement takers have a basis for crying "foul!" to such inflexible pronouncements from nutritionists. The revelation that a majority of Washington State dietitians use supplements seems to make this a clear case of professionals recommending to their clients, "Do as I say, not as I do."

Under the circumstances, it is gratifying to see a few nutritionists like Susan Male Smith urging their colleagues to be more open-minded on the subject, pointing out that the public wants information and advice, not reprimands, on supplement use.

We intend our chapter to give neither reprimand nor advice, but essential information that should be part of any decision about whether or not to pill. We can offer no formula for deciding how much of what nutrients anyone ought to take. That couldn't be done right now, given, among other things, differing philosophies about the goals of nutrition, and major gaps in our understanding of how nutrient requirements vary under differing life conditions. Our intention is simply to help make anyone's decision a more informed one.

It is the nature of the scientific method that it separates things into their smallest parts in order to learn how they work. This means that a highly developed society like ours becomes very knowledgeable about parts, although sometimes less wise about wholes. Where nutrition is concerned, the nutrients (especially the vitamins and minerals) are the parts we have learned most about. They can be isolated, purified and used in specified amounts for experiments on animals and humans.

Such experiments have in the past enabled us to learn how much of which nutrients were absolutely essential to "normal functioning"—as best we could define it. But once we had isolated these marvelous substances, it seemed inevitable in a country given to fads that they would come to be viewed as cures for our ills. As Arthur Vander pointed out, iodine became such a fad soon after its discovery, as did thiamine during World War II, as did vitamin E time after time after time.

As we write this at the beginning of 1986, calcium supplements are hot items (even meriting a cover story in *Newsweek*), riding the wave of suggestive evidence that they help prevent or treat osteoporosis in women, and may protect against the development of colon cancer and high blood pressure in all of us. Vitamin C was the rage throughout the 1970s, and zinc, selenium and chromium had their turns at popularity a while back. Authors Durk Pearson and Sandy Shaw were responsible for the American fascination with nutrient antioxidants when their book, *Life Extension* (and its sequel), monopolized the best seller lists in the early 1980s. And the sagas of "MaxEPA" and "Daily Greens" show us that the savvy promoters and exploiters are still with us.

So fads *are* a problem. But as the articles in this section make clear, if one is concerned about public health, it is probably just as

333

dangerous to ignore or denounce the public's concern with supplements as it is to risk encouraging it by open discussion.

In deciding whether supplements are advisable, you have first to contend with the fact that many (most?) nutrition scientists don't recommend them. Individuals eating diets that include reasonable variety, their argument goes, should be meeting their nutritional requirements easily. Dr. Harper finds little evidence that current eating habits are leading to nutrient deficiencies, even when intakes are somewhat below the Recommended Dietary Allowances, and concludes that most diets are probably nutritious enough. Supplements, he believes, tend to encourage a potentially dangerous "self-medication" philosophy, and should be considered only when diets are frankly inadequate or when illness raises nutritional requirements.

On the other hand, experts like Dr. Krehl argue that routine use of supplements at moderate levels is a "practical and economic" means to insure an adequate intake of nutrients, especially for members of certain groups — people of low income, adolescent girls, adults consuming less than 1600 calories per day — who often show dietary inadequacies.

Unfortunately, it is easy for many of us to jump to the conclusion that we need supplements even if we don't fall into one of the at risk groups Dr. Krehl mentions. Most of us have friends who take supplements and claim to feel better as a result. It's hard to resist such claims. We'd all like to feel better and more energetic — especially without a lot of effort. And many of us don't eat as well as we should all of the time. Wouldn't supplements help?

Before jumping to answer such a question for yourself, you need to check up on the quality of your diet. You can do that by occasionally keeping a record of everything you eat or drink over a period of several days and then comparing your intake to one of the available food guides (see Chapter 2). For greater accuracy, have your diet analyzed by an experienced nutritionist, who can calculate the nutrient composition of what you've eaten and interpret it in relation to your "requirements" (usually the RDAs). You can do this yourself if you've had some nutrition training.

This is a far from perfect system, however, since humans need more than 50 nutrients, and nutrient composition data for many foods is incomplete or inadequate. Moreover, too little is known about many nutrients to establish RDAs for them, and there are additional health-promoting factors in food that we know even less about.

In theory, you could get a better idea of your true nutritional status by having analyses done of your various tissues. But there are limits to what can be learned even from this relatively expensive approach.

334

From a purely practical standpoint, then, a crude dietary analysis can probably give you some indication of whether any kind of supplement makes sense for you. In an introductory nutrition course both of us have taught at our university, we routinely have students analyze their diets using food composition tables and common food guides. Most are surprised to discover that their diets are reasonably nutritious, even when they had believed otherwise because their hectic lifestyles interfered with "proper" eating. It probably helps that many of them are young and very active.

Regular exercise raises food requirements, and as long as the food is reasonably nutritious, the more food you take in, the more nutrients come with it. Our point is that you may be eating better than you think, and a dietary analysis, crude as it is, will put you in a better position to evaluate your need to supplement.

If you do decide to supplement, the next question is: What should you buy? A helpful way to think about the issue is to consider three possible kinds of supplement use. For convenience, we'll call them the insurance, optimal, and megavitamin approaches.

Let's assume for the moment that you, like most people, are interested in the insurance approach. A dietary analysis has showed you which nutrients you may not be getting enough of. Or perhaps you simply want to take a general multi-vitamin and mineral supplement to compensate for occasional shortfalls in your diet. Both Dr. Krehl and pharmacist David Roll view this as an acceptable practice.

But it will be difficult for you to choose an appropriate supplement even for insurance because, as the Tuft's newsletter article shows, most products are not well "balanced." That is, they provide relatively large amounts of some nutrients and not enough of others, or they don't contain all the nutrients for which there are official recommendations.

However, even if some compromises are required in selecting an "all-in-one" supplement, the alternative — taking each of these nutrients at RDA amounts in separate pills — would be both more expensive and lots more complicated.

The theory behind the second approach to nutritional supplement use, what we have called the optimal approach, is that extra vitamins and minerals can help individuals attain improved health and efficiency, and reduce their risks of developing the major degenerative diseases. The idea is to "optimize" one's nutritional status, to find a level of nutrient intakes where an individual feels and functions best, somewhere between deficiency and toxicity.

Unfortunately, nutrition science, at its present level of development, is quite unable to provide you with guidance on either

335

the kinds or quantities of nutrients any individual should be getting to be at his or her best.

As physician Arthur Vander points out, each step in determining what would be optimal nutrition for an individual presents problems (some of the same ones we touched on in the chapter on RDAs). These include: first, figuring out what end points you have in mind (that is, what does optimal nutrition mean in practical terms?); second, figuring out how to measure for those end points (e.g., what do serum levels of vitamin C have to do with a feeling of well being?); and third, actually doing the enormously time-consuming and expensive experiments that would be necessary.

Vander used the controversy over vitamin C and the common cold to illustrate the dilemma, but there is a further problem pointed out by Dr. Mertz: interactions between the nutrients may affect their absorption and availability to the cells of our body. Because of this, as Hegsted observed in his article in the RDA chapter, it may be almost impossible to determine specific amounts of individual nutrients necessary for health.

One almost insurmountable obstacle to studying optimal nutrition is the level of cooperation required of the human participants. Subjects would have to be maintained on many different types of dietary and supplement programs, while their health status and other indicators were monitored from birth to death to see which programs offered continual advantages over others. Few individuals would be likely to volunteer as "guinea pigs" in such a lifetime study, nor would many investigators be willing to devote their lives to such a task.

Imagine the difficulty of regularly getting lifestyle and dietary information, blood and urine samples and other measurements from groups of people living active lives, many of them likely to be moving about the country or the world at some time during the study. And imagine the costs! Even relatively simple studies that collect such information over time from groups of people living in a single community cost tens of millions of dollars.

Certainly the attempt (or "quest," if you see this goal as visionary) to determine how humans can achieve optimal nutrition will be among the most challenging problems facing nutrition science in the decades to come. And, as the above discussion makes clear, there is no guarantee that success will *ever* be achieved, if success is measured by the ability to provide individually tailored recommendations. The problems of defining optimal diets for people of various sexes and ages, hereditary endowments, lifestyles, adaptabilities to change and stress are enormous. We're a long way from being able to give precise advice on optimal diet to anyone, despite the claims of those who offer (for a price) to tailor such a diet for you with the help of a computer, a little information, and some blood, hair and urine.

336

Given all these limitations, our best information to date about what an optimal diet might look like comes from comparing the eating habits of different cultures, and measuring selected parameters of health status. Such studies usually conclude that a diet composed largely of a variety of natural foods, relatively low in fat, refined sweeteners and salt, and relatively high in fiber and complex carbohydrates offers health advantages. You've already heard about this type of eating plan if you read our Goals and Guidelines chapter.

There is no evidence that nutritional supplements added to such a dietary pattern will confer additional health advantages, but admittedly that possibility has not been studied. Some have proposed that any sort of "optimal diet" would be necessarily "unnatural," requiring both nutrient-dense foods and supplements. (See, for example, Mark F. McCarty. Point of view—a role for "nutritional insurance" supplementation in preventive medicine. *Medical Hypotheses.* 7:171–185, February 1981). But until such a rather surprising contention is proven scientifically (if it ever is), little use can be made of it.

The third approach to using nutritional supplements is the megavitamin approach. The term "megavitamin" has no precise definition, but it commonly refers to the use of any nutrient in amounts greater than ten times the RDA. While an individual might end up using one or more nutrients at megadose levels in the optimal approach, the more usual megavitamin (or megamineral) approach is to use nutrients as you would use drugs to deal with particular illnesses or health conditions, e.g., taking megadoses of vitamin C to reduce the severity of cold symptoms, taking megadoses of vitamin E for leg pains, or using a variety of B vitamins in megadoses to treat various mental disorders.

In regard to such doses, Vander insists that any nutrient used as a medication should be able to pass the same tests that a drug must pass before it is allowed to be marketed: that it works for what it is supposed to work for, and that it is relatively safe for its intended purpose. At present, despite numerous anecdotal accounts of treatment successes, there are few reports in the medical literature of well-conducted research studies assessing the usefulness of nutrients as "drugs" in the treatment of diseases.

Why this is so remains a matter of speculation. Some assert that researchers refrain from investigating possible relationships between particular nutrients and diseases because they fear being tarred with the brush of faddism. Others claim that pharmaceutical houses will not fund such research because nutrients can't be patented to make money for the firm that holds the patent.

Whatever the truth of such allegations, the fact is that most high dose nutrient claims have not been subjected to careful study. Therefore we don't know if these "treatments" work.

337

The importance of knowing that something will work before using it cannot be overemphasized. Some time ago, Dr. Wilfred Shute, who used vitamin E extensively in his practice to treat heart disease, was asked why he didn't "prove" his claim to the medical world by conducting double-blind studies where his patients randomly received either vitamin E or a placebo. He replied that such studies were unethical since he was personally convinced of the importance of vitamin E to the recovery of his patients.

Unfortunately, his unwillingness to prove his case to the satisfaction of his peers keeps us from knowing whether the vitamin is useful in the treatment of some forms of heart disease. The few well-conducted studies done by other investigators suggest that it is not. If appropriate studies proved his case, many more physicians would be recommending it to appropriate patients, and many more lives would be saved than Dr. Shute alone can claim.

Those who decide to "optimize" their health by taking nutritional supplements or therapeutically megadosing will be faced with even more problems in choosing what they want than if they just settled for "insurance." There are hundreds of different supplement products available, in various combinations and potencies. Many health food stores look like drugstores, with a large assortment of pills, capsules and powders filling the shelves and reducing the foods to second-class status.

Megadosing is also risky, and may over time result in consumption of toxic amounts of one or more nutrients. While pharmacist Roll urges professionals not to "scare the hell out of people by publicizing isolated reports of vitamin toxicity," it is also a fact that large doses of nutrients are not risk-free. We've included a chart that compares nutrients in terms of their margins of safety. Clearly it's much less hazardous to take large doses of vitamin C (for which the toxic dose is probably at least 30 times the recommended one) than large doses of selenium, which has a safety factor one-sixth as large.

In making decisions about whether to take or recommend nutritional supplements and in what potencies, there are some points we hope you'll keep in mind.

Decisions about whether supplements are necessary should be based on decisions about whether diets are adequate. The more people know about what they get from their food, the less likely they are to spend money for unneeded nutrients. Most people are probably eating better (or worse) than they think. Instead of ads proclaiming "Don't take chances — Take a supplements," we'd like to see ads saying "Don't take chances — Eat regularly and nutritiously."

Nutritional supplements are heavily advertised, usually in ways that suggest we'd *all* benefit from using them. Who among us never eats "junk foods," never skips a meal, and never suffers stress? Who doesn't have *some* lifestyle quirk — occasional drinking, smoking or dieting, for example — for which supplements are urged as compensatory? Who wouldn't want "nutritional insurance," when we have insurance on ourselves, our autos and our homes? Where is the lucky person (who even Paavo Airola would agree doesn't need supplements) who lives in other than a "polluted, chemicalized and very unnatural environment?"

Physicians Victor Herbert and Stephen Barrett caution us to beware not only of ads, but also of nutritional advice, really thinly-veiled product promotion, often volunteered by untrained people. Denise Hatfield further advises us to hang on to our skepticism in evaluating supplement claims made by even reputable manufacturers.

Even the best available information will be difficult to handle, because there are at least 50-odd nutrients to know something about. It's hard to figure out how much of each is enough, how much is too much, and how much is just right. And if you decide to take someone's advice, keep in mind there's a lot of scary advice out there. The American right to freedom of speech means that almost any claim can be made about this or that nutrient for this or that purpose (as long as it isn't on the label). There are nutrient claims based on personal beliefs and philosophies, self-experimentation and anecdotal information, and there are apparently experimental studies where nutritional supplements seem to confer health benefits. You can get yourself into trouble if you blindly accept any claims that come your way, without at least a little skepticism and interest in fact-finding.

Supplements should not be used as a substitute for good eating for any length of time. There's a great deal we don't know about factors in food beyond traditionally defined nutrients, that might influence our health. In the final selection in this chapter, Dr. Mertz mentioned some such factors found in meat, yogurt and garlic. Food factors of this sort are quite unlikely to be present even in "naturally" formulated supplements, despite the frequent claim that they are. If we don't know what these supposedly enhancing substances are, there is little reason to believe that they survive the processing necessary to reformulate a food into a concentrated supplement. Taking "Daily Greens" is clearly not a quick way to heed the advice of the Diet, Nutrition, and Cancer panel about consuming more vegetables!

Indeed, the amount of processing required to manufacture nutritional supplements is remarkable. As our excerpt shows, the process of making "natural" vitamin E from deodorizer sludge left from purifying crude plant oils has much in common with the process used to produce refined sugar. In both cases the desired substance (vitamin E or sucrose) is concentrated by removing other

339

substances found in the source materials (deodorizer sludge or sugar cane). Since in both cases the final concentrates are present in the source materials, the final products can both be said to be "natural." Yet many who supplement their diets with natural vitamin E debunk refined sugar as "unnatural" because of the severity of its processing.

What sort of distinction can be made between "natural" and "synthetic" supplements? The usual understanding is that natural supplements are those whose active ingredients were present in the original source material, while synthetic supplements are those whose active ingredients were manufactured by chemical synthesis from non-nutrient precursors.

Since all mineral supplements are commonly concentrated from bones, foods, or mineral-containing products, they are by definition natural. Vitamin supplements are more problematic since they can, by the definition given above, be natural or synthetic. Our excerpt on vitamin E makes clear, however, that a lot of what most people would think of as "unnatural" goes into the production of even a "natural" vitamin.

There are, moreover, no labeling definitions, so manufacturers can use the terms natural and synthetic pretty much as they wish to in describing their products. Natural vitamin C, for example, is usually synthetically produced (by our definition) with glucose as a starting material. But since one of the steps by which glucose is converted to ascorbic acid involves bacterial fermentation, the end product is described as "natural." Even vitamin C supplements said to be concentrated from rose hips or acerola cherries (both rich sources of the nutrient) may be composed almost exclusively of glucose-derived vitamin C.

Anyone who intends to take nutritional supplements should, by all means, buy those free of questionable additives such as artificial colors. But as Jim Schreiber warns, remember that manufacturing truly natural supplements from organically-grown foods is not presently possible.

The reality is that even the most expensive supplement labelled "natural" in bold letters is a poor substitute for nutrient-rich foods. Nutritionists prefer to emphasize foods because, to begin with, the whole (about which we know little) is more than the sum of the parts that we know something about. The broccoli you might have had for dinner is more than a collection of nutrients such as vitamins A, C and calcium. It also contains water, fiber and some potential carcinogens as well as anti-carcinogens. It is, in fact, a whole set of chemicals, the sum total of which we do not understand at all. There is much more in food relevant to health than its nutrients.

We also teach people about food rather than nutrients because it's much harder to hurt yourself with carrots than it is with concentrates. Once you concentrate anything in the food chain, whether it is vitamin A or selenium or salt or fat, it is easy to make mistakes. That's why nutritionists are generally wary of recommending the use of supplements, and focus instead on nutritious dietary patterns.

Nutrients and other non-nutrient substances relevant to health are readily available in familiar and attractive packages called fruits, vegetables, grains and animal products. And they come in concentrations and in combinations with which humans have had long cultural familiarity. Moreover, traditional knowledge throughout most of human history also enabled people to avoid or deal with the poisons available in the environment. But culture has not taught people who have trouble converting milligrams to micrograms how to handle and balance more than 50 nutrients, and it probably won't. It is much easier for us to become familiar with some useful generalities about food.

And finally, at the risk of sounding preachy, we'll conclude by stating our belief that it's a good idea for people, before searching for better health through food supplements, to make certain they're eating well, exercising regularly, and refraining from risky health behaviors such as smoking. Those changes alone might very well produce the health improvements they're looking for.

The "Great Vitamin War," as it has been called (Joe Graedon. 1980. *The People's Pharmacy-2.* New York: Avon Books), is still fought with great fervor, and no end seems in sight. As the debate over the role of nutritional supplements in American diets continues, we can only hope that the "psychic wounds" are minimized. We'll have to learn to talk to each other more respectfully about this nutrition controversy before it will have any chance of being resolved.

7

Food Safety: Is it Really Safe at the Plate?

A sk most food technologists and nutrition scientists, "Is our food supply safe?" and you would probably get a vigorous reassurance that our food supply is as safe as it's ever been — not only safe, but abundant, cheap and astonishingly varied. Yet quite another view of food safety is popular among lay nutrition counselors and their followers: namely that the food supply is growingly unsafe, that it is increasingly riddled with intentionally and unintentionally added poisons that cause much human illness and disease. Between these extremes are the rest of us, confident or uneasy, wondering whether our food supply could (and should) be better than it is.

All of us have the same goal. Ideally we want to optimize our consumption of the *good* substances in food (e.g., the nutrients and dietary fiber) and minimize our intake of the bad substances in food (naturally occurring toxins, pesticide residues, contaminants and so on). Depending on whether we think the food supply is safe or hazardous, we may view this task as either hard or easy. But in selecting foods to eat, all of us are constantly making largely unconscious decisions, trying to deal with the anxieties, whatever they are, that we personally experience around the issue of safe food.

In this section we try to offer you some help in making safety-related decisions about food. Here we deal with the "bads" all of us seek to avoid. We look at the safety of the food supply and at threats to that safety that some people believe may come either from the activities of food technologists or from the contamination of the food producing environment by farmers or industry — some of which we discussed in Chapter 4 on vegetarianism. The issue of the "goods" in our food is partially considered in our "Goals and Guidelines" chapter.

The subject of food safety is so broad that we cannot spend much time on specific processes or chemicals, or even in discussing specific sources of food contamination. But that would, in any case, only get us into the "carcinogen of the week" trip that we would like to help you avoid. We will deal with the issue of food safety in a general way, giving you a background for making personal decisions about specific substances in food that may concern you now or in the future.

Our selections begin with factual excerpts on the number and extent of non-nutritive substances in our food supply, and on how they are evaluated to determine their potential danger to human health. Following these are several opinion pieces that debate whether or not it is even sensible to worry about food safety in the U.S.

The final selections focus on the nature, extent and relative potential harm of the risks in our lives, as well as on the factors that affect which specific risks we attend to and how we behave toward them. We suspect that our treatment of this controversy, **343** like the others we have discussed in this volume, will raise more questions for you than it answers. That's the way things are right now. There are no fixed answers — only intelligent questions. Those are what we hope to help you to ask.

- E.M. Foster, Ph.D.:

  As far as the American food supply is concerned there is no evidence whatever of a safety crisis. Activists and skeptics argue otherwise, but not from facts or knowledge. Americans are living longer, healthier and more satisfying lives than ever before. *

- Charles J. Bates, Ph.D., President, Institute of Food Technologists, 1985 – 86:

  As the food supply has become ever more nutritious, safe, and convenient, it has also become more complex. This has made it ever more incomprehensible to those who lack the background and training to understand how and why the changes that are being made really are improvements. **

- Donald Kennedy, Ph.D., former Commissioner of the Food and Drug Administration:

  Analytical chemistry has developed more rapidly than the science of toxicology, so we find ourselves in a position to detect more than we can evaluate, and to measure more than we can understand. ***

- Charles Perrow, Ph.D.:

  . . . sensible living with risky systems means keeping the controversies alive, listening to the public, and recognizing the essentially political nature of risk assessment. Ultimately, the issue is not risk, but power; the power to impose risks on the many for the benefit of the few. ****

---

*E. M. Foster. How safe are our foods? *Nutrition Reviews (Supplement).* 40:28 – 29, 32 – 34, January 1982

**Food Technology.* 38:10, July 1984

***Oversight of Food Safety* hearing record, U.S. Senate, June 8 – 10, 1983. Page 33.

****Charles Perrow. *Normal Accidents: Living with High-Risk Technologies.* (1984). New York: Basic Books, Inc. Page 306.

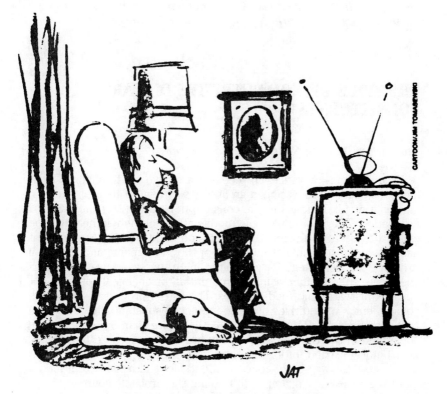

"... and the federal Food and Drug Administration warned today that
watching the evening news when seated in your favorite chair, while your dog lies
sleeping next to it, may be a possible source of cancer ... "

Just what is the problem where food safety is concerned? Or what is it some people think is the problem? An essential first step in understanding what the fuss is about is to learn what actually is in our food. This selection, from the 1982 report on Diet, Nutrition and Cancer from the National Academy of Sciences, briefly summarizes the substances (other than naturally occurring ones) that may be found in the U.S. food supply. It then provides an overview of what we know about their hazard potential—where cancer is concerned.

THE ROLE OF NON-NUTRITIVE DIETARY CONSTITUENTS*

Committee on Diet, Nutrition, and Cancer

... Technological advances in recent years have led to changes in the methods of food processing, a greater assortment of food products, and, as a result, changes in the consumption patterns of the U.S. population. The impact of these modifications on human health, especially the potential adverse effects of food additives and contaminants, has drawn considerable attention from the news media and the public. Advances in technology have resulted in an increased use of industrial chemicals, thereby increasing the potential for chemical contamination of drinking water and food supplies. The use of processed foods and, consequently, of additives has also increased substantially during the past four decades. Roberts estimates that more than 55% of the food consumed in the United States today has been processed to some degree before distribution to the consumer.

Clearly, the degree of concern about the health risks from food additives varies. For example, in ranking the probable sources of health hazard in the U.S. diet, the Food and Drug Administration (FDA) has consistently listed food additives in fifth or sixth place, well below microbiological contaminants and nutrient deficiencies. In contrast, consumers surveyed in five cities recommended that the FDA give high priority to assessing the safety of food additives.

Food Additives

In this report, the term "food additives" is often used generically to refer to *all* substances that may be added to foods. However, in the

*Section B: "The Role of Non-nutritive Dietary Constituents". *Diet, Nutrition, and Cancer,* 1982, pp. B1–B17. National Academy Press, Washington, DC. Used with permission.

1958 Food Additives Amendment to the Federal Food, Drug, and Cosmetic Act, the term has a more restricted legal definition:

" 'Food additive' means any substance the intended use of which results or may reasonably be expected to result, directly or indirectly, in its becoming a component or otherwise affecting the character of a food. . . ."

The 1958 amendment changed the rules under which food additives were regulated. Until then, a substance added to food was presumed safe until someone (usually the government through the FDA) could prove it otherwise; after 1958, FDA approval of safety was required prior to use. Because this change in the law would have placed an unmanageable burden on the manufacturers to conduct the tests required to prove the safety of the many hundreds of substances then added to foods, the definition of "food additive" was modified for regulatory purposes to exclude many classes of substances. The term now covers approximately 400 of the 2,600 to 2,700 substances intentionally added to foods. Not included are approximately 500 food ingredients termed GRAS (Generally Recognized as Safe) substances; about 100 other "unpublished GRAS substances;" approximately 1,650 flavoring agents, most of which are classified as GRAS; prior-sanctioned food ingredients, consisting of about 100 substances approved by the U.S. Department of Agriculture (USDA) or the FDA prior to 1958; and approximately 30 color additives. It would be difficult to prepare a list of all the compounds in these categories. . . .

Contaminants

. . . It is estimated that approximately 12,000 substances are introduced unintentionally during processing, and an unknown number of other contaminants are inadvertently added to the food supply. The first group (also called indirect additives) includes by-products of processing (e.g., caustics used in potato peeling, machinery cleaners, packaging components), as well as residues of permitted pesticides and of drugs given to animals. There are regulations restricting the concentrations and types of these compounds in food and the purposes for which they can be used. Contaminants in the second group, classified as unavoidable "added" constituents, are regulated when found. For example, after an accidental contamination by a hazardous chemical, the concentration of the chemical is compared to established "action levels" to determine if the foods are fit for human consumption.

The Delaney Clause and Other Regulatory Actions

The regulation of carcinogens has been a matter of special concern because it is covered by the Delaney Clause of the Federal Food, Drug,

347

and Cosmetic Act. The amendment prohibits the FDA from approving the use of any food additive found to cause cancer in animals or humans. It has been criticized as being too restrictive by setting a zero level of risk. In fact, it applies only to approximately 400 of the 2,700 substances intentionally added to foods, many of which are GRAS. If any GRAS substance is found to be carcinogenic, it would no longer be considered GRAS and would fall under the legal definition of a food additive, thereby becoming subject to the Delaney Clause.

In addition to the Delaney Clause, numerous amendments to the Federal Food, Drug, and Cosmetic Act have been made since the early 1960's. It appears that the statutory provisions governing food safety are a patchwork of divergent, sometimes carefully considered, but sometimes offhand, legislative policies that invite uneven monitoring of different substances in foods and inconsistent treatment of comparable risks from different categories of food additives. . . .

Exposure of Humans

To determine the risk of carcinogenesis from food additives and contaminants, it is necessary to know the extent to which humans are "typically" exposed, the degree of exposure in subgroups of the population, the carcinogenic potency of the compound, and the quantity and quality of the data concerning its toxicity and carcinogenicity.

Although humans are exposed to various additives and contaminants at levels ranging over several orders of magnitude, some generalizations can be made about exposure to different classes of substances. The National Science Foundation estimated that 0.5% (by weight) of the U.S. food supply consists of intentional food additives, and the per capita intake of food additives has increased approximately fourfold in the past decade. Currently their use amounts to approximately 5 kg per capita annually, although as a measure of the average intake of food additives this may be misleading because approximately one-half of these additives are used in amounts of 0.5 mg or less. . . .

Information about the use of indirect additives by the food industry is much less precise. Consequently, exposure of humans is difficult to estimate. It would depend to a large extent on the physical and chemical characteristics of the additive. For example, packaging materials can migrate into food. . . . Most pesticides and industrial chemicals are ingested in trace amounts, resulting in a daily intake of only a few milligrams or less of each compound per capita. . . .

The FDA's Market Basket Surveys conducted since the mid-1960's have monitored only a few substances and have excluded convenience foods. However, they have provided information on the levels of some pesticides, industrial chemicals, and heavy metals that are ingested as contaminants in the diet. . . . With a few exceptions, information about

348

the exposure to other classes of additives is estimated indirectly from the amount produced or used in the processing of foods rather than by direct measurement of actual consumption. . . .

Assessment of Effects on Human Health

Lack of adequate data on a large number of substances precludes a comprehensive assessment of the risk to humans exposed to food additives and contaminants. . . .

> *How is the safety of all those chemicals that can turn up in our food evaluated? In this excerpt from the 1985 edition of his popular book,* Eater's Digest, *consumer advocate Michael Jacobson of the Center for Science in the Public Interest provides an overview of just what it is that scientists do when they want to understand whether a chemical may harm us. Although his discussion focusses on intentional additives, it should be clear that the kinds of tests he describes are those we would want to have done on any chemical that might be added, intentionally or otherwise, to our food.*

HOW ARE FOOD ADDITIVES TESTED?*

Michael F. Jacobson, Ph.D.

. . . A manufacturer who wants to introduce a new food additive bears the responsibility for conducting scientific tests to establish its safety. The FDA then evaluates the tests. The substance must be shown to be free from hazards before it may be used in foods. This process is of remarkably recent origin, having been incorporated into law only in 1958 (1960 for color additives). Prior to 1958 the situation was reversed: manufacturers could put anything they pleased into food; the FDA could ban a chemical only after it had proved that the chemical was dangerous. Millions of people would be consuming the additive while the FDA built its case. . . .

---

*Excerpts from *The Complete Eater's Digest and Nutrition Scoreboard* by Michael F. Jacobson, Ph.D. Copyright © 1972, 1976 by Michael F. Jacobson. Reprinted by permission of Doubleday & Company, Inc. Pgs. 186–198.

349

For chemicals that are not "generally recognized as safe," a manufacturer must conduct tests on animals and then petition FDA to permit the chemical in foods. The petitioner must state the composition of the additive, its function, the amount to be used in food, the types of foods in which it would be used, the testing procedures, and the results of the tests. FDA scientists evaluate the petition and, if the chemical appears safe, approve the additive and specify the conditions of safe use. The public has a brief period in which to object to FDA's decision, after which time food makers can use the new additive. Note that the FDA's role is usually limited to evaluating the manufacturer's data. The FDA does not ordinarily perform its own tests to verify the information that the petitioner has submitted.

As we have become more aware of the range of harmful effects a chemical may have, the FDA has required manufacturers to conduct more extensive tests. Prior to the 1950s, most toxicological studies involved only a few dozen animals, lasted several months, and could detect only out-and-out poisons. In the last thirty years, we have become concerned about subtle and long-range effects of chemicals, and the sophistication of testing has improved markedly. Scientists test more animals for longer periods of time and look for a wider variety of effects.

The most difficult effects to detect are those that show up only months or years after a person is exposed to a chemical. A food additive that had no immediately toxic effects, but that causes birth defects, cancer, or mutations, might escape detection indefinitely, because there is no simple way of associating the ingestion of a chemical in 1985 with the birth of a deformed child in 1986, the occurrence of liver cancer in 1999, or a case of hemophilia in 2052. Extensive testing on laboratory animals and microorganisms is the only practical means of weeding out dangerous food additives before they cause subtle or long-range damage in people. Even though laboratory animals are not physiologically or anatomically identical to humans, they are similar enough to permit fairly accurate predictions of the effects of a chemical on humans.

Testing usually begins with brief (one to six months) studies. Scientists examine animals' growth, blood, urine, and liver function. Once they know an animal's approximate tolerance to a chemical, they can select the most appropriate dose levels for the crucial lifetime feeding studies.

Feeding studies demonstrate the effects of a chemical on the animal; biochemical experiments reveal the effects of the animal on the chemical. By learning how an animal's body handles a chemical, one can frequently estimate a substance's toxicity. For instance, some chemicals, such as the thickening agents carboxymethylcellulose and karaya, are not absorbed by the body and are likely to be harmless when present in moderate amounts. Additives that are identical to chemicals occurring in the body, or that are converted to such chem-

350

icals in the digestive tract, are generally also safe. Some chemicals may themselves be harmless, but biochemical experiments can reveal that they are converted by bacteria living in the intestine or by liver enzymes into toxic agents. In other cases, potentially poisonous substances may be detoxified in the liver and then harmlessly excreted.

The way in which a chemical is administered to animals greatly influences the results and interpretation of studies. Ordinarily, scientists expose animals to a chemical by adding it to their food or water or by administering it through a stomach tube. The oral route is the most meaningful way of testing food additives, because additives enter the human body through the mouth. A stomach tube insures that the animal actually consumes the chemical, rather than scattering it around the cage. Administering the chemical by tube also increases the sensitivity of a test by exposing the animals to a sudden, high dosage of chemical. This type of exposure is similar to a person gulping down a can of soda pop or cup of coffee. When the chemical is mixed in with the food, the animal consumes it gradually throughout the day and is never exposed to a high concentration.

While feeding studies are generally the most informative, some information can be obtained by applying the additive to the skin or injecting it under the skin (subcutaneously), into a blood vessel (intravenously), or into the body cavity (intraperitoneally). Injecting a chemical with a syringe bypasses the animal's digestive enzymes, stomach acids, and intestinal bacteria, any of which may alter the substance under study, and also exposes the animal to sudden, exceedingly high levels of the agent. The results of this kind of experiment must be interpreted in light of metabolic studies that show whether the substance, when ingested, is absorbed into the bloodstream or is converted into a second substance by the digestive system. Otherwise, the conclusions drawn from injection studies are likely to be erroneous.

The most important test used to evaluate food additives is the chronic, or lifetime, feeding study. This test is designed to detect chemicals that cause cancer or are toxic when ingested over long periods of time. In a chronic feeding study, researchers feed animals a diet that contains ten times to one thousand or more times as much of the additive as a person might consume. These studies typically employ fifty animals of each sex of two species of rodent, usually mice and rats. As a control, an equal number of animals is fed identical food, except that the additive is left out. The animals are maintained on the diets for their entire lives, usually about two years. In the best tests, animals are first exposed to chemicals while they are still in their mothers' womb. Thus, an animal will be exposed from the very moment of conception, just as a person might be.

Technicians monitor the animals' weight, consumption of food, and blood composition. Special tests may be performed to measure the health of the liver, kidney, or other organs. After the animals die or are sacrificed, pathologists examine the major organs, first by eye and

351

then microscopically, for evidence of tumors or other harm. The highest dosage that has no harmful effect is determined. FDA then sets a safe level for human exposure by applying a one hundredfold safety factor to the "highest no-observable-effect level." A chemical is unacceptable as a food additive if low dosages are harmful or if any amount causes cancer.

In interpreting the results of animal studies, it is crucial to keep one eye fixed on the chemical's effects and the other on the dosage levels used. Disregarding the quantity of chemical that causes a toxic effect all too commonly leads to groundless fears. Large enough doses of *any* chemical, even water, are injurious to animals and humans. Some substances upset the water balance, causing chronic diarrhea or increased production of urine; others taste so bad that animals would rather starve than eat their food; still others may overwork and damage the kidneys or liver. These effects do not arise when animals consume the small or moderate amounts that would likely be added to food. Thus, just because extremely high dosages of a chemical are harmful does not mean that normal dietary levels will be harmful and that the chemical should be prohibited as a food additive.

Cancer

Cancer, however, does *not* appear to be one of the effects that occur at high dosages, but not at low dosages. The scientific evidence strongly indicates that, if large amounts of a chemical cause tumors, we should assume that small amounts will also cause tumors, though less frequently. . . . Despite this general agreement, however, it is conceivable that large dosages of some chemicals might disrupt an animal's metabolism to such an extent that only high dosages, but not low dosages, would cause cancer. If such chemicals are found, they would deserve to be regulated as exceptions to the general rule. . . .

Cancer tests that employ some method other than feeding (or stomach tube) must be interpreted cautiously. When a chemical is injected subcutaneously, local tumors (fibrosarcomas) often develop at the site of injection. Scientists argued for years over whether these tumors reflect a hazard to humans or are simply due to nonspecific physical irritation caused by repeated injections. Sometimes local tumors can be induced by implanting bits of inert plastic or by repeatedly injecting harmless chemicals under the skin. Many cancer specialists are not concerned about tumors that arise only at the site of injection, but view with suspicion chemicals that cause tumors far from the point of injection — in the liver, lung, bladder, etc. . . .

Lifetime animal studies designed to detect cancer-causing agents typically take three to four years to conduct and cost several hundred thousand dollars. These two factors stimulated scientists to seek quick, inexpensive tests that could identify cancer-causing chemicals.

352

In the 1970s, Bruce Ames, a molecular biologist at the University of California at Berkeley, made the first real breakthrough. The "Ames test" takes just a few days and costs just a few hundred dollars.

The Ames test measures a chemical's ability to cause mutations in bacteria. The researcher mixes the chemical with enzymes from a rat's liver. The enzymes convert the chemical to some of the metabolites that might form in the body. (Sometimes the basic chemical will be safe, but its metabolites harmful.) Bacteria are then exposed to the chemical mixture. The number of mutant bacteria that form is compared to the number of mutants that form in the absence of the chemical. The more mutants, the more mutagenic is the chemical. The ability to cause mutations correlates closely with the ability to cause cancer.

The Ames test and other similar microbiological tests are good, but not perfect indicators of carcinogenicity. Some cancer-causing chemicals do not cause mutations in bacterial tests. Other chemicals that do cause mutations in bacteria have not been identified in animal tests as being carcinogenic. Because the short-term tests are still not foolproof, food additives and other chemicals to which humans may be exposed still need to be subjected to the more expensive and lengthy animal tests before they can be considered safe.

Many chemical companies are now using the quick mutagenicity tests to routinely screen newly synthesized chemicals. The manufacturers can save enormous amounts of money by not developing chemicals that show up "positive" in the screening.

Birth Defects

. . . In the 1960s, the FDA began asking manufacturers of proposed additives to conduct animal reproduction studies. These studies are usually integrated into lifetime feeding experiments. A good reproduction study spans four generations and reveals a chemical's effect on fertility, lactation, and the development of the embryo. . . .

Most good reproduction studies take great pains to expose pregnant animals to only one chemical at a time. That keeps the experiment easy to interpret. However, such as experiment does not bear much resemblance to a pregnant woman's lifestyle. The average pregnant woman consumes dozens of food additives, may smoke cigarettes and drink alcohol, breathes scores of air pollutants, and may take a dozen different prescription and over-the-counter drugs. It should hardly surprise us, if some combination of all these chemicals multiplied the risk to the developing fetus. . . .

A key problem with teratology studies is that scientists do not agree on how to interpret the results. For cancer studies, most experts agree that if large amounts of a chemical cause cancer in animals, a **353** small amount would also cause cancer, but much less frequently. In other words, there is no "threshold" level below which a carcinogen is safe. This may or may not be the case for chemicals that cause birth defects. The reproductive process is so complicated and sensitive that huge amounts of otherwise safe chemicals could often cause birth defects or infertility. Thus, there may be threshold levels below which a chemical does not cause birth defects.

Also, cancer experts agree that a chemical that causes cancer in animals should be assumed to be a carcinogen in humans. By contrast, some birth defect experts question the relevance of animal studies to human beings. . . .

In the late 1970s, federal officials were developing a uniform, governmentwide policy on interpreting animal reproduction studies. . . . According to FDA's Dr. Frankos, ". . . a thousandfold safety factor would be applied in those cases where there is evidence of serious developmental effects in two species." For minor or temporary birth defects, FDA would use its standard hundredfold safety factor.

Mutations

. . . Biologists have known for decades that radiation or chemicals can cause changes — or mutations — in the genes of plants and animals. Genes in a woman's egg cells and in a man's sperm carry, in chemically encoded form, the instructions for the proper development of the next generation. Mutations in these genes may garble the precisely inscribed instructions and cause such "mistakes" as hemophilia, extra fingers, heightened need for certain nutrients, reduced intelligence, mongolism, and decreased resistance to disease. The mutations — and their effects — may persist from one generation to the next. . . .

Mutation studies involving live animals are relatively expensive, time-consuming, and insensitive. They have been largely superseded by the Ames test, described earlier, which uses bacteria. Similar tests have been developed involving other microorganisms or cultured animal cells. These quick, inexpensive tests have made it possible to routinely screen all new chemicals for their ability to cause genetic mutations.

How Good Are the Studies?

Testing a proposed food additive for carcinogenic, teratogenic, and mutagenic effects and conducting metabolic studies is a major undertaking. But even after this great investment of time and money in what would appear to be a thorough investigation, an apparently safe additive could still cause trouble.

354

Food additives that cause only very occasional cancers, mutations, or birth defects would probably not be detected by current testing methods. In fact, the reason we are justified in being alarmed when an additive is found to cause cancer is that current methods are so coarse and insensitive. The primary weakness of feeding tests is that only a small number of animals are used. The results of these relatively small experiments are inevitably blurred by spontaneously occurring tumors or malformations, random variations, and the premature death of some of the animals. For instance, a typical reproduction study involves only twenty parent animals at each dosage level. A chemical would have to increase the incidence of malformations in the range of five to twelve times above normal before it could be positively identified as a teratogen. In a typical long-term feeding study involving one hundred animals, at least about five to twenty animals would have to develop cancer before the chemical being tested could, with any confidence, be identified as a carcinogen. Using doses one hundred to one thousand times greater than amounts to which humans would be exposed compensates somewhat for the small number of animals, but the studies are still not all that sensitive. Even assuming that animals and humans are equally sensitive to a chemical, a "rigorous" experiment could detect only those carcinogens that cause more than about one cancer death in two thousand to twenty thousand persons. This means that a "safe" food additive could cause cancer in as many as ten thousand to one hundred thousand Americans.

It should be emphasized that feeding studies, which because of costs inevitably involve a limited number of animals, are as sensitive as they are only because massive amounts of chemical are fed to the animals. Even strong carcinogens might escape detection if a hundred rats were fed a chemical at the level at which it occurs in a human diet. Food industry officials sometimes argue that experiments in which huge doses of chemical-caused cancer are [involved are] invalid because enormous amounts of *any* chemical will cause cancer. In fact, . . . extremely high doses of most chemicals do *not* cause cancer. They may destroy the liver, or damage the heart, or cause continuous diarrhea, but they do not cause cancer.

In virtually all toxicologic studies only one or two species of animals are treated with the chemical. Yet we know that sensitivities to chemicals that cause birth defects and cancer vary greatly from one species to another, and it is impossible to know which species' reaction would be most similar to human's. . . .

In addition to the markedly different sensitivities of different species to a chemical, there are significant variations between strains of animals within a species. Animals used in experiments are not field mice or sewer rats recently captured in the wild, but rodents that have been highly inbred over many generations in the laboratory. Different strains of the same species may be extremely sensitive to or uniquely resistant to a specific carcinogen or teratogen. Usually only one strain of a species is used in a feeding study. In contrast, the entire extraordinarily diverse American population ingests food additives. Americans of African or European ancestry may react differently to an additive than a person of Asian descent. Moreover, subcultures within the United States — blacks, adolescents, vegetarians, suburbanites, etc. — have distinctive eating habits and lifestyles that may increase or decrease their sensitivity or exposure to a certain chemical.

Laboratory experiments are almost always conducted with well-fed, pampered animals, the kind that might be most resistant to the effects of marginally toxic chemicals. Humans, on the other hand, suffer infections and diseases and are frequently malnourished. Diabetes, alcoholism, hypertension, food allergies, and dozens of other problems could increase the toxicity of a chemical. . . .

Another difference between laboratory conditions and real life is that typical toxicity tests measure the effects on animals of one food additive in an otherwise "pure" diet. Most Americans consume a rich assortment of synthetic antioxidants, thickening agents, emulsifers, coal tar dyes, and preservatives, as well as drugs, air pollutants, water pollutants, and pesticides. The possibilities are endless for two otherwise harmless chemicals to interact and cause a problem. . . .

Still another of the inadequacies of current testing procedures is that only a limited range of effects is monitored. Rarely studied are possible effects on the brain. A chemical that causes impaired eye-hand coordination, a slight reduction in memory, or hyperactivity would never be identified by current test procedures. Government and other scientists have developed special tests that can evaluate a chemical's effects on behavior, but the FDA does not require food additives to be so tested.

One of the biggest problems is that most testing of food additives is done by the manufacturers themselves. Companies either test chemicals in their own facilities or contract the work out to private testing laboratories whose financial solvency may depend upon delivering favorable results to its clients. One would not be surprised if companies used lax experimental protocols or overlooked an occasional tumor. At the subtle end of the spectrum, industry scientists might unthinkingly interpret ambiguous results in a way that absolves the chemical of any harmful effect. At the other end of the spectrum, are the horror stories about lying, cheating, greedy laboratories. . . .

> *In the face of all this scientific uncertainty, is the food supply safe or not? Food microbiologist E. M. Foster, Director of the University of Wisconsin's Food Research Institute, believes there is little cause for worry. Our present food supply is free of significant hazard, he argues, and the public needs to be taught to focus on the more important risks they face in their lives.*

IS THERE A FOOD SAFETY CRISIS?*

Edwin M. Foster, Ph.D.

A hundred years ago . . . there was a concern for food safety in the United States no less intense than the concern Americans face today. Urbanization of America following the Civil War brought a complete change in the nation's food supply system. No longer could each family produce its own food or buy it from a nearby farmer. A food industry became necessary to supply the growing cities.

During that time Americans were facing new health problems. In 1869 . . . *Harper's Weekly* complained that "The city people are in constant danger of buying unwholesome meat; the dealers are unscrupulous; the public uneducated." This was only five years after Louis Pasteur had disproved the theory of spontaneous generation, and even before Robert Koch showed that microbes cause disease.

The milk supplies in the cities were even more hazardous than the meat. According to Otto Bettmann, "Bacteria-infected milk held lethal possibilities of which people were unaware. The root of this problem was in the dairy farms, invariably dirty, where the milch cows were improperly fed and housed."

"It was not unusual for a city administration to sell its garbage to a farmer, who promptly fed it to his cows. Or for a distillery to keep cows and feed them distillery wastes, producing what was called 'swill milk.' This particular liquid caused a scandal in the New York of 1870 when it was revealed that some of the cows cooped up for years in filthy stables were so enfeebled from tuberculosis that they had to be raised on cranes to remain 'milkable' until they died."

On top of that "It was common knowledge to New Yorkers that their milk was diluted. The dealers were neither subtle nor timid about it; all they required was a water pump to boost two quarts of milk to a gallon."

*"Is There A Food Safety Crisis?" by E. M. Foster. *Nutrition Today* 17:6 – 13, November/December 1982. Used with permission.

Unscrupulous manufacturers adulterated coffee with charcoal, cocoa with sawdust, olive oil with coconut oil, butter with oleomargarine, honey with sugar, and candy with paraffin. They preserved milk with formaldehyde, meat with sulfurous acid, and butter with borax.

The American people had something to complain about in those times. The result, of course, was passage of the Pure Food and Drug Act in 1906. . . .

"Is There a Food Safety Crisis?" This title implies that there is one, or there may be; but the answer is no. We don't have a food safety crisis except, perhaps, in the minds of people who are prone to worry and believe everything they hear. What we do have is a giant controversy with conflict between various factions of society over what we as a nation ought to do about food safety. . . .

Historical Perspective

Twenty years ago Americans never even thought about the safety of our food. Safety was assumed. Now we question nearly everything. Had it not been for the quick action of Congress a few years ago, both nitrite and saccharin would have disappeared from the American food supply. Our nation's top regulatory agency, the Food and Drug Administration, felt legally obliged to ban both nitrite and saccharin. The agency was overruled by a body of politicians, the United States Congress.

Needless to say, the American people are worried and confused by the mixed signals they are receiving from the many voices that speak on safety issues. Over and over again we hear that our foods are being poisoned with unsafe preservatives, unnecessary additives, toxic pesticides and all manner of dangerous chemicals. We hear that our diet is composed of non-nutritious junk filled with empty calories. . . .

. . . Why has food safety become a national issue? Why are so many people worried and confused about the safety of the foods they eat?

Nature of the Hazards

Before we consider answers to questions such as these let us identify the hazards that have been associated with food. A convenient starting place is the list prepared by Dr. Virgil Wodicka when he was at the Food and Drug Administration about ten years ago. Named first and considered the greatest danger to consumers were foodborne toxigenic and pathogenic microorganisms. Next, in order of decreasing seriousness, were malnutrition, environmental contaminants, toxic natural constituents, pesticide residues and finally, in last place, food additives.

358

To this list I would now add reaction products that are formed during processing or preparation for eating. Nobody knows if they represent a significant hazard to man, but I have elected to list them in fifth place after naturally occurring toxicants. I reserve the right to move them to another place at some future time as more evidence accumulates. . . .

Overall Assessment

The real problems, the ones we know about and the ones we have a valid basis to fear, are the biological agents — pathogenic and toxigenic bacteria, foodborne viruses and parasites, fungal toxins, and toxic natural components of edible plants and animals. We know how to prevent all of these.

Everything else is either hypothetical or it is rare, accidental, and preventable with reasonable care, just as auto accidents are. There is absolutely no evidence that we are using unsafe food additives, yet concerns about foodborne hazards seem to be inversely proportional to how much we know about them. The less we know, the more we worry.

Many Americans are confused, scared, and concerned about food safety because they don't know what to believe nor whom to believe. . . .

It is difficult to understand how we got into this state of affairs until we recognize the unique, almost mystical properties of food. Food has the largest burden of symbolic, ceremonial, and religious overtones of any component of our daily lives. Food is something special. We feel comfortable with food and nervous without it. Concern about our food supply can make us irrational. We are seeing that today.

Food scientists have been modifying, manipulating, and improving our food since the time of Nicholas Appert. Wars accentuate the need for preserved food, and World War II in particular provided an environment for technological innovation that carried over into the post-war civilian food supply. The late 1940s and the decade of the fifties were the heyday for food technologists interested in developing new goodies to please the American palate and ease the housewife's job of food preparation.

Then came the consumer movement — or it might better be referred to as the anti-industry movement — of the 1960s with a ready-made opportunity to attack the food industry for adding, in the words of a well-known former U.S. senator, "all those unsafe, untested, unnecessary chemicals to our food supply."

The consumer movement was made up of a loose federation of activists from many and varied backgrounds who shared antipathy for the food industry. They had a simple and effective mode of action.

359

First, they would seize the high moral ground as defenders of the individual consumer against his monolithic foe, the food industry. From this vantage point the activists would attack industry for manufacturing and selling unsafe and unwholesome food. Anyone who did not agree with the activists was dismissed and discredited as a toady of industry.

Coincident with their attacks on industry, the activists mounted a campaign to change people's food habits. They urged us to eat less processed food, avoid food additives, and cut down on animal products. They recommended that we eat a "natural" diet with more whole grain cereals and other unrefined foods obtained from plants.

How successful have the activists been? I have no specific figures, but news reports and observations tell me that their efforts have not been in vain. In every group one finds people who have changed their food habits. They are cutting down on salt, or they have quit eating bacon, or they have given up beef, or they eat only one egg per week, or they avoid sweets. Far more people now are reading labels, looking for the name of additives they want to avoid. The phenomenal growth of the so-called health food industry attests to the magic of the word "natural," which nobody can define but everybody, including beer advertisers, uses to lure a gullible public. Natural is supposed to mean pure and safe, neither of which it does. . . .

How did industry react to its attackers? I would characterize the response as very quiet. With a few notable exceptions, industry went about its business without public utterance. There was occasional wringing of hands in boardrooms and plenty of complaining and worrying in private, but that was as far as it went. In typical marketer fashion, most companies were determined to give the customer what he wants. If he wants "no additives" and "everything natural," that's what he will get. Meanwhile, the same companies usually sell other products containing a full quota of chemical additives. The hypocrisy doesn't seem to bother them a bit. That is called opportunism in the marketplace.

In retrospect it is not difficult to see why the activists have been so successful in elevating food safety to a national issue. It is because they had no opposition of consequence and because we are so ignorant. As a modern philosopher once said, one cannot counter anecdotal data with no data. Claims that something *might be* unsafe cannot be laid to rest by a simple retort that it *might not be* unsafe. As a friend of mine said recently, we don't know enough to solve the food safety problems, but we know too much to ignore them.

Well, what can we do about the controversy over food safety? I have four suggestions:

1. Let's get our priorities straight. Let's put our efforts on the *real* hazards in life and quit dissipating our energies on hypothetical and imaginary dangers. . . .

The figures tell us that smoking kills 150,000 people every year. That is almost three times the number of Americans killed during the entire Viet Nam War. Alcohol kills 100,000 people every year; motor vehicles kill 50,000. . . . Drunk driving kills an average of 70 people *every day*. These are real numbers, and these are real dead people.

. . . Not a single fatality is attributable to the much-criticized food constituents, pesticides, antibiotics and spray cans.

2. The second thing we might do is use a little common sense. At the height of the nitrite controversy critics of the food supply were demanding that nitrite be banned from cured meats on the grounds that it may cause cancer. They were willing to jeopardize a $12 billion industry and allow the consumer to take the risk of botulism knowing full well that the ban would reduce his exposure to nitrite by less than 10 percent. . . .

3. The third and by far the most difficult thing we need to do is identify the real dangers in our food supply and learn how to control them. Unfortunately we do not have the basic information required to do this, and a great deal more research will be necessary before we can reach valid conclusions. Calling for more research is a typical reaction from a scientist, but that is the only way to get the facts we must have. The alternative is to continue as we are. Who is going to do the research, and who is going to pay for it? Recently [the] FDA Commissioner urged the food industry to step up its research efforts in food safety. I wish him well in this approach, but I am not sanguine about his chances.

4. My fourth suggestion is to develop a mechanism for getting the facts about food safety to the public. Up to now people have been subjected to a great deal of misinformation and supposition that was based not on fact but simply on the biases of the communicator.

Things are not nearly as bad as they look. There is very little evidence of hazards in our food supply, and the ones we know about we can control. In spite of all the claims about carcinogens in food, the death rates from cancer for all organs except lungs are declining or remaining level. Life expectancy is increasing. The average American now lives twenty-one years longer than he did when I was born. That is an entire generation gained in one lifetime.

We must be doing something right.

361

> *Some of Dr. Foster's arguments would likely be echoed by Dr. Bruce Ames, chairman of the biochemistry department at the University of California at Berkeley. This selection from* American Health *magazine discusses Dr. Ames' contention that if reducing our risks of developing cancer is the goal, then natural substances, rather than man-made ones that sometimes turn up in foods, are what we should be worrying about.*

DIET AND CANCER — ROUND 2*

Janet Hopson and Joel Gurin

It's the about-face of the decade in cancer research. Bruce Ames, the renowned biochemist who once shed harsh light on manmade chemicals, has now declared that a different set of substances may be the major causes of cancer. We don't need to worry so much about traces of all those toxic synthetic chemicals, says Ames. The key to cancer is much more likely in our diet.

According to Ames, food may not explain just *part* of the cancer problem, as other scientists have suggested. What we eat, together with cigarettes and the aging process, may be virtually *all* of it.

The idea is that natural substances in food may have a much greater effect on cancer risk than synthetic chemicals do. Lab tests have shown that everyday food — health food as well as junk food — is riddled with potential carcinogens. Mushrooms, peanut butter, burnt toast, charbroiled hamburgers, bruised celery and potatoes, and alfalfa sprouts, among other common foods, all contain vastly more carcinogens than do the doses we get of manmade pesticides, says Ames. Ames' goal in presenting his argument has been "not to pinpoint particular foods and say don't eat celery or alfalfa sprouts, but simply to show how widespread natural mutagens and carcinogens are in the diet, and how much greater the background level of these compounds is than of manmade compounds."

At first the argument has a preposterous ring. After all, if foods as ubiquitous as celery and pepper contain dangerous chemicals, why don't we all get cancer?

Clearly, the answer isn't simple. But just as he believes we've paid too little attention to natural carcinogens, Ames — like many other scientists — also thinks we should accelerate research into the natural substances that may *protect* us from cancer. Many foods contain "anti-

---

*"Diet and Cancer — Round 2," by Janet Hopson and Joel Gurin. Reprinted from American Health: *Fitness of Body and Mind*, November, 1984. Copyright, 1984, American Health Partners.

carcinogens" that actually seem to lower cancer risk. The key to avoiding cancer may not be just shunning potential dangers; it may also be to eat enough of the foods that appear to protect us.

There's a surprising, and controversial, corollary to this new theory. If we get such big doses of naturally occurring carcinogens from just eating, says Ames, the traces of manmade chemicals we get should be insignificant. EDBs, PCBs and all the other manmade carcinogens of the month aren't worth a lot of worry unless you get big doses in your job, he says, and most of us don't.

It's this last point that many of Ames' colleagues have found the most troubling. Ironically, Ames is the scientist who in the past 15 years did more than almost anyone to focus attention on the cancer-causing potential of *synthetic* chemicals. So some colleagues view his dramatic turnaround as scientific heresy, and several have attacked his reasoning and questioned his motivation. For starters, they believe Ames' new stance gives far too much aid and comfort to the chemical and food industries.

The debate began when Ames published a major article in *Science*, a scientific journal, that summarized studies done in laboratories throughout the world over the past few years. But soon the argument spilled beyond the boundaries of the scientific community. . . .

Despite all the publicity, Ames' hypothesis is not new. What *is* new is that a scientist of his stature has supported it publicly.

A slightly built, energetic man whose narrow face and wire-rimmed spectacles make him look a bit like a Dickens character, Ames has impeccable scientific credentials. The 55-year-old chairman of biochemistry at the University of California at Berkeley was the inventor of a fast, simple test that vastly simplified the search for hazardous industrial chemicals.

The now-famous "Ames test" determines whether a substance is a mutagen — a chemical that mutates DNA, causing the genetic damage many believe may lead to cancer. Mutagens aren't always true carcinogens (cancer-causing chemicals) but they are prime suspects. The test uses *Salmonella* bacteria, takes a day or two to complete, and costs about $500 — a fraction of the time and resources needed to test a substance in a rat, mouse or rainbow trout.

Ironically, the test may have been too good. Thousands of researchers round the world, using the Ames test to discover mutagenic chemicals, find them almost wherever they look — in natural chemicals as well as synthetics. This trend set Ames thinking and he began to change his ideas about human cancer. Why he wondered, is so much attention paid to manmade chemicals instead of those in food?

Of course, Ames himself was part of the answer. In those days, he was pointing fingers at a lot of manmade chemicals, and there are a lot of them to point at. About 50,000 synthetic chemicals are used commercially, and 500 new ones are introduced into the market each year, many of them mutagenic and carcinogenic.

363

So, a few years ago, Ames and many others feared that industrialized society was running straight into a huge cancer epidemic. But we should have seen the start of the epidemic by now. Cancer takes 20 to 30 years to develop, and precisely that period has elapsed since we began to live better through chemistry after World War II. Nonetheless, no obvious epidemic has materialized.

Ames cites a major study published in 1981 by Oxford University epidemiologists Richard Doll And Richard Peto. They compiled and analyzed hundreds of studies and concluded that the incidence of only one type of cancer — lung cancer — has increased dramatically in the past 50 years. And the rise of cigarette smoking — first among men, then women — seems to explain it almost entirely. . . .

. . . If Doll and Peto are right, and Ames believes they are, something present in the old-fashioned "natural" days, before synthetic chemicals began to take over, must play a role as large as tobacco in causing the disease that kills one of five Americans. Something like food.

"Of all the compounds that attack DNA," says Ames, his rapid-fire speech accelerating as he discusses the subject, "my guess is that 99% occur naturally, many of them in the common foods we eat. On this basis, I"ve come to the same conclusion Peto and Doll did with epidemiology — the *really* important factors in human cancer, in addition to carcinogens made by aging, are smoking and diet."

In his *Science* article, Ames published a list of foods that contain natural compounds that are mutagens in the Ames test. (For a few examples, see the box) Many of these same natural chemicals have also proved carcinogenic in lab animals. As a result, they are suspected — though not proven — to cause human cancer. "Every meal you eat is full of mutagens and carcinogens," says Ames.

Why do plants produce carcinogenic chemicals? Mostly to fight marauding insects. Ames calls them "natural pesticides." He also offers a startling thought: To avoid excessive use of manmade pesticides, we are now breeding plants that are increasingly insect-resistant — and are sharply boosting the doses of natural pesticides and carcinogens that we eat.

"There is a feeling here in America that nature is benign, but that's not true," says Ames. "Plants have to protect themselves from predators, and every plant in nature is 2% to 10% toxic chemicals. We're eating grams and grams of the stuff every day."

Ames' roster, which reads like a malevolent grocery list, makes planning dinner something of a problem. It might be easy enough to swear off false morels and peanut butter, but the list covers most hot drinks and a good many popular vegetables. To make matters worse, Ames has described dreadful chemical changes that take place when you cook protein or when fat goes rancid. But it's hard to avoid "burnt stuff" entirely unless you like a steady diet of sushi and steak tartare — which has its own problems. . . .

364

But even if all the chemicals on Ames' grocery list are true carcinogens, that still doesn't necessarily mean you should shun celery and potatoes. The chemicals, purified from food, may cause cancer in animals — but the whole food itself may not cause cancer in people. Ames himself still feels far too little is known to change his own diet (except to cut back in fat). For this reason, he reassures one and all that *he* still cooks his food, *he* isn't calling for a ban on peanut butter or burnt toast, and *his* taste for celery and the rest remains unabated.

However, Ames does like to make sure his diet isn't deficient in nutrients that may help *protect* us from cancer, the so-called anticarcinogens. They include the antioxidants vitamin E, beta-carotene, selenium, vitamin C and one that Ames' own research uncovered — uric acid.

Interestingly, mutagens and anticarcinogens like beta-carotene are often present in the same foods — parsley, celery, lettuce and spinach. The balance between "good" and "bad" factors in these foods may determine their effect on health. . . .

Ames' list of toxins in food may make it harder to come to any firm conclusions, at least for a while. "It's very confusing to the general public," says T. Colin Campbell — a Cornell University professor of nutrition biochemistry, who was on the National Academy of Sciences diet-cancer panel.

But Campbell feels that some of the confusion is coming from the way nutrition research is being done. The problem, he believes, is that scientists studying diet and cancer are trying to find the effects of single nutrients — like vitamin A, or a toxin in potatoes — and ignoring the complexity of nutrient interaction. . . .

Ames, for his part, agrees that the precise links between diet and cancer remain to be worked out. But he is now confident that the biochemical mix of free radicals, natural mutagens and antioxidants is where "the main action in cancer and aging research" will be for years to come.

It may turn out, he adds, that "the cheapest, easiest way to cut cancer rates is to cut down on fat or feed people beta-carotene instead of making our highest priority the removal of a little bit of trichloroethylene from the drinking water."

The "Bad" Stuff in Food . . .

Though Ames doesn't recommend giving up these foods, he has cited several with carcinogens that need more study. The government's National Toxicology Program — which now does 30% of its testing on natural substances — is looking at several of these chemicals.
- Some spongy mushrooms contain hydrazines. Common table mushrooms have a carcinogen called phenyldiazonium that causes mouse tumors.
- Celery, parsnips, figs and parsley contain psoralen derivatives, which can

become potent mutagens and carcinogens when activated by light. Bruised or rotting celery contains 100 times more psoralens than the vegetable does when fresh.

- Black pepper contains 10% by weight of piperine, which has caused tumors in mice.
- Red wine contains mutagens called quercetins — members of the flavonoids family, common in many foods.
- Quinones, the pigments that make apple skin red, can mutate DNA.
- Theobromine (a relative of caffeine) in tea and chocolate, though not a direct carcinogen itself, can interfere with the repair of DNA damage due to carcinogens in cells.
- Alfalfa sprouts, a mainstay of health food enthusiasts, contain a highly toxic compound, canavanine, that seems to cause an autoimmune-like disease in monkeys.
- Molds that contaminate peanut butter, bread and apple juice can secrete highly carcinogenic compounds, such as aflatoxin.
- Beets, lettuce, spinach and radishes contain nitrates, which are converted in the body to nitrosamines, suspects in cancer of the esophagus and stomach.
- High levels of dietary fat are linked to breast and colon cancer — the biggest killers after lung cancer.
- Allyl isothiocyanate, a major flavoring in mustard oil and horseradish, is a carcinogen in rats.
- The burnt or browned layer on cooked or charcoal-broiled meats, toasted bread or roasted coffee beans is highly mutagenic in the Ames test, and some of the compounds in "burnt stuff" cause cancer in rats and mice.

. . . And the Good Stuff

According to one leading theory, carcinogens cause cancer by producing highly reactive oxygen atoms (which also promote aging). And anticarcinogens may protect us by being antioxidants: They disarm the renegade atoms. These "free radicals" — oxygen molecules with "free," unpaired electrons — are created in the body through a number of processes, from sugar metabolism to immune system function. Many of the natural mutagens on Ames' list produce oxygen radicals. Fats can, too, when they're stored, cooked or digested.

Free radicals have the potential to attack and alter a cell's DNA, perhaps leading to cancer. But oxygen radicals are usually short-lived, and an antioxidant molecule can often trap the radical and absorb its excess, destructive energy. Several kinds of antioxidants are now being studied as potential anticarcinogens.

- Vitamin E is a normal component of cell membranes, and has been shown to protect animals from the DNA damage caused by quinones, hydrazines and other "natural pesticides."
- Beta-carotene is a natural component of orange, yellow and green plant pigments. It protects rats and mice against some carcinogenic compounds. One widely publicized Japanese study — now being validated by an American study — suggests that smokers who eat large amounts of green and yellow vegetables are less likely to get lung cancer than smokers who pass up the salad bar.

- The mineral selenium occurs in most soils, and we usually get plenty of this trace element in seafoods, wheat germ and whole grains. Like vitamins A and E, it is toxic in high doses. Given to animals in proper amounts, however, selenium inhibits the skin, liver, colon and breast tumors induced by various carcinogens.
- Vitamin C in foods protects rodents from the carcinogenic effects of ultraviolet light and nitrites.
- Finally, there's uric acid, present in human blood and saliva at high levels. Although it hasn't been shown specifically to protect animals from cancer, uric acid is an antioxidant, and Ames and others are studying it.

While neither Foster nor Ames seems concerned about the substances that may get into our food (as opposed to those that are there "naturally"), some scientists are concerned—at least partly by our level of ignorance about the chemicals in the food environment. The chart reproduced here is from a report called Toxicity Testing *published by the National Academy of Sciences.*

Do we know enough about the chemicals in our environment to determine how safe they are? Look especially at the top line, "pesticides and inert ingredients of pesticide formulations," and at line four, "food additives." The black and dotted segments are the percentage of that category about which we know enough, or almost enough, to assess how hazardous these substances might be to human health.

[Please see table on the next page]

Steering Committee on Identification of Toxic and Potentially Toxic Chemicals for Consideration by the National Toxicology Program

Category	Size of Category	Complete Health Hazard Assessment Possible	Partial Health Hazard Assessment Possible	Minimal Toxicity Information Available	Some Toxicity Information Available (But below Minimal)	No Toxicity Information Available
Pesticides and Inert Ingredients of Pesticide Formulations	3,350	10	24	2	26	38
Cosmetic Ingredients	3,410	2	14	10	18	56
Drugs and Excipients Used in Drug Formulations	1,815	18	18	3	36	25
Food Additives	8,627	5	14	1	34	46
Chemicals in Commerce: At Least 1 Million Pounds/Year	12,860	11	11			78
Chemicals in Commerce: Less than 1 Million Pounds/Year	13,911	12	12			76
Chemicals in Commerce: Production Unknown or Inaccessible	21,752	10	8			82

Legend:

Complete Health Hazard Assessment Possible	Partial Health Hazard Assessment Possible	Minimal Toxicity Information Available	Some Toxicity Information Available (But below Minimal)	No Toxicity Information Available

Toxicity Testing: Strategies to Determine Needs and Priorities. National Academy Press, Washington, DC., 1984, p. 118. Used with permission.

> *Why do we know so little about the safety of what is in our*
> *food environment? One of the authors of the present volume*
> *argues that rapid changes in the food supply have made it dif-*
> *ficult for the regulators to keep up.*

FOOD SECURITY IN THE UNITED STATES:
A NUTRITIONIST'S VIEWPOINT*

Joan Dye Gussow, Ed.D.

. . . If we leave . . . "added" substances aside, it is obvious . . . that no
one has any idea what has been happening to the chemical composition of the food supply — additives aside — just as a consequence of
the processing foods undergo. That is, even if all the additives were
proven safe, how do we know whether the novel sorts of compounds
produced by novel sorts of processing are equally safe? . . .

. . . The extent of the actual information gap is . . . illustrated by
reference to a document put out in 1980 by the Food and Drug Administration — the agency most responsible for assuring the safety of the
food supply. The document is called The Bureau of Foods Research
Plan, and it is, in a sense, the research wish list of the Head of the
Bureau of Foods [now the Center for Food Safety and Applied Nutri-
tion]. It lays out the research which the Bureau scientists believe to be
necessary to assure that the nation's food is safe and wholesome.

The document lists 719 research needs, grouping them into a
series of overall goals such as "Nutritional Requirements" and "Toxicological and Epidemiological Testing." Goal C, "to isolate, purify and
identify potentially hazardous food and cosmetic constituents and
adulterants." includes research needs number 117 through 286 inclusive. Item 133, "Survey natural plant extracts for mutagenic/estrogenic
properties; isolate and identify the responsible toxic agents," reminds
us again that plants contain certain natural toxicants.

This is item 124 under Goal C: "Determine products formed as a
result of chemical modification of foods. e.g., bleaching of flour with
chlorine dioxide, chlorine, peroxides, and oxides of nitrogen." Flour is
simply used as an example — and a relatively uncomplicated one.
What is suggested here is . . . [that] we know almost nothing about the
chemical compounds formed from natural foods in the course of

*Chapter 10: "Food Security in the United States: A Nutritionist's Viewpoint" by Joan
Dye Gussow. *Food Security in the United States*, Westview Press, © 1984, pages 207 –
230. Lawrence Busch and William B. Lacy, editors. Edited portions used with permission.

manufacturing the extraordinary array of products in the supermarket.

Finally, item 128, "Determine from literature on production, volume and uses, and laboratory research in chemical and physical properties, which chemicals of the more than 43,000 commercially produced have the greatest potential to enter the food chain and present a human health hazard." Those are two of the 719 things the Bureau of Foods thinks it needs to know, and — more importantly — *does not currently know* in order to assure us that our food supply is safe. This is the "universe of knowledge needed by the Bureau," in the words of its director, "to fulfill its responsibilities to protect the national food supply."

Many people seem to believe that someone is already on top of all this. No one is. And, what is more, no one will be. Even given the propensity of scientists to exaggerate the amount of research that needs to be done, what is outlined here is mind-boggling. The research plan contains 719 items, a large number of which are, like those quoted, each a giant research plan of its own. Clearly the FDA is desperately behind in its work. . . .

What is going on? In a recent article in the *Ecologist*, Kauber makes it clear why we cannot get the knowledge we need. Contemporary technology, he observes, is "dominated by the process of innovation. . . . The appearance of wholly new substances" testifies "to the increasingly swift introduction, diffusion and turnover of things and ways of doing. Increasingly too 'unnatural synthetic' substances are being injected into the environment . . . compounds of all sorts previously unknown in nature." This rapid innovation, he points out, "undermines the experimental nature of empirical evaluation by radically increasing the number of variables required to be taken into account (43,000 chemicals, for example) as a result of prior innovations." Trouble arises "at the very start of the evaluative process. The data which ordinarily set the parameters for experimentation must arise out of prior experience with the elements from which the object or process in question is composed. But under conditions of extreme innovation, we often do not possess that kind of knowledge. Thus under conditions of rapid innovation we find ourselves encountering new substances whose combinations are poorly understood."

Ideally, therefore, one would extend the testing process, but marketplace forces urge haste; market forces also work against a slow introduction of the product, although inadequate background data and "hurried and incomplete" testing would make slow diffusion prudent. As a consequence, persons responsible at the later post-testing stages (the Food and Drug Administration, for example) "are faced with an awesome task . . . to assess on a continuing basis, the long-term effects of an innovation which, we recall, has been injected into an environment already overloaded with novelties. Such testing, were it responsibly carried out, could swallow up a quantity of resources which would dwarf that of the original implementaions, while the 'correction of undesired conditions' could conceivably become the sole occupation of an entire society of technicians." Or the entire staff of a score of FDAs.

. . . Let us assume that individuals (or a nation of individuals) can only have food security by knowing how to select wisely from among the foods available to them; and assume further that they are faced — in the future as they are now — with a marketplace containing some 12,000 items, most of them bearing little resemblance to anything their neolithic ancestors might have eaten, many of them unfamiliar even to immediately preceding generations. (Many of them unfamiliar even to *this* generation; between January and June of 1982 — a not atypical period — manufacturers introduced, among other new products, 103 new frozen foods, 48 new snacks, crackers, and nuts, 33 new beverages, and 27 new cakes, cookies, and breads.) . . .

To select among items like Tang, Start or Count Chocula, the modern consumer cannot use what one observer has called "craft skills" — the knowledge of how spoiled meat smells or how a ripe fruit feels. Therefore, the consumer cannot make personal judgments about whether these foods are safe and nutritious, but must trust someone else — presumably the food manufacturers, the nutritionists, or the Bureau of Foods of the FDA. The fact is that increasing numbers of shoppers appear not to trust any of these people; and, as the FDA research plan suggests, they are probably wise not to do so.

What, then, can consumers do? They can't make independent judgments and they aren't sure they can trust anyone. All they can really do is avoid. And that is precisely what some of them are doing. Research done on food labeling for the FDA shows that of all persons who pay attention to the list of ingredients on the label (that is, 54 percent of *all* food shoppers). 70 percent do so to *avoid* one or more substances. They are avoiding sugar and salt; they are avoiding "preservatives/chemicals." They are turning to foods labeled "natural" and "organic" even though the government has persistently refused to define these terms in such a way as to ensure that they mean anything. The authors of the FDA study call the information about label readers "disturbing." Nutrition professionals tend to denounce such behavior as superstitious, faddist, irrational, and so on, terms that are difficult to defend when no rational counterstrategy is readily available. . . .

. . . If we want to ensure nutritional security, our concern ought to be to bar the introduction of and encourage the phasing out of chemicals that are both highly toxic and persistent, and to discourage the excessive processing of foods and the proliferation of highly engineered food products. These solutions, of course, raise difficult economic and political questions.

371

So that you can better understand the food safety debate, we now move away from a direct discussion of food to a more general discussion of risk. How do we make decisions about what to eat or how to act when we don't really know enough to make the ideal choice among alternatives? Cathy Popescu, a researcher with the American Council on Science and Health, argues in this selection that we need to keep in perspective the numerous health risks we face in the course of everyday life. Risk assessment experts, she believes, can help us to deal with those risks in a way that minimizes personal harm.

In the piece that follows, Yale sociologist Charles Perrow argues that expert risk assessments contain such fundamental flaws that they cannot provide us with useful guidelines about comparative risks to our well-being. As you read these selections, try to decide for yourself where food risks fall on the spectrum of frequent or infrequent, avoidable or unavoidable, voluntary or involuntary, and whether we have enough control over our own food so as not to need government regulation to protect the food supply.

RISK AND REASON*

Cathy Becker Popescu, M.S.

Risk. Once reserved largely for epidemiologists, statisticians and the like, this word is becoming an integral and emotionally-charged element of everyone's vocabulary.

Turn on the television and you are likely to hear of the "still unknown risks" associated with the latest discovery of dioxin contamination. Pick up a newspaper and you may read of the "risk of a meltdown" at a nearby nuclear power plant, or of the alleged "cancer risk" posed by chemicals in our food or environment.

America has developed an obsession with risk, and with the idea that modern man has created a world which is inherently more risky than ever before. Yet, risk has always been with us, although its form has varied over the ages.

Our distant ancestors faced the risk of being eaten by predators. Our more recent ancestors risked death by plague or starvation. At the turn of this century, tuberculosis, diphtheria, tetanus, and frequent

 *"Risk and Reason", by Cathy Becker Popescu. *ACSH News & Views*, 4:8–10, November/December 1983. American Council on Science and Health.

physical injury from farm implements and industrial machinery were among the most important risks Americans faced. They also faced risks from sources that many people are concerned with today, such as food chemicals, and those risks were of a magnitude which we no longer tolerate. Fruits and vegetables were sprayed with "Paris Green", a toxic lead arsenate. Teas, candies and other foods were colored with lead chromate, which today's chemists would prefer not to touch, let alone eat. But few citizens were aware of these particular risks at the time.

The average life expectancy in the U.S. in 1900 was 47 years; today it is more than 74 years. Obviously, the sum of all the risks to which we are exposed must be less now than it was then. Yet, we are led to believe that the opposite is true.

Technological development has certainly brought with it its share of risks, but we must keep in mind that modern day risks have largely *replaced* the risks of yesteryear. Modern technology has not introduced an unprecedented burden of risk into a previously risk-free world. In fact, technology had played an important role in eliminating the risks of the past.

The Nature of Risk

... Risk can be *measured* — sometimes directly and relatively precisely, sometimes indirectly and theoretically.

For example, statistics tell us that commercial aircraft in the U.S. carry passengers 100 billion passenger-miles per year. They also tell us that only about 100 people are killed in airplane crashes per year. Therefore, the risk of dying in an airplane crash is about one in a million for every thousand miles of flight.

Other risks are not so easy to assess. The yearly risk of an individual living near a nuclear power plant being killed in a large accident (estimated to be 1 in 2,000 million) cannot be calculated from statistics on past incidents, because none have occurred. Rather, these estimates are based upon complex theoretical analyses, which rely upon both human judgment and probability figures.

To put the risks associated with nuclear power and flying in perspective, it might be helpful to glance at Table 1, which lists some common activities that increase the risk of death by one in a million.

Weighing the Risks

People constantly estimate risk in their daily lives. What is the risk that I will get cancer from the asbestos ceiling tile in my workplace? What are the chances of developing Toxic Shock Syndrome from using tampons? What is the risk of being injured or killed if I cross this busy

373

street against the light? We ask ourselves questions such as these and adjust our behavior according to the answers.

People rarely have adequate information on hand to answer such questions accurately. Nevertheless, they routinely make judgments about risk, based upon limited information and certain psychological principles. In many cases, these risk assessments correlate little with the actual probability of harm. . . .

Table 1. You Will Increase Your Chance of Death by One in a Million if You. . . .

Risk	Cause of Death
Spend 1 hour in a coal mine	Black lung disease
Spend 3 hours in a coal mine	Accident
Travel 6 minutes by canoe	Accident
Travel 10 minutes by bicycle	Accident
Travel 300 miles by car	Accident
Travel 1,000 miles by jet	Accident
Travel 6,000 miles by jet	Cancer caused by natural radiation
Live 2 months in Denver on vacation from New York	Cancer caused by natural radiation
Live 2 months in an average stone or brick building	Cancer caused by natural radiation
Have one chest X-ray taken in a good hospital	Cancer caused by radiation
Eat 40 tablespoons of peanut butter	Cancer caused by aflatoxin
Drink Miami drinking water for 1 year	Cancer caused by chloroform
Live 5 years at site boundary of typical nuclear power plant	Cancer caused by radiation
Drink 1,000 24 oz. soft drinks from recently banned plastic bottles	Cancer from acrylonitrile monomer
Live 20 years near a PVC plant	Cancer caused by vinyl chloride (1976 standard)
Live 150 years within 20 miles of a nuclear power plant	Cancer caused by radiation
Eat 100 charcoal broiled steaks	Cancer from benzpyrene
Live within 5 miles of a nuclear reactor for 50 years	Cancer caused by radiation from large accident
Work for 1.5 weeks in typical factory	Accident
Rock climb for 1.5 minutes	Accident
Spend 20 minutes being a man aged 60	Mortality from all causes

Based upon a table in "Analyzing the Daily Risks of Life," by Richard Wilson in *Technology Review*, Feb. 1979.

Another Way of Looking at Risk

Even if people have accurate information on the risk associated with a particular activity or technology, the importance of that risk may be difficult to comprehend. How significant is a risk of one in a thousand?

Is it something worth worrying about? Is there really that much of a difference between a one in a million and a one in five million risk?

A more useful way of looking at risk might be to translate it into everyday terms, as Physics Professor Bernard L. Cohen of the University of Pittsburgh has done. Dr. Cohen has calculated the number of days of expected life lost due to exposure to some risks, based upon the probability that any given individual will die as a result. For example, a 40 year-old man could expect to live another 34.8 years according to average life-expectancy figures. If he takes a risk that has a one percent (1 to 100) chance of causing death immediately, then his life expectancy is reduced by .348 years (one percent) or 127 days.

Obviously, some people will not lose any days of life as a result of exposure to a particular risk factor, while others will die several years prematurely. Dr Cohen's estimates merely represent the average number of days of life lost, taking both extremes into account.

As indicated in Table 2, exposure to some commonly feared risks, such as nuclear power and oral contraceptives, is actually responsible for the loss of no more than a few days of life. Other risks, which the public seems willing to accept placidly, such as cigarette smoking and overweight, are responsible for an average of several *years* of lost life. . .

Table 2. Average Life Expectancy Reductions Associated with Various Risks

Risk	Avg. Days of Life Lost
Cigarette smoking — male	2250
Being 30% overweight	1300
Being a coal miner	1100
Cigar smoking	330
Pipe smoking	220
Dangerous job — accidents	300
Motor vehicle travel	207
Alcohol (U. S. average)	130
Legal drug misuse	90
Average job — accidents	74
Job with radiation exposure	40
Being a pedestrian — accidents	37
Safest jobs — accidents	30
Illicit drugs (U. S. average)	18
Exposure to natural radiation	8
Medical x-rays	6
Oral contraceptives	5
Nuclear reactor accidents	0.02 – 2
Exposure to radiation from nuclear industry	0.02

*Excerpted from a table by Bernard L. Cohen and I-Sing Lee, in "A Catalog of Risks," *Health Physics* 36:707, 1979

Consequences

. . . Safety cannot be guaranteed or even empirically determined. While scientists or the proponents of a new technology can measure its risks, the public and its representatives bear much of the responsibility for the more complex and subjective decisions about safety. They also have a responsibility, however, to make such decisions based upon information which is as accurate, realistic and complete as possible, and to consider the benefit side of the equation.

When safety decisions are based upon distorted or disproportionate perceptions of risk, or inaccurate assessment of benefits, the consequences may be far-reaching.

When such misconceptions are responsible for blocking the development or implementation of useful technologies, all of society may suffer. The economy, social structure, environment or public health may be adversely affected.

Overestimating some risks, while underestimating or discounting others, may engender misplaced fear and misallocation of resources. . . .

Risk, in some form, is an intrinsic part of life. It always has been; it always will be.

Reason dictates that we take heed of risks, but that we keep them in perspective and concentrate our efforts on those that matter.

LIVING WITH HIGH-RISK SYSTEMS*

Charles Perrow, Ph.D.

. . . When societies confront a new or explosively growing evil, the number of risk assessors probably grows — whether they are shamans or scientists. I do not think it is an exaggeration to say that their function is not only to inform and advise the masters of these systems about the risks and benefits, but also, should the risk be taken, to legitimate it and reassure the subjects. With the increase in risk and public concern today, a new field of risk assessment has grown up, giving advice and (usually) legitimating the decisions of elites in the private and public sectors. At the behest of Congress, regulatory agencies have appeared in large numbers, and another function of risk assessors is to second-guess these agencies' awkward attempts to do a very difficult job. Risk assessors, interestingly enough, usually call for less

---

*From *Normal Accidents* by Charles Perrow. Copyright 1984 by Basic Books, Inc., Publishers. Pgs. 304–315. Reprinted by permission of the publisher.

regulation and are severe in their criticism of the agencies.

The professionals in this field are generally engineers, scientists, and social scientists; they are based in universities, research organizations, government regulatory agencies, military establishments, and industry trade groups. . . .

This is a very sophisticated field. Mathematical models predominate; extensive research is conducted; and the esoteric matters of Bayesian probabilites, ALARA principles (as low as reasonably achievable), "discounted future probabilites," and so on are debated in courtrooms as well as academic conferences. Some of the best scientific and social science minds are at work on the problem of "how safe is safe enough."

Yet it is a narrow field, cramped by the monetarization of social good. Everything can be bought; if it cannot be bought it does not enter the sophisticated calculations. A life is worth roughly $300,000, one study concluded; less if you are over sixty, even less if you are otherwise enfeebled. After taking into account age and potential earning power, a life is a life. Death by diabetes should have the equivalent impact on people as death by murder, is the implication of a study that deplores the public's unawareness that the former is a cause of many more deaths than the latter. "Unfortunately," they say, "there is evidence that peoples' perception of risks are subject to large, systematic biases. . . . Such biases may misdirect the actions of public interest groups and government agencies resulting in less than optimal control of risk." This bias in reasoning is due largely, they imply, to sensationalism of the media. But consider how a murder death affronts human values such as dignity, and the desire for security and predictability; the researchers themselves note it is not to be equated with a diabetes death, and public estimations of death rates reflect that, but the public is still held to be "biased." To take another case, for some economists and risk assessors (often the same people) there is no difference between the death of fifty unrelated people from many communities and the death of fifty from a community of one hundred. Social ties, family continuity, a distinctive culture, and valued human traditions are unquantified and unacknowledged. Fifty thousand highway deaths a year are equivalent to a single catastrophe with fifty thousand casualties for these experts, and they deplore the fact that the public protests nuclear plants and estimates highway deaths to be only half of what they are.

The field acknowledges the difference between voluntary risks such as skiing and hang-gliding, and involuntary ones such as leaching of chemical wastes. But it does not acknowledge the difference between the *imposition* of risks by profit-making firms who could reduce the risk, and the *acceptance* of risk by the public where private pleasures are involved (skiing) or some control can be exercised (driving). All are bundled up in a vague reference to market principles, as if we would not have heat and light without X number of dead   377 miners or irradiated nuclear glow boys. The literature reflects a rational, calculative marketplace theory of cost-benefit analysis. The technical literature is fond of pointing out that we spend millions of dollars in safety devices to save one nuclear power worker, but refuse to spend $80,000 to save the driver of an automobile. . . . It is thus irrational to spend that much money on the nuclear plant; we should spend it on seat belts, highway guardrails or anti-smoking literature. It is as if there were a fixed budget category for safety, regardless of whether corporation profits or private needs are involved, and the budget, being fixed, cannot be enlarged when new risks come along. . . .

Risk-benefit analysis, with its monetarization of cultural goods and values, has been succeeded by cost-benefit analysis, with its more open concern with the dollar as the ultimate solvent for all things social. Baruch Fischhoff, in a thoughtful examination of cost-benefit analysis, . . . notes another consequence of the monetarization of social good by economists. Cost-benefit analysis is "mute with regard to the distribution of wealth in society," he notes. "Therefore, a project designed solely to redistribute a society's resources would, if analyzed, be found to be all costs (those involved in the transfer) and no benefits (since total wealth remains unchanged)." Risks from risky technologies are not borne equally by the different social classes; risk assessments ignore the social class distribution of risk.

Cost-benefit analysis also relies heavily upon current market prices for evaluating costs and benefits. Yet these reflect current economic arrangements that many might question and wish to change. For example, people with low earning power can receive lower prices on their lives. The current market price for temporary nuclear workers is quite low, given a long recession; when calculated, the costs of replacing steam generator tubes reflects this. This can mean that the cost of an accident is low only because the economic system places a low value on some people. Property values near a chemical plant are likely to be low because of odors, fumes, and fire and explosion risks. When an accident takes place, the damage to the environment is calculated in terms of values already depressed because of the accident potential, rather than what the land would be worth if an electronics plant were there, or a nice park.

Another consequence of the prevailing assumptions is the argument that new risks should not be any higher than existing ones we have "already accepted" (Have we really had much choice?), and the corollary that if other industries get much riskier, the safety levels of nuclear plants or chemical plants can be lowered. . . .

Another argument that we hear much of these days is that we must push ahead with risky endeavors or other companies or nations will beat us in the competitive race to the marketplace. This line of reasoning notes that our country was founded in risk and grew powerful by taking risks, and the social benefits have been enormous. We

378

should, for example, push ahead with genetic engineering or the Japanese will beat us. . . .

There are those who argue that we are losing our moral fiber because we no longer want to take risks with technologies. But it is striking that those who feel we have abandoned risk in our search for security are speaking only of technological risks associated with large corporations and private profits, or aggressive military postures. The corporate and military risk-takers often turn out to be surprisingly risk-averse (to use the jargon of the field) when it comes to risky social experiments which might reduce poverty, dependency, and crime. . . .

The risks that made our country great were not industrial risks such as unsafe coal mines or chemical pollution, but social and political risks associated with democratic institutions, decentralized political structures, religious freedom and plurality, and universal suffrage.

Nor do the risk-assessment and risk-benefit studies distinguish between addiction and free choice in activities. . . . Along with high-way fatalities, lung cancer from smoking is the favorite referent of the new body-counters. It is treated as a voluntary activity, like hang-gliding. But most of us who smoke today do so because we were barraged with advertisements and inducements that soon addicted us. . . . This is not a matter of free marketplace decisions made by informed consumers, to be ridiculed and compared to these same people's "irrational" attacks on nuclear weapons, nuclear power, or Love Canals. Smoking is a government-supported program of addiction, for immense private profit. An individual's addiction to smoking should not be compared to the costs industry must be forced to incur to reduce brown lung disease or make safer Christmas toys.

We could say the same of alcoholism and other forms of drug abuse. These also are the referents of the risk assessors, cited to show that the public is incapable of making sensible choices between the cost of more airline safety and the cost of "substance abuse." Liquor advertising is substantial; the willingness of physicians to prescribe tranquilizers and other drugs is well known, and their abuse is said to far outdistance the use of illegal substances. There is little free market choice at work here.

Finally, the risk-assessing field only infrequently distinguishes between those activities over which the person has some control, however illusory it may be, and those where she or he does not. Driving is a key one. We appear to accept risks more readily when we think our skill will play some part in avoiding the hazard. We fear and reject risks where we are passive recipients of harm. The plant, we feel, not unreasonably, should not blow up, the dam break, the air controller goof, the Ford executives fail to protect a gas tank from exploding; over these risks we have little control. But we are willing to take our risks with driving, skiing, and parachuting. Risk assessors treat the difference as one of voluntary or involuntary risk, but I think that misses **379** a key point. Driving to work for many of us is about as involuntary an activity as there is, but at least we have some control over it. On the other hand, although we voluntarily fly in an airliner to a distant vacation, we have no control over the aircraft or the airways. We voluntarily attend large events at stadiums that sometimes burn or collapse, but we have no control over the architects or the construction firms, or the owners who always seem to lock the safety exits. Furthermore, "active risks," as we might call them, are generally not pursued for someone else's private profit; "passive risks" generally are.

For active risks, those that the individual performing the activity has some control over, the marketplace provides at least a rudimentary, though imperfect, way of addressing safety issues. Safer skis sell better; people stopped buying Corvairs and Pintos. Though there are exceptions, people make sensible choices when they have meaningful choices, and in time manufacturers respond. . . .

For such activities as nuclear waste disposal, brown lung disease, toxic contamination of Times Beach, Missouri, or the Midland area of Michigan, or the Teton dam, we cannot count on any "market" to automatically incur the costs of more safety. These activities are beyond our control. For these, the government must step in.

In more and more areas of our life the government must step in. This is not the result of the cancerous growth of government, but rather is essential because our personal control over our environment and our activites is being steadily eroded by systems that we participate in, or are passively affected by. In some cases Congress recognizes this danger. . . . Nevertheless, one frequent refrain in the risk assessment literature is lamenting over-regulation. . . .

The risk assessors, then, have a narrow focus that all too frequently (but not always) conveniently supports the activities elites in the public and private sectors think we should engage in. For most, the focus is upon dollars and bodies, ignoring cultural and social criteria. The assessors do not distinguish risks taken for private profits from those taken for private pleasures or needs, though the one is imposed, the other to some degree chosen; they ignore the question of addiction, and the distinction between active risks, where one has some control, and passive risks; they argue for the importance of risk but limit their endorsement of the approved risks to the corporate and military ones, ignoring risks in social and political matters. . . . Risk assessment is not as risky as the systems being assessed, but it has its unfortunate consequences for our society nevertheless.

One unfortunate implication of quantitative risk assessment is that the public should be excluded from discussions that affect them. Few of the risk assessors call for this outright, most imply it; some state that the public must be involved, but only on the risk assessor's terms, and a few reject the implication and genuinely think the public has something to contribute. . . . Most seem to take the middle position: bring the public in but control them. This is to be done by "closing the gap between the expert and the public" (that is, them and us); but the gap almost always is to be closed in one direction only — by bringing the public over to the experts' side through education. . . .

> *We drive our cars without using seatbelts, yet worry about saccharin. We light our cigarettes as we walk away from the polling place where we voted against a nuclear power plant. Are we stupid in balancing the real health risks we face? In this selection,* Science 85 *staff writer William Allman describes research that suggests we may not be as dumb about risk as we are sometimes made to feel.*

STAYING ALIVE IN THE 20TH CENTURY*

William F. Allman

. . . The . . . general public . . . smokes billions of cigarettes a year while banning an artificial sweetener because of a one-in-a-million chance that it might cause cancer; the same public that eats meals full of fat, flocks to cities prone to earthquakes, and goes hang gliding while it frets about pesticides in foods, avoids the ocean for fear of sharks, and breaks into a cold sweat on airline flights.

In short, we the general public are irrational, uninformed, superstitious, even stupid. We don't understand probability, are biased by the news media, and have a fear of some technolgies that borders on the primeval.

And we have no business, say many professional risk assessors, trying to force our unscientific worries into policy decisions about the hazards of modern living. Many hazards involve sophisticated technologies, statistics, and economic and political considerations. Assessing how such hazards threaten society is a task many believe is better left to experts. Why should the public have a say about the risk of a technology like nuclear power — which some experts believe poses a lesser threat than bicycles — when we don't have enough sense to put on a seat belt?

The experts have a point: When it comes to numbers, news, and neutrons, we're numskulls. But a few scientists are beginning to ask if

---

*"Staying Alive in the 20th Century", by William F. Allman. *Science 85,* 6:30–37, October 1985 © 1985 The American Association for the Advancement of Science. Used with permission.

technical savvy is the only qualification needed to be a legitimate worrier. They are finding that, while our behavior often appears irrational and confused, perhaps we're not so dumb after all. We may be lousy with mortality statistics, but our fears may tell us a lot about how a risk affects society as a whole.

One problem with the way we deal with risk is that our decisions can be influenced by the way a situation is presented. . . .

According to Amos Tversky and Daniel Kahneman, that makes all the difference. The two psychologists discovered one of the fundamentals of our flip-flops about risks: "When it comes to taking risks for gains, people are conservative. They will take a sure gain over a probable gain," says Stanford University's Tversky. "But we are also finding that when people are faced with a choice between a small, certain loss and a large, probable loss, they will gamble". . . .

Our inability to cope with probabilities, says Tversky, makes certainty appealing. In one study people who were asked to play a simple game of chance were given the opportunity to pay to increase their chances of winning. The researchers found that people were willing to pay more to increase their chances from 90 to 100 percent than they would pay for a 10-percent increase from 60 to 70 percent. This desire for absolutes goes beyond games. Former Food and Drug Administration commissioner Alexander Schmidt, looking forward to an upcoming scientific evaluation of cyclamates, said, "I'm looking for a clean bill of health, not a wishy-washy, iffy answer." When asked about the health effects of pollution, Edmund Muskie responded by asking for a "one-armed" scientist who does not say, "On the one hand, the evidence is so, but on the other hand. . . ."

Our desire for absolute certainty makes a high probability, such as 85 percent, seem insufficient. Likewise the desire for impossibility sometimes makes a five percent probability seem like a lot. The result is that low probabilities seem greater than they are and high probabilities seem less. This is perhaps the reason some of us feel comfortable buying a lottery ticket — even though there is an extremely low chance of winning — at the same time that we purchase a pack of cigarettes and dismiss the health risks as improbable.

If we can't be certain about the risks we face, we at least want to have some control over the technologies and activities that produce them. It has long been known, much to the frustration of some risk experts, that we may be much more willing to accept higher risks in activities over which we have control, such as smoking, drinking, driving, or skiing, than things over which we have little control, such as industrial pollution, food additives, and commercial airlines. . . .

A feeling of control can actually make a risky technology even more dangerous. That's because we often have inflated opinions of ourselves. Most of us consider ourselves above-average drivers, safer than most when using appliances and power tools, and less likely to suffer medical problems such as heart attacks. "Such overconfidence is

382

dangerous," says [psychologist Paul] Slovic. "It indicates that we often do not realize how little we know and how much additional information we need about the risks we face."

Unfortunately, when we want additional information, we often turn to the news media, and the media are more chroniclers of the extraordinary than a bank of information. . . .

This media emphasis on the sensational may be responsible for some of our skewed worries about the world. Slovic and his colleagues asked people to estimate the frequency of various causes of death such as tornadoes, heart disease, and homicides. Most people overestimated the number of deaths from causes that were sensational and underestimated more common causes of death that were less dramatic. Homicides, for example, were incorrectly estimated to take more lives annually than diabetes, stomach cancer, and strokes. Strokes actually take 10 times as many lives as homicides. . . .

Because things that recently occurred or are easy to imagine tend to stick in our minds, we can be difficult to educate about risks. A nuclear engineer, for example, talking of the many low-probability events that must happen in succession to cause a nuclear waste site to leak, may actually alarm someone into thinking, "I didn't realize there were so many things that could go wrong."

Which is not to say that we don't want to know more about the risks we face, especially if they concern medicine. Surveys show that most of us want as much information as possible when making a decision to have surgery or to take a certain drug. But according to one study, confusion can arise when doctors try to inform us about medical risks. Physician Barbara McNeil at Harvard University and her colleagues asked a group of radiologists, graduate students, and patients to imagine that they had lung cancer and to choose between surgery or radiation treatment. The researchers presented actual statistics, telling one group that 10 out of 100 people die during surgery, and 66 out of 100 die within five years. With radiation no one dies during treatment, but 78 out of 100 die within five years. Fifty-six percent of the group chose surgery. The group was then told there was a new study of the risks. The number of deaths during surgery remained the same, but the study showed the life expectancy of surgery survivors is 6.8 years, while the life expectancy of those treated with radiation is 4.7 years. While in fact, the statistics are based on the same death and survival data as in the first example, the number of people choosing surgery rose to 75 percent.

"There are no neutral ways to present information," says psychologist [Baruch] Fischoff. Perhaps the best way to inform people about risks, he says, is to give them the information in several different ways. . . .

Many risk assessors . . . have honed their models of technical failure, designed sensitive tests for screening new drugs and chemicals, and held countless symposia on how to save the lives of people who, **383** by and large, pay their salaries. But we — the American public — often seem intent on making a mess of their work. We ignore their advice, killing ourselves by the thousands because we find seat belts uncomfortable. We disregard their scientific findings, preferring to risk cancer rather than give up cigarettes. . . .

When we think about risk, says Slovic, we are not only concerned that a technology has the potential to cause deaths. We also worry about more subtle aspects: How well do we understand the risk? How will it affect society? Could it wipe out an entire community? Make a particular area uninhabitable for a long time? Would it affect future generations or some members of society more than others?

Slovic and his colleagues found that when people were asked to apply these societal concerns to the risks of some 90 different activities and technologies, each took on a profile that was broader than a simple death statistic. Some items, like dynamite, were considered deadly, but also fairly controllable. Others, like microwave ovens, were thought to involve risks that were delayed in their effects and not well known, but were also voluntary and unlikely to cause catastrophes. The respondents overwhelmingly regarded the risks of nuclear power as involuntary, uncontrollable, unknown, inequitably distributed, likely to be fatal, potentially catastrophic, and evoking feelings of not just fear but dread. Automobiles, which kill far more people per year, evoked few of these concerns.

According to Slovic, we are also concerned about the inherent riskiness of assessing risks. Part of our worry about technologies such as nuclear power, toxic wastes, and genetic engineering, for example, stem from the knowledge that the assessments of these risks are not based as much on the experience of a proven track record as on scientific analysis which, like some scientific analyses, might be in error.

That's because scientists, while good at solving problems, are not always as good at determining the limits of their expertise. . . .

In a study, seven highly respected engineers were asked to predict at what height a particular embankment with a clay foundation would collapse and were told to include a margin of error large enough to have a 50-percent chance of containing the correct answer. None of the estimates, including the margins for error, contained the correct height.

Since many new technologies are understood by few people in the first place, says Fischhoff, the experts are left to assess the quality of their own judgments, which can lead to problems. "Many risk problems force experts to go beyond the limits of the available data," he says. "In doing so, they fall back on intuitive processes much like those of lay people and are capable of making the same types of mistakes."

The fact that the public is keenly aware that scientists can be wrong is at the root of the concern about the nuclear accident at Three Mile island. Before the accident, scientists had said confidently that the chances of a serious reactor breakdown were quite remote.

384

But when a potential disaster occurred relatively early in the history of nuclear power, even though the safety systems worked and the disaster never materialized, the mishap sent out a signal that the overall assessment of the risks of nuclear power might be in error. . . .

. . . Says Slovic, "With the accident at Three Mile island, the health and safety consequences were insignificant; no one was killed, and there is probably no latent cancer. But the costs to society were enormous. Because the accident was a signal of potential problems, the ripple effect shut down reactors all over the world at a cost of billions of dollars. That's an expensive signal."

The big question, says Slovic, is whether our worries and fears, which are sometimes the result of faulty logic and misinformation — but also stem from a broader concern for how risks affect society as a whole — should be considered when making decisions about risk. "The dilemma is that if you give extra weight to nonstatistical factors such as catastrophic potential, inequity, and dread, and therefore choose an alternative — coal-fired power plants, for example, over nuclear-powered plants — you may actually be harming more people," he says. "The crux of the problem is finding the proper way to look at risk. One person might believe that rational decisions should be based solely on death, injuries, and damage. Another might say there are other important, hard-to-quantify feelings and values that we need to consider when making a risk decision."

And because these feelings include concerns for society at large, we can add a different perspective to risk debates. The scientists are better at seeing the trees, perhaps, but maybe we're better at seeing the forest. "We come down real hard on the public because they seem uninformed and irrational," says Slovic. "But their behavior may tell us something important about the essential elements of a humane society. In a sense there is real wisdom in people's reactions."

This wisdom depends less on understanding the details of scientific risk assessment than understanding the limits of what that science can do. "People are often more scientific in watching the processes of science than scientists themselves," says Fischhoff. "If the public looks at us with a skeptical eye, maybe they know something we don't."

*If consumers worry about different things than the experts,
and if consumers are sometimes right because they have taken
concerns other than death into account, what things about
food worry consumers? A recent survey by Louis Harris
Associates for the Food Marketing Institute, a trade association,
confirms Foster's statement that people don't worry about the
things experts think they ought to. As you read the responses
of the consumers, ask yourself how the articles on consumer
perception of risk you have just read apply to the things consumers do worry about with regard to their food.*

PESTICIDES AND FOOD: PUBLIC WORRY NO. 1*

Chris Lecos

For years, various surveys have documented the continued confidence
of most American consumers in the safety of the foods they buy and
eat. But what happens to the public's trust in food safety after a series
of widely publicized incidents such as product tamperings, recalls of
foods, controversy over chemical residues in foods, and publicity about
a relationship between the foods we eat and cancer?

The Food Marketing Institute (FMI), an organization of food retailers and wholesalers, including most big supermarket chains and many
independent supermarkets and regional firms, sought the answers in a
telephone survey of 1,008 shoppers last January. The Washington, D.C.,
organization's report, "Public Attitudes Toward Food Safety," was
issued in late March. . . .

The 1,008 participants — 60 percent of them women — were interviewed on behalf of FMI by Louis Harris & Associates Inc., New York,
between Jan. 17 and Jan. 30. EDB already was on the front pages,
although media coverage was more extensive afterward, FMI's report
noted. EDB specifically was not mentioned in FMI's survey. The survey
concluded that there is a persistent public concern over chemical residues in foods but that there has been no general decline in overall
"confidence" in the food supply. . . .

Of those surveyed, 77 percent said that chemical residues such as
pesticides and herbicides are a serious hazard, and 18 percent described them as something of a hazard. The second highest level of
concern was over cholesterol content of food; 45 percent cited it as a
serious hazard and 48 percent as something of a hazard. Salt in food

*"Pesticides and Food: Public Worry No. 1", by Chris Lecos. *FDA Consumer*, 18:12–13,
15, July/August 1984. U.S. Food and Drug Administration.

was viewed as a serious hazard by 37 percent, additives and preservatives by 32 percent, sugar 31 percent, and artificial coloring agents by 26 percent. Only 2 percent did not view chemical residues as a hazard.

"The response toward residues is significant," the FMI report said, "because it outstrips the others by such a wide margin". . . .

The report noted that FMI's continuing research "has shown a tendency for the public to be somewhat skeptical of new scientific findings about health hazards. The reaction to the proposed saccharin ban is a case in point. The public has become used to conflicting scientific opinion on health issues and position reversals on topics ranging from dietary recommendations to the depletion of the ozone layer. . . .

"However, the findings on residues in this study indicate that the public is not taking a wait-and-see attitude. Residues seem to be a pervasive concern. This leads us to believe that residues should not be thought of in the same category as previous food controversies of scientific debate with little public constituency."

Consumer Food Concerns

Q": How concerned are you about the following items being in food? Would you say that (Read Each Item) (is/are) a serious health hazard, somewhat of a hazard, or not a hazard at all?

	Serious Hazard (%)	Somewhat Of a Hazard (%)	Not a Hazard at All (%)	Not Sure (%)
Residues, such as pesticides and herbicides	77	18	12	3
Cholesterol	45	48	5	2
Salt in food	37	53	9	1
Additives and preservatives	32	55	8	4
Sugar in food	31	53	15	1
Artificial coloring	26	53	17	5

(Some figures are rounded out so not all lines will add up to exactly 100%.)

Source: Food Marketing Institute survey, "Public Attitudes Toward Food Safety," by Timothy Hammonds, senior vice president, Washington, D. C.

Another part of the FMI survey covered concerns about the nutritional content of food. Of those responding, 95 percent said they were either "very concerned" or "somewhat concerned," up 3 percent from the previous year. When asked what concerned them most about what **387** they ate, one-fourth named chemical additives, and 22 percent mentioned sugar content of food. Vitamin/mineral content of food, second in 1983, slipped to third and was mentioned by 19 percent of those interviewed. Although cholesterol was considered the second most serious concern of the six subject areas, only 8 percent mentioned it in terms of nutritional content of food.

Although pollsters and food professionals distinguish between nutritional content and food safety, the public doesn't. Many consumers mix food safety and nutrition issues, the report noted. . . .

The FMI report said the various concerns do not detract from the general finding that public trust in the overall safety of food remains high: "Although we know that consumers tend to lump nutrition and food safety issues together in their minds, the best news is that there has been no general decline in overall confidence in the food supply. . . .

Nutritional Worries

Q: What is it about the nutritional content of what you eat that concerns you and your family the most? What else?

	1983 (%)	1984 (%)	Percent Change
Chemical additives (e.g., flavoring, MSG, steroids)	27	25	−2
Sugar content, less sugar	21	22	+1
Vitamin/mineral content	24	19	−5
Food/nutritional value	10	19	+9
No preservatives	22	17	−5
Salt content, less salt	18	17	−1
Freshness, purity, no spoilage	14	12	−2
Making sure we get a balanced diet	10	9	−1
Calories, low calories	6	9	+3
Fat content, low in fat	9	8	−1
Cholesterol levels	5	8	+3
As natural as possible, not overly processed	12	6	−6
No harmful ingredients, nothing that causes illness/cancer	10	6	−4
Protein value	5	6	+1
Quality of food	3	5	+2
Excess food coloring/dyes	6	4	−2
Empty calories, junk food	4	4	0
Carbohydrate content	1	2	+1
Fiber content	2	1	−1
Starch content	1	1	0
Other	2	4	+2
Don't know/refused	5	5	0

388   Source: Food Marketing Institute survey.

> *OK,OK, you might now be saying. . . . But I can't worry about everything. What should I actually do? We close our chapter on the food safety controversy with three pieces meant to help you worry rationally and act effectively.*
>
> *The first selection contains a figure you have seen before in this book's Introduction. It lists 39 "health and safety factors" ranked by over 100 health professionals in terms of their ability to actually harm our health. If you have forgotten seeing it the first time, you may be surprised by the results. You will in any case learn more about those results and how they were arrived at by reading some excerpts from the text of the study.*

PREVENTION IN AMERICA: THE EXPERTS RATE 65 STEPS TO BETTER HEALTH*

A survey by Louis Harris and Associates

Introduction

This survey of health experts across the United States was commissioned by *Prevention Magazine*, published by Rodale Press, as part of its larger project to establish the Prevention Index. The Prevention Index will measure on an annual basis what America is doing to prevent disease and accidents and to promote good health and longevity. . . .

Louis Harris and Associates interviewed 103 health experts between October 6 and October 18, 1983. We asked them to rate the importance of each of 65 health and safety factors affecting adults and children. The average importance rating for each factor becomes the weight to be used in The Prevention Index in conjunction with key data on the actual behavior of the public.

The ratings given to the 65 health and safety factors are also of interest in their own right. They indicate which health behaviors the experts consider most important and which they consider less important. . . .

The sample included Medical School Chairmen of Preventive Medicine, Public Health School Deans, Chairmen of Health Education, government officials, journal editors, spokesmen for medical organizations

---

*"Introduction" (and) "The Findings". "Prevention in America: The Experts Rate 65 Steps to Better Health," conducted by Louis Harris and Associates, Inc. (Study #830411) *Prevention Magazine* © 1983. Edited portions used with permission.

and other experts. We do not necessarily assume that the experts are always correct — only that their collective view is likely to provide an indication of current professional understanding and practice. . . .

Experts' Weighting of Health and Safety Factors for Adults

Thirty-eight of the 39 health and safety factors for adults are rated by the experts in the top half of the 1-to-10 importance scale. Thus, in absolute terms, the experts consider almost all of the 39 factors to be of importance. Figure 1 shows the 39 rankings.

The top ranked factor is non-smoking; it receives a mean importance rating of 9.78 from the 103 health experts. Four other factors also receive mean ratings above the level of 9.0; they are: avoiding drug dependency (9.41), never smoking in bed (9.24), using seatbelts all the time (9.16), and never driving after drinking (9.03).

Six of the top 9 factors relate to safety and accident prevention. . . .

Thus, there is a tendency for the experts to rank most highly those factors that have immediate or direct or clear life-saving consequences. Other critical factors whose consequences for life and health are longer-term or less direct in nature tend to be ranked somewhat lower. Examples are: regular exercise (8.20), moderation in alcohol use (8.15), not eating too much fat (7.82), keeping close to the recommended weight (7.71), and taking steps to control stress (7.58). These factors — requiring regular repetition over long periods of time to produce their consequences — rank toward the middle relative to other factors (although still high in absolute terms.)

One nutrition factor (not eating too much fat) ranks higher (7.82) than genetic inheritance. Somewhat lower in the distribution of the 39 adult behaviors are most of the other nutrition factors: getting enough fiber (7.41), calcium (7.28), vitamins and minerals in general (7.12), and not getting too much cholesterol (7.15), sodium (7.04), and sugar (6.90). What these factors may have in common in the experts' minds is that they make their impact on health through an even longer-term and even less-direct process, requiring day-in-day-out and year-in-year-out repetition. Almost all the nutrition factors are still ranked over 7.00 on the 1-to-10 scale, indicating that in absolute terms they are all considered important.

These are the most striking general patterns in Figure 1. In addition, there are several more particular patterns that are of interest. One is the relatively high ranking given to the three social or psychological factors. Feeling happy with one's life (8.53) is seen by the experts as the seventh most important factor in its effect on health. Having friends, relatives, and neighbors to socialize with (8.31) is also ranked in the top dozen factors. Feeling happy with one's job (8.06) is in the top half. None of these factors would usually be considered as immediate or direct in its effect on health, and yet the experts see them as relatively important. . . .

Figure 1. Experts' Weighing of Thirty-nine Health and Safety Factors
for Adults

Thinking about the overall health of the general population, how important
is it for adults to . . .

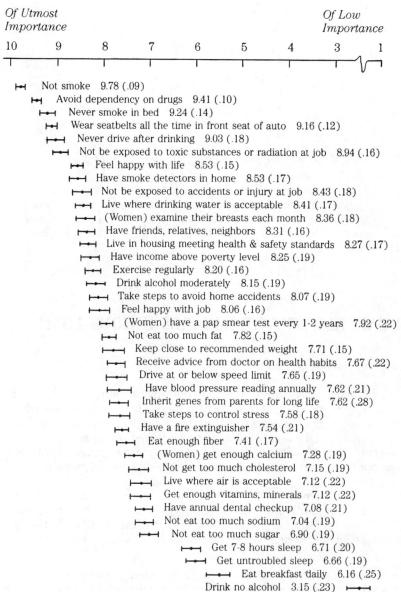

Of Utmost Importance							*Of Low Importance*	
10	9	8	7	6	5	4	3	1

Not smoke 9.78 (.09)
Avoid dependency on drugs 9.41 (.10)
Never smoke in bed 9.24 (.14)
Wear seatbelts all the time in front seat of auto 9.16 (.12)
Never drive after drinking 9.03 (.18)
Not be exposed to toxic substances or radiation at job 8.94 (.16)
Feel happy with life 8.53 (.15)
Have smoke detectors in home 8.53 (.17)
Not be exposed to accidents or injury at job 8.43 (.18)
Live where drinking water is acceptable 8.41 (.17)
(Women) examine their breasts each month 8.36 (.18)
Have friends, relatives, neighbors 8.31 (.16)
Live in housing meeting health & safety standards 8.27 (.17)
Have income above poverty level 8.25 (.19)
Exercise regularly 8.20 (.16)
Drink alcohol moderately 8.15 (.19)
Take steps to avoid home accidents 8.07 (.19)
Feel happy with job 8.06 (.16)
(Women) have a pap smear test every 1-2 years 7.92 (.22)
Not eat too much fat 7.82 (.15)
Keep close to recommended weight 7.71 (.15)
Receive advice from doctor on health habits 7.67 (.22)
Drive at or below speed limit 7.65 (.19)
Have blood pressure reading annually 7.62 (.21)
Inherit genes from parents for long life 7.62 (.28)
Take steps to control stress 7.58 (.18)
Have a fire extinguisher 7.54 (.21)
Eat enough fiber 7.41 (.17)
(Women) get enough calcium 7.28 (.19)
Not get too much cholesterol 7.15 (.19)
Live where air is acceptable 7.12 (.22)
Get enough vitamins, minerals 7.12 (.22)
Have annual dental checkup 7.08 (.21)
Not eat too much sodium 7.04 (.19)
Not eat too much sugar 6.90 (.19)
Get 7-8 hours sleep 6.71 (.20)
Get untroubled sleep 6.66 (.19)
Eat breakfast daily 6.16 (.25)
Drink no alcohol 3.15 (.23)

The weight for each factor is the mean importance rating given by 103
experts using a 1-to-10 scale. Given in parentheses is the standard error of
the mean. An indicator of the variability of individual ratings around each
mean is graphically displayed as a band or range consisting of ± two standard
error values

391

Another interesting pattern is for some commonly accepted rules to be less highly rated by the experts. Getting seven to eight hours of sleep most nights (6.71), getting untroubled sleep (6.66), and eating breakfast almost every day (6.16) — while not unimportant in absolute terms — are placed near the bottom of the experts' list of priorities. . . .

> *Our second expert, consumer advocate Michael Jacobson, offers his ranking of health risks, attempting to counter our feelings of helplessness with specific advice about concentrating our constructive energies on the risks that are actually most important. As an old friend used to say, in the face of too many things to worry about, we need to practice selective apathy.*

DEALING WITH THE HAZARDS IN YOUR LIFE*

Michael Jacobson, Ph.D.

Scientists are discovering hazards in our environment far more rapidly than people are learning to cope with them. Most of us wonder what we can do or if we should just throw up our hands in despair and go down smiling. Like a general devising measured responses to various levels of battlefield aggression, so technology-age citizens need to understand how to react to health risks of very different magnitudes. . . .

. . . The warnings have come fast and furious: nitrosamine in beer causes cancer, formaldehyde in toothpaste and many other products cause cancer, salt causes high blood pressure, saccharin in diet soda causes cancer, caffeine causes birth defects, Tris flame retardant

---

*"Dealing with the Hazards in Your Life", by Michael Jacobson. *Nutrition Action*, 7:3 – 6, March 1980. Copyright, Center for Science in the Public Interest. Edited portions used with permission.

causes cancer, food additives cause hyperactivity, hair dyes cause cancer, fat causes cancer, new cars contain cancer-causing nitrosamines. DDT, PCB, PBB, DBCP . . . the list of dangerous chemicals and their attendant horrors gets longer and longer. Are deranged scientists determined to find something wrong with *everything* in our environment . . . and turn us all into cancerphobiacs?

. . . I admit to sometimes sharing the public's feeling of dismay and helplessness. When out of the clear blue sky, someone warns that hamburgers or new cars pose a cancer risk, I, too, notice my mind hitting the "off" switch. . . .

While the grey cloud of bad news refuses to drift away, we should not overlook the real silver lining in that cloud. Because citizens and government have become sensitized to the hazards in our environment, industry can no longer market or dump into the river whatever it wants without being required to do some rudimentary safety studies and take some elementary precautions. For the first time in the industrial age scientists in government, universities, citizen's groups and even industry are systematically searching for hazards in our environment. The glare of publicity is forcing industries to change their products and practices instead of shoving their problems under the rug or into the fathomless depths of obscure journals.

The sometimes loud and combative public debate about health hazards is slowly producing a safer environment. Indeed, the debate has had the effect of making it part of conventional wisdom, especially and most deeply among the young, that we should have a clean, healthy planet. What a change from the 1950s when hardly anyone thought about such matters!

We should also gain some satisfaction from the fact that, despite frequent grim headlines in the paper, *most* chemicals are safe. Most chemicals do not cause cancer, birth defects, mutations, or other irreversible harm. Several years ago the National Cancer Institute tested 120 pesticides and other toxic chemicals. Surely, if any chemicals caused cancer, it would be these. Animals were fed high dosages of the chemicals, but only 11 caused cancer. The sky is not yet falling.

But to return to the main point, what is a citizen to do about the flood of information concerning dangerous products and chemicals? Should one with equal dedication stop smoking, stop drinking beer, stop riding in new automobiles, and stop drinking tap water? Must one, to survive in this day and age, subscribe to a hundred scientific journals? Or should one just ignore all the warnings?

It is absurd to think that people could, would or should organize their lives in accordance with each and every health warning, some of which are even contradictory. Clearly, some things are more important than others. And some environmental dangers — like sitting in the sun or smoking — are pretty much under an individual's control, while others — like pollutants in air and water — are less so.

393

Some health problems can be solved by each of us as individuals, while others need to be addressed politically. If we learn only one thing from the kepones, Love Canals, red dyes, tars and nicotines, and foul air that have sickened and killed millions of us, it should be that informed citizens, organized into effective groups, are an absolutely essential prerequisite to the solution of our nation's problems. This applies not only to health, but to all other issues, from saving the family farm to promoting equality of opportunity. You cannot avoid every little carcinogen in the environment, but you can support groups that are promoting public policies aimed at producing a safer, healthier environment.

Congress has established regulatory agencies like the Food and Drug Administration and the Environmental Protection Agency to control those risks that are beyond the general knowledge and control of the average person. . . .

Of course, oftentimes the distance between theory and practice is proportional to the size of the economic interests affected, and regulatory agencies have not always lived up to the public's expectations.

Despite their criticisms of regulatory agencies, advocates for improved health and a safer environment see them as allies and are frequently their only supporters when Congress plays political football with agency budgets. After all, if regulatory agencies were even weaker than they are today — as many powerful business interests desire — who could do anything about the multitude of agents that are jeopardizing our health and environment? . . .

The other side of the coin is personal action. Obviously, you should worry *most* about the things that pose not a one-in-a-million chance of harming you, but a one-in-two, -ten, or -hundred chance of harming you. We can not rate with precision all the risks we encounter, and there will be substantial variations from individual to individual due to genetic factors. But we can surely identify some of the major priorities. My list of things that individuals should be *most* concerned about is:

- Cigarette smoking. All the organic food in the world will not protect a smoker from heart disease and cancer. The cigarette is the biggest killer around.
- High fat and cholesterol diet. Heart disease is the natural outcome of a diet rich in fatty meat, hard cheeses, eggs, butter and saturated vegetable oils (coconut and palm oils). Bowel and breast cancers appear to be promoted by diets high in fat, regardless of the source.
- Polluted workplaces. Occupational health problems and accidents kill about 100,000 people a year. If your employer won't clean up the workplace, contact your union and the occupational Safety and Health Administration. Demand or obtain a safer job if the problem persists.
- Alcohol abuse. Excessive drinking destroys families as well as indi-

394

vidual lives. Auto accidents, liver disease, and oral cancers are
caused by the bottle.
- Salt. High salt diets promote high blood pressure and stroke. You
  can eat significantly less salt (or, to be more precise, sodium) by
  switching from processed to natural foods and by using less salt in
  cooking and at the table.
- Sedentary lifestyle. Sitting at a desk or in front of a TV set all day
  promotes obesity, which in turn may cause diabetes, stroke, or heart
  disease. Exercise also provides a great release for mental and
  physical strain — and it's fun.

Sugar and food additives are generally less important than the above
causes of health problems, though they have received an enormous —
perhaps disproportionate — amount of publicity. . . .

All the other harmful chemicals that we can do something about in
our food and environment certainly cause some premature injury and
deaths, but any single agent is probably not a major killer. The risks
posed by most of these agents to an *individual* are miniscule — and
should not dictate the way we spend our lives. But even a miniscule
risk, multiplied over our population of 225 million, is often large
enough to justify a *social,* if not individual, response: regulatory or legislative action. In other words, when industry spokespersons say that a
risk is too small for you as an individual to worry about, they may be
right. Nevertheless, the risk may *not* be too small to trigger a response
by society. Hundreds of small risks lurking in all facets of our lives
may quickly add up to a sizable cumulative risk to the population.
Here is my rough (I emphasize *rough*) guideline on ranking the risks:

1. Serious risks (e.g. 1 in 5,000 chance or greater of harming you):
   make changes in your own buying or living habits; personal behavioral changes should be supported by educational campaigns,
   product recalls, prohibitions when appropriate, and other health-
   and safety-promoting regulations.
2. Smaller risks (e.g. between 1 in 5,000 and 1 in 5 million chance of
   harming you): support regulatory or legislative actions to reduce or
   eliminate the risks; personal changes optional.
3. Trivial risks not only to you, but to the population as a whole (e.g.
   less than 1 in 5 million chance of harming anyone): don't worry
   about them.

Yet, is it pointless to avoid very "small" and "trivial" risks? No, of
course not. If even one percent of the public shunned a product because of a questionable ingredient or impurity, manufactuers would be
quicker to make changes. And there might be health gains for the individuals, but in most cases the health gains would be tiny — or even
non-existent, if the substitute product or activity poses a greater risk
than the one being avoided.

395

So, get rid of that look of despair on your face. Identify the biggest risks to your health and change the way you live in these several regards. In an equally determined fashion, urge legislators and regulatory officials to take swift, strong action against the smaller risks and those that are impossible for individuals to control themselves. . . .

> *Our final expert's co-author insisted she be given the final word on this topic. Should we worry about the food supply or shouldn't we? Are we sicker or healthier? Nutrition educator Joan Gussow, speaking to the Massachusetts Public Health Association, suggests that one way to solve this dilemma is to look beyond ourselves and devote some of our energies to making our food and our overall environment safer for all life — now and in the future.*

OVERVIEW; POLLUTION AND THE FOOD CHAIN*

Joan Dye Gussow

. . . It is very hard to make a case for our health having gotten generally worse as we have increased our exposure to man-made chemicals. . . . Our overall health statistics show us that life expectancy is constantly increasing (although we do not rank internationally where we ought to). . . . Morover, heart disease mortality has been steadily declining over a decade or so, and . . . as far as we can presently tell, there is *not* an epidemic of cancer.

So the apparently good news that I want to begin with is that we do not presently have clear evidence that the industrialization of food, or of other parts of our lives, is harming our health — *no matter how profoundly we believe that it is*. This is not to say that there are no toxic chemicals and that they are not causing harm to the people who work with them. It is to acknowledge, however, that there are no epidemiologic or other studies which demonstrate that we are in poorer health than our less industrialized forebears, despite our acknowledged chemicalization of the food environment. . . . My students don't like to hear that because it makes it harder for them to be self-righteous about the food supply — but it's true.

---

*"Overview: Pollution and the Food Chain" by Joan Dye Gussow. Speech to the Massachusetts Public Health Association. Inc., May 23, 1984. Used with permission.

But as the National Academy of Sciences Diet, Nutrition, and Cancer report acknowledges, "This is not to say that industrial exposure is harmless but simply that relatively few of the middle aged and older members of our current population have been exposed to great occupational hazards. . . . In addition, we have to remember that the time course of carcinogenesis commonly extends over 20 years or more. This means that we have to be very concerned about the possible long-term effects resulting from exposure to novel hazards."

One of the significant dilemmas we face today, in many fields, is that much of what we need to know is scientifically unmanageable — yet we have been conditioned to look to science for answers to our questions. Can we control nuclear weapons without accidentally setting off a war? Will continued cutting down of forests in the poor countries and the continued heavy use of fossil fuel in the industrialized ones (both of which raise CO_2 levels in the air) result in global warming and hence the flooding of the coastlines — or might it result in a new ice age? And will either happen soon enough to worry about? (And when is soon enough?) What will be the effects on us and on the biosphere of continuing to add to the 53,000 novel chemicals we have already put into the environment?

None of these questions is answerable with the degree of certainty that scientists demand. Hence scientists are very uncomfortable dealing with them, or in dealing with other than very little parts of them. . . . And many scientists tend to deal contemptuously with anyone who tries to look at the larger picture and act on it, as an astrologer or futurologist — or philosopher. . . .

I know it would be easier to fight the polluters of our food chain if we *knew* what they were doing was killing us. And I am personally terrified about what our careless dumping into the environment is doing to the whole biological world that supports us.

We may not be able to prove that people get cancer from eating contaminated fish, but the fish are getting cancer, at staggering rates, and that has a lot of scientists scared. And we may not be able to prove that pesticide residues are really harming us, but we already know that heavy use of pesticides has caused a marked increase in the number of insects that are pests, as well as an uncontrollable resurgence of malaria in poor countries (due to the emergence of pesticide-immune mosquitoes). We cannot wish for, and in a broader sense *we do not need,* an upturn in that cancer rate to prove the need to change what we are doing to the food-producing environment. . . .

In early 1984 a National Academy of Sciences panel brought out a report on toxic chemicals, which concluded that "for vast numbers of chemicals used in commercial products and processes, food, cosmetics, pesticides and drugs, there are little or no toxicity data available and even less information . . . on the extent of human exposure to them." In short, we don't know whether what's out there is hazardous if we were exposed to it, and we don't even know if we are exposed to it in significant amounts. Said the toxicologist who led the study, "This report does not prove there is a health hazard . . . but I find the results scary. There's a potential for some real major health problems out there, something totally unexpected . . . The lack of data is very worrisome."

So you have to worry. But how? . . .

Until now nutrition educators have assumed that the role of nutrition education . . . was to produce healthy individuals who ate well enough to become well-functioning members of society — students, parents, workers. The extreme of this sort of individual emphasis is, I believe, what we have now — a culture in which some of the brightest people are obsessed with caring for their own bodies while the world around them falls apart for lack of mutual caring. What we have is a fanatic concern for individual health, healthy individualism, people who jog and grow vegetables and lift weights and worry about their own longevity while exhibiting little concern over the longevity and well being of the earth from which their food derives and of which they are a part. . . .

I believe it is our individualism that ultimately depresses us, since all we can do as individuals worrying about our own health is to try frantically to keep up with the latest scientific alarms, or reassurances, and try to avoid (or counteract with mega-somethings) whatever threatens in the short or long term to harm our apparently increasingly beleaguered bodies. Everything I have said today is intended to make it clear that such an approach is *utterly pointless* whether or not pollutants are there and whether or not they are harmful. We cannot know what to avoid, since we do not know what we are being exposed to or whether it is capable of injuring us.

Of course there are some actions one can take, personally and politically. There is first the clearly sensible one of eating fewer animal products and less fat generally, because such diets will reduce our exposure to substances that concentrate as they move up the food chain, will cause us to eat more grains, fruits and vegetables (the benefits of which have been demonstrated), and will put less demand on the ecosystem. But mostly we need to worry about bigger issues, political issues. It is not enough to worry about keeping ourselves healthy unless we are keeping ourselves healthy with a purpose.

I believe that in a large sense we ought to be scared about the long-term safety of the food supply, since the fabric of the earth is threatened by everything from thermonuclear winter to soil erosion, but our response to these things ought not to be to obsess about each bite of food we ingest. Food is the product of a complex ecosystem, a life-support system dependent on the continued occurence of multitudes of natural events which are daily threatened by our activities. Real concern about the safety of our own food requires that we be concerned about the safety of everyone's food — as well as the health of the environment. We all need to turn some of the energy we devote to private health to public action.

Afterword

You've now been exposed to the major points of view about food safety. What's your verdict? Is our food supply safer or more dangerous than you thought it was before you read this chapter?

You should understand, to begin with, that we have not invited any of the shrillest voices to speak; there are partisans camped at both extremes. In one of these camps are those who maintain that our food supply is so safe that any public concern is pointless. In the other camp are those, often laypeople and their gurus, who contend that our food supply is leached of nutrients and laced with poisons as a result of the malefactions of profit-hungry agribusiness corporations.

In the middle, where most of the authors in this chapter would fall, are thoughtful participants in the food safety debate, who agree that we don't know enough about how much of which chemicals we are exposed to — or what they are doing to us. These groups differ mainly in their judgments of just how much we do know, how to interpret the facts we have, and what sorts of eating adjustments these facts demand of us.

Whether or not you believe our food supply to be essentially safe has a lot to do with which facts you attend to. A focus on gaps in our knowledge inevitably leads to concern. As you have seen, the Diet, Nutrition, and Cancer Committee of the National Academy of Sciences estimated that 2,700 chemicals are intentionally added to our foods, another 12,000 sneak in during growing and processing, and an unknown number contaminate it.

The National Academy of Sciences report on Toxicity Testing makes clear that for the vast majority of all these substances, we are able to make only very incomplete assessments of possible long-term health effects.

If other facts are chosen, a far rosier picture of our food supply emerges. With rare exceptions (e.g., sulfite sensitivity has caused death in several people who consumed foods containing sulfites), there is no evidence to indicate that our overall health has been compromised by the processed foods in our marketplace. Death rates from heart disease and stroke in the United States have declined significantly, while cancer rates remain steady (aside from those lung cancers attributable to smoking). In fact, as both Foster and Popescu observe, our food supply a century ago posed many more obvious dangers to health. "Additives" then included toxic lead salts and formaldehyde, and markets contained meat and milk from diseased animals.

One of the major sources of controversy in the food safety debate is how to interpret the animal testing that determines whether an additive will be permitted in foods. Time after time we're warned by headlines that, on the basis of animal tests, one

399

or another substance in food has been judged harmful. We share with Dr. Foster and Ms. Popescu a concern that this "carcinogen of the week" phenomenon encourages in the general public either skepticism on food safety issues or excessive worry about putting anything into our mouths.

Most scientists and regulators agree that current food chemical testing procedures, described here by Jacobson, represent a compromise between the ideal and the practical. Animals are used in food safety tests as surrogate humans, so the results almost always excite differences of opinion about the applicability of the findings to humans. How well can genetically pure strains of mice and rats, given doses of an additive much greater than humans could consume, stand-in for a human population of different sexes, ages, susceptibilities to diseases, dietary patterns, and states of health?

The assumption has generally been that, within certain limits, they can stand in well. That is, food additive test results in animals probably hold true for at least some people. But when the Food and Drug Administration proposes to ban an additive based on animal feeding studies, that underlying assumption is almost always challenged by one or another interested party.

Concern about food additives and contaminants has focused especially on fears that their long-term ingestion might increase our risk of cancer. Congress addressed this concern in 1958 when it added the Delaney Clause to our patchwork of food safety laws — specifying that no additive shown to cause cancer in humans or animals would be allowed into our food supply.

Now the increasing sophistication of our technology has complicated enforcement of the Delaney Clause. We are able to detect ever smaller traces of chemicals in foods, so that, as former FDA Commissioner Donald Kennedy observed, "we find ourselves in a position to detect more than we can evaluate, and to measure more than we can understand."

If a substance found in food at the parts per trillion level (one drop of water in 36 Olympic-size swimming pools) proves harmful to test animals when fed in very large amounts, does that substance pose a risk to humans? The Delaney Clause says the answer is "yes" if the risk posed is cancer. According to our present food safety laws there is no threshold level, below which a carcinogen no longer acts as a carcinogen.

However, as we write this in early 1986, the FDA has felt justified in reinterpreting the intent of the law. They are allowing a few food chemicals known to be carcinogens — methylene chloride used to decaffeinate some brands of coffee; the artificial food color Red No. 3; and a few livestock drugs that can leave residues in meat — to remain in foods on the grounds that their presence poses an insignificant (de minimus) cancer risk to humans. It remains to be seen whether such a regulatory interpretation will hold up to legal challenges and the weight of public opinion. (It is ironic to note here, as we mentioned in the Afterword to Chapter 4, that many animal drugs that could leave residues are not being regulated, and for most of them there is not even a detection procedure to find residues — at any level.)

Taking all this into account, however, it must be kept in mind that there is no evidence to date that our cancer rates have been affected by the increasing industrialization of our food supply. And although caution is certainly warranted, it is important not to allow a focus on cancer to distract us from other potential health problems. For example, a National Academy of Sciences panel, re-evaluating data on the banned artificial sweetener cyclamates, found testicular atrophy of male rats of more potential concern than carcinogenicity. Similarly, the debate over the safety of the currently popular artificial sweetener aspartame focuses appropriately not on cancer, but on the chemical's possible role in causing behavioral disturbances in sensitive individuals. Where overall food safety is concerned, cancer distracts.

In theory, many interpretational problems, at least where added chemicals are concerned, would be overcome if we could test additives on humans first, before adding them to foods. But such studies are obviously neither practical nor moral. Would you volunteer to eat foods containing a questionable additive to see whether your health would suffer as a result?

The first and last such studies were conducted at the turn of the century by Harvey Washington Wiley of the Department of Agriculture and his "Poison Squad," 12 healthy young men who consumed measured amounts of suspect additives with their meals. He got reform, but his methods have gone out of fashion. The problems of testing potentially harmful substances in humans are multiples of the problem of testing nutritional supplements that we outlined in the preceding chapter.

One of the most complicating aspects of the food chemical controversy is our increasing knowledge about substances that occur naturally in foods. It has become startlingly clear that almost every food contains some naturally-occurring chemicals that, when isolated, will flunk the tests we use for assessing food safety. Some scientists argue that these substances ("nature's pesticides," as Dr. Ames calls them) are more likely to be hazardous to our long-term health than any man-made substances that get into our foods, since they are consumed in much larger amounts. These scientists believe that the Delaney Clause maintains an unfair double standard, because natural substances are presumed to be safer than those produced industrially.

The work of biochemist Bruce Ames has played a major role in the public emergence of this argument. Should natural foods be **401** banned if one of their components is shown to pose some risk to our health in very high doses? Even leaving aside the fact that this could lead to banning most of the foods we eat, Ames says "no." He is quick to point out that even though natural foods are full of nasty chemicals, especially when cooked, they also contain substances, including nutrients, that seem to reduce the risk of cancer.

The 1982 report of the National Academy of Sciences' Diet, Nutrition, and Cancer panel noted, for example, that even though citrus fruits and cruciferous vegetables (cabbage, broccoli, etc.) contain several known mutagens, the consumption of those foods is associated with a *lowered* risk of cancer. Foods are complex mixtures of chemical substances, including carcinogens and anti-carcinogens, mutagens and antioxidants; the finding that an extract of a single food is a carcinogen may have no bearing on whether there is a health risk to humans from consuming that food whole in a mixed diet.

Advances in biotechnology will undoubtedly lead to another set of food safety concerns related to the natural components of foods. Genetic engineering and more sophisticated plant breeding techniques will allow technologists to alter food crops in a variety of ways — for example, to manipulate their nutrient content, to increase their yields, to make them more resistant to herbicides or more amenable to mechanical harvesting, or to improving their pest resistance by increasing their levels of "nature's pesticides."

Our knowledge of plant composition is very limited. All plant breeding reduces some chemicals and increases others — some of which are unknown, many of which are unmeasured — and biotechnology is likely to speed up this process substantially. The fear is that such manipulations might alter levels of these naturally occurring substances in ways that subtly threaten our health.

Although the possibility of such an outcome may seem remote, the development of the Lenape potato in 1969 was just such an event. This potato variety, destined for use as potato chips, was discovered to contain unusually large amounts of a naturally occurring poison that caused chills, vomiting and headaches. The strong association between consumption of these potatoes and the symptoms kept the Lenape potato from retail food markets, but the lesson is an important one. As Dr. Walter Mertz reminded us in Chapter 6 on Nutritional Supplements, food has important influences on our health "that cannot be totally explained on the basis of our present knowledge of nutrients."

Biotechnological modifications of food crops will obviously need to be conducted cautiously and with frequent monitoring of the results. We predict that consumer advocates will be at odds with regulatory agencies over how much caution and monitoring is prudent.

Despite all the problems that food chemical testing presents, no one involved would argue for the abandonment of current methodologies. But there is a growing consensus that when test results are equivocal, or seem at worst to indicate a minor risk, common sense must temper conclusions about the human hazard involved. And we ought at a minimum to be as concerned with the overall quality of our dietary patterns as we are with specific foods or their chemical components.

With so many questions unresolved, how does the public decide what to worry about? Are people as irrational in their rankings of food hazards as some of our selections suggest? Not really, although the evidence suggests that there are things in food—the saturated fats, cholesterol, sugar and salt content, for example—that have a greater impact on the public's health than the chemical residues that the public is most concerned about. However, the public does rank cholesterol and salt as major worries, and even the FDA, as Foster reminds us, ranked environmental contaminants as the third most important hazard consumers face from their food.

Looking at citizens' concerns about food tends to confirm the conclusions of some of the readings in this chapter that people are smarter in their evaluation of health risks than many experts give them credit for. Both experts and the public use cost-benefit analyses to reach conclusions, although the public makes such calculations much less consciously. But the calculations of both groups are often questionable because of what each side chooses to focus on.

When experts conduct risk (or cost-benefit) assessments, they measure both costs and benefits in dollars and in numbers of people likely to die or be injured. Popescu's ranking of various risks according to their ability to shorten life or cause death reflects this point of view. Sociologist Perrow finds such calculations flawed by their narrowness of focus. "Unquantified and unacknowledged" in such calculations, he asserts, are "social ties, family continuity, a distinctive culture, and valued human traditions." According to the Louis Harris survey excerpted in this chapter, even in ranking important health behaviors, experts "rank most highly those factors that have immediate or direct or clear life-saving consequences."

Ordinary people view the situation differently. They evaluate health risks according to whether those risks are voluntarily undertaken (like eating "junk food") or involuntarily imposed (like eating chemical residues), and whether the risks are well understood (like short-term toxicity) or poorly understood (like carcinogenesis).

People also seem to evaluate health risks in terms of their catastrophic potential, irrespective of odds. Therefore, even though most experts believe there is little risk of harm from consuming a variety of industrially produced food products, many people intuitively feel that consuming unprocessed foods grown with as few chemicals as possible is superior. Although such a belief has not been supported scientifically, a diet of wholesome foods, appropriately selected, can be both nutritious and health-promoting, and may contain fewer questionable chemicals.

No food supply can ever be made entirely risk-free. Although attention to what we eat and how it is produced is warranted, there is little reason to fear eating an occasional additive-laden or processed food.

We are, however, not comforted by the words of food technologist Bates, quoted at the beginning of this chapter, that only lack of knowledge keeps people from viewing the growing complexity of our food supply as a series of improvements. It is precisely because of our knowledge, limited as it is, that we are concerned. While many food products in our supermarkets are wholesome, we might be better off, as Gussow suggests in her piece on food security, if many others were simply unavailable, and if the economic imperative to continually market food novelties were somehow voluntarily controlled.

Since this is unlikely to happen, our food choices will continue to be made from among the more than 12,000 items available in supermarkets. Assuming that you, like us, desire to minimize potential risks to your health from natural as well as added substances in food, we leave you with the following pointers we use to aid our food purchasing decisions.

- Eating a wide variety of foods is the key not only to obtaining adequate amounts of nutrients, but also to minimizing risks from consuming any unwanted chemicals. There is much less reason to fear foods containing artificial sweeteners or food dyes, for example, if they are consumed only occasionally.
- Eating low on the food chain minimizes the consumption of potentially toxic agricultural chemicals whose levels usually increase as they are transferred from plants to animal products, and reduces intake of animal drug residues. This involves eating plenty of whole grains, legumes, fruits and vegetables, along with smaller amounts of animal products.
- Many manufactured foods depend for their very existence upon the multitude of additives that grant them their color, flavor and shelf life. These products are often high in fat, sugar or salt as well. Minimizing consumption of them not only improves the diet, but helps minimize intake of many questionably safe food chemicals.
- Convenience foods are not only often expensive for their food value (and not as time-saving as they promise), but they usually

contain unwanted additives. Spend your discretionary money instead on cookbooks that teach quick preparation of fresh foods in nutrient-conserving ways.

- Any health benefits to be attained from eating fewer questionable food chemicals can be offset by other health compromising behaviors. Do you buckle up when driving? Refrain from smoking? Have a working smoke detector where you live? According to many experts, health risks from the food supply are much less worrisome than those from other sources. Reasonable people may disagree with their rankings, but it seems sensible to work toward minimizing *all* the health risks one faces. Popescu and Jacobson sensibly urge us to concentrate our efforts on the risks that are most important to reduce.

- Personal food concerns have a greater likelihood of being addressed by government officials when people of similar interests band together and make themselves heard. Consumption of pesticide residues, for example, is more likely to be minimized by groups urging Congress to support research into sustainable agriculture than by individuals acting separately, each hoping that the organically labelled foods they purchase in health food stores are truly organically grown. Gussow suggests that we turn some of the energy we now devote to obsessing about food toward public action.

Our food supply today is at best a mixed blessing. Products of little nutritional value, containing food chemicals of questionable safety are often the foods most heavily promoted. Nevertheless, the sheer variety available allows us to eat as well or as poorly as we desire, in keeping with our personal level of concern. The American food supply is, appropriately, still the envy of most of the world.

So, what will you eat for your next meal? We hope this chapter has made your decision easier. Bon appetit!

Epilogue

A number of colleagues who were asked to look over this manuscript before we sent it to the publisher protested that we hadn't really lived up to our own subtitle, *Sorting Out Some Answers*. One of them even accused us of "near nutritional nihilism," which sounded intellectually impressive, but alarming. She meant, as she explained, that we kept ending our chapters with lines like "so there is no answer," or "decide for yourself." She feared that the ordinary looking-for-answers reader who encountered that sort of statement seven times might just throw up her hands and say "What's the use? Nutritionists can't agree on *anything*, so I might as well do whatever I feel like."

We do not want to be misunderstood: you can't *afford* to do whatever you feel like. But we're afraid our critic may be right in accusing us of having been too equivocal. It's true we didn't really tell you whether you should take nutritional supplements or avoid certain foods for your safety's sake. It's even occurred to us that by raising questions about things that you probably thought were non-controversial — like RDAs and food guides — we may have left you more confused than you were when you started.

Our emphasis on the fact that there are experts on all sides of every issue surely hasn't helped your state of mind either. Just whom *should* you believe? If you were to conclude, as did a recent headline in the *New York Times*, that "1 Expert Plus 1 Expert = 0," then you may think you're not much better off than you were when you began this book. (Worse off, maybe. Maybe beforehand you thought you *knew* the answers.)

We can't deny that we intended to shake up your convictions. The nutrition debates we've tackled *are* debates precisely because there are disagreements among experts about interpreting the known facts. If the nutrition community were, for example, of one mind about whether every food on the supermarket shelves was inarguably safe, then precise advice could be given without fear of contradiction. But there's simply no escape from the reality that experts don't agree about what to avoid, to maximize longevity and good health. Meanwhile, of course, you need to choose *something* to eat at least by your next meal; you will starve to death if you wait for everyone to agree on what mix of foods (and supplements?) is ideal.

We felt we could not preach our beliefs and be true to our purpose, which was to encourage thinking. We had hoped that if you studied all sides of controversies that often erupt only in one-sided headlines, you might be able to make food selections more confidently, knowing that you had taken account of all the best arguments. Now, however, based on the early returns from reviewers, we have come to suspect that you want something more from us than options. You may want to know what decisions about these controversies would look like translated into everyday activities.

We've decided to accommodate. Having studied what we believe to be all arguments, we have both developed points of view about the issues covered in this book. You've undoubtedly picked up some of our convictions in our "Afterwords," and in occasional selections from J.G. scattered throughout the chapters. (You *may* have caught on to our viewpoint, but again you may not; one of our early readers accused us of being "too fair" in our presentations!)

You've probably concluded (correctly) that we're supporters of the Dietary Guidelines, that we're not big on unprescribed supplemental nutrients other than (perhaps) a low dose pill for "insurance," and that we think our food supply can (and should) be made safer. Based on these and other comparable decisions, we have each developed a personal food policy — the net effect of which is to make our everyday eating decisions easier.

We believe everyone needs to develop such a personal policy for him or herself. In fact, we believe most people unconsciously operate out of such policies, and that many of these policies, if articulated, would appall their owners. Making your food policy explicit is often a first step toward improving it.

Though by doing so we risk encouraging you to imitate our choices instead of our decision-making process, we've decided to outline our own food behaviors. They reflect, of course, our personal food policies. Our dietary habits are quite similar. We both try to eat a variety of foods every day, basing our selections largely on whole grains and fresh fruits and vegetables, along with legumes, nuts and seeds, low-fat dairy products, and some animal flesh. (This means, in practice, that we eat lots of whole grain breads, lots of pasta, lots of stir-fried rice, combined in various ways with a variety of vegetables — raw or lightly cooked.)

Unavoidably — a word we use for those who think of cooking as a life-denying chore — our diets require knowing something about cooking. We believe that every man, woman and child ought to know enough about food preparation to feed him or herself — it's part of being a self-reliant individual. But cooking need not mean "slaving for hours over a hot stove." Because we've learned to cook in time-saving ways, we seldom spend more time preparing a meal than it would take to heat up a prepared one. We often prepare foods like brown rice and dry beans in quantity so that they can be quickly incorporated into future meals.

One of us (J.G.) has a home in the suburbs and gardens organically; the other (P.T.) lives in a New York City apartment and often buys fresh fruits and vegetables from a local farmers' market which handles some produce that is organically grown. We like "organic" produce primarily because we like the environmentally-conserving agricultural practices it represents. As for store-bought fruits and vegetables, we believe it's more important to buy and eat them for health than not to buy them out of concern over pesticide residues. (Residue concerns can best be addressed by working with groups seeking to reduce pesticide use on the farm.) We also try to use fruits and vegetables in season and to encourage local agriculture by buying locally-grown produce.

Now you may have concluded from the preceding few sentences that we had some considerations other than nutrition in mind when we adopted our personal food policies. You are correct. Both of us have some strongly held social-justice and environmental concerns that affect what we choose to buy. Without trying to lay out all our concerns (J.G. has written extensively on these issues elsewhere), we will simply note here that we believe thoughtful people should take into account more than their own health in making eating decisions in a food abundant country.

Those who wish their eating decisions to promote not merely their own well-being, but the well-being of the entire globe and its inhabitants, should begin to find out why countries whose own people are hungry are sending an agriculturally-rich country like ours so much food. Learning to purchase tropical products (like bananas) so as to increase not only your own potassium level but global well-being is a complex and interesting task.

We hasten to add, however, that we ourselves are not always true to our ideals. We sometimes eat in restaurants where the food is richer than it ought to be; we sometimes succumb to "convenience" when we're traveling, and we've been known to indulge in potato chips and ice cream (though not *together*!). We also find we can't resist charcoal broiled burgers at picnics. (P.T. also can't resist hotdogs on these occasions. J.G.) Obviously our personal food policies accommodate such deviations from what some consider "sound nutrition." But because we feel our overall policies are sound, we also believe that we can "indulge" from time to time — if only to show the world that nutritionists are humans.

We find it relatively easy to make good eating part of our everyday life because of policy decisions we have made about where to shop, what sorts of foods *not* to buy, what to keep on hand, what sorts of things it's worth *learning* to like. Most of the time we evaluate our diets not by the RDAs or by whether our selections meet the quantitative standards of a particular food guide, but by a rule of thumb once offered by nutritionist John Yudkin: "It's what you don't eat that matters." We consider that we've done well by ourselves in terms of the day's nutrition if we've eaten a variety of whole foods with few if any low-nutrition, highly processed products, and if we have taken care not to dilute our nutrients with too many fats and sugars. On most days, but not all, we find we have eaten well. In addition, we get some regular exercise, don't smoke, and support with our money and time several organizations working for a future food supply system we see as

409

more desirable than the present one.

We can recommend our eating pattern to you without hesitation — assuming you have no allergies or other disorders that prevent you from eating one or another of the food types we emphasize. We recommend it because it's practical, incorporates sound nutrition principles, and is one that our ancestors have, for millenia, eaten and prospered on.

Future research may show it not to be the ideal pattern (in which case we'll modify our policies), and you may decide on a different set of choices. That's fine, but keep a few general points in mind as you develop your food policy. All the experts represented here, whatever side they take on the controversies, would recommend that you eat as large a variety of foods as you can. (This means *real* variety, biological variety, not 20 different snack foods.) Following this guideline alone will improve your chances of meeting your nutritional needs, and will reduce your chances of consuming harmful quantities of undesirable substances (whether natural or added). We'd also recommend that you decide on a general dietary pattern that reflects some thought and flexibility — and then let yourself relax and live with your decision for a while. Revising what you put in your mouth every time a new report hits the press is a sure recipe for anxiety. Most new information will not justify a policy change.

Nutrition is not the only factor affecting your state of health, or necessarily the most important one. Being happy with life also makes a difference, as we mentioned way back in the Introduction, and you're more likely to be happy if you're not brooding over whether today's food decisions are perfect. If you adopt a general policy of eating for health, rather than for convenience or just to fill up your stomach, you are likely to find yourself making increasingly healthy food choices.

Recognizing that our food choices aren't the only things that influence our health should make it easier for all of us to stop brooding over whether our personal food policy is flawless. There are lots of problems out there in the world that need our attention. It's a shame to spend all our time tending to our own bodies.

We hope you'll use this book positively to reach some decisions about how to live your eating life, after which we'd like you to fit eating into your life and get on with helping save the world.

Our last word is a practical one. We're hoping to make this volume a perennial, so we'd like you to send us any speeches, testimony, articles or reports you find have clarified your own thinking and might, therefore, be useful to include in a future edition of this book. We're sure the controversies discussed in the preceding chapters will be with us for a long time, and that new controversies are sure to emerge. We believe that the community of those interested in nutrition can only be strengthened by careful and open discussion of the things we disagree about. None of us can wait to eat until the controversies are resolved. All of us should try to be rational policy makers.

Eat well. We hope we've helped you to eat thoughtfully.